THE ASTHMATIC CHILD

in play and sport

The Asthmatic Child
in play and sport

Edited by

S Oseid MD
Associate Professor, The Norwegian College of Physical
Education and Sport, and Children's Asthma and
Allergy Institute, Voksentoppen, Oslo, Norway

and

A M Edwards MA MB BChir MRCGP Dip, Pharm. Med.
UK Medical Director, Fisons plc, Pharmaceutical Division
Loughborough, Leicestershire

PITMAN

First Published 1983

Catalogue Number 21.0020.80

Pitman Books Limited
128 Long Acre
London WC2E 9AN

Associated Companies:
Pitman Publishing Pty Ltd, Melbourne
Pitman Publishing New Zealand Ltd, Wellington

© Fisons plc 1983

British Library Cataloguing in Publication Data
The Asthmatic child in play and sport.
  1. Asthma in children—Congresses
  2. Exercise therapy for children—Congresses
I. Oseid, S.   II. Edwards, A. M.
618.92′238062   RJ436.A8
  ISBN 0-272-79692-1

Printed and bound in Great Britain
at the Pitman Press, Bath

PREFACE

The basic defect in bronchial asthma appears to be an altered state of the bronchial tissues with hyperreactivity to a number of different trigger stimuli. Particularly in young individuals immunological hypersensitivity is an important aetiological factor, but infection, emotion, cold air, wind and temperature variations, air pollution, tobacco-smoke, hyperventilation and hormonal factors may also trigger obstruction.

It has been known since the 17th Century that physical exercise can also precipitate an attack of asthma in susceptible individuals. However, it is only during the last 20 years that exercise-induced asthma (EIA) has been subjected to rigorous scientific investigation.

Extensive studies have been performed to elucidate the mechanisms of EIA. Several theories and hypotheses have been put forward, reflex bronchoconstriction secondary to activation of airway vagal receptors and direct narrowing as a result of the release of mediators being the most amenable to investigation. The 'heat-flux' theory presented by Deal, McFadden and co-workers threw new light on the understanding of triggering factors, but the basic mechanisms of EIA are yet not fully understood.

Bronchial obstruction triggered by physical exercise represents a major clinical problem and a severe handicap to young asthmatic children, restricting not only their physical but also their normal social and psychological development.

At Voksentoppen, the Children's Asthma and Allergy Institute in Oslo we have for several years been interested in studies on different trigger factors of bronchial obstruction, and also how these factors may interact through biochemical and physiological mechanisms. In addition, we consider sport and physical exercise to be very important factors in the habilitation and rehabilitation of the child with chronic asthma. In the above, sport is taken to mean all forms of physical activity, including individual exercise, TRIM activities and competitive sport organised to meet individual demands. Through studies on EIA we have worked out a model for the use of physical training in this context.

Although exercise provokes bronchoconstriction in most asthmatics, the severity of EIA can be reduced by several factors:

Control of exercise intensity and duration

Prolonged warm-up periods

Intermittent work (interval training)

Higher temperature and humidity of the inspired air

Increase on aerobic fitness and the use of drugs

These factors and their influence on physical training programmes were reported during the International Symposium 'The Asthmatic Child in Play and Sport. Habilitation and Rehabilitation of Asthmatic Children' held in Oslo 20–23 May 1982. The aim was to discuss in detail not only the scientific basis of EIA, but also to present data on the use of exercise programmes for these children. Several groups of asthmatic children from Norway, United Kingdom, Sweden and Denmark demonstrated different activity programmes on the last day of the symposium, and small inter-group competitions were also arranged. The children had trained regularly for several months to prepare for this event. These demonstrations, the last three papers and the final discussion took place at The Norwegian College of Physical Education and Sport in Oslo.

On behalf of the organising committee I would like to express my thanks and admiration for this valuable contribution to the symposium, not only to the children, but also to all their helpers, physical instructors, nurses and doctors who were involved in the preparation and fulfilment of these programmes.

I would also express my gratitude to all the speakers who contributed so professionally through their papers and discussions. The success of the symposium was a result of hard work and excellent presentations, scientifically and practically.

I would also take the opportunity to express special thanks to Fisons Pharmaceuticals, and particularly to Dr Alan Edwards. Without Fisons' financial support and administrative help it would have been impossible to arrange an international symposium of this magnitude. In this respect Fisons has shown great interest in prophylactic work and rehabilitation programmes through sport and physical training. This — in my opinion — is becoming increasingly important in modern society, and I am impressed by Fisons' engagement in this field.

Last, but not least, I want to express my thanks to Betty Dickens and Pitman Books Limited for their professional work with all the typescripts and discussions, making possible the high quality of this Symposium book. I am sure the published Proceedings will be of interest not only to those working with asthmatic children, but also to anyone interested in the use of physical activity in preventive medicine and rehabilitation throughout the world.

Svein Oseid, MD
Associate Professor
Chairman, Organising Committee

ACKNOWLEDGMENTS

We would like to acknowledge the invaluable help given by Dr Robert Richardson in the day-to-day editing of the abstracts and contributions to the book, and proof reading the finished results.

S Oseid
A M Edwards

CONTRIBUTORS

K Aas

Associate Professor (Pediatric Medicine), Children's Asthma and Allergy Institute, Voksentoppen; and Pediatric Research Institute, Rikshospitalet, University of Oslo, Oslo, Norway

S D Anderson

Principal Scientific Officer, Department of Thoracic Medicine, Royal Prince Alfred Hospital, Missenden Road, Camperdown, 2050 NSW, Australia

R H Andrasch

Hochgebirgsklinik Davos-Wolfgang, 7299 Davos-Wolfgang, Switzerland

A Backman

Associate Professor, Allergy Hospital and II Department of Pediatrics, Helsinki University Central Hospital, Helsinki, Finland

O Bar-Or

Professor of Pediatrics and Director, Children's Therapeutic Exercise and Fitness Centre, McMaster University, Hamilton, Ontario, Canada, L8N 3Z5

R Bolle

Department of Pediatrics, University Hospital of Tromsø, Norway

A Bundgaard

Laboratory for Respiratory Physiology, Department of Medicine B, 2011 Rigshospitalet, DK-2100 Copenhagen, Denmark

R Dahl

Department of Thoracic Medicine, Aarhus Kommunehospital, Denmark

T-Ø Endsjø

Prinsensgt 22, Oslo 1, Norway

M-J Finnilä

Jorv Sjukhus, 02740 Esbo 74, Finland

K D Fitch

Department of Human Movement and Recreation Studies, The University of Western Australia, Nedlands, Western Australia 6009, Australia

I Gillam

Lecturer, Department of Health, Physical Education and Recreation, Victoria College, Burwood, Victoria, Australia

J M Henriksen

Paediatric Department, Aarhus Kommunehospital, 8000 Aarhus C, Denmark

H Hildebrand

Paediatrician, Department of Allergy, Children's Hospital, Länssjukhuset, S-301 85 Halmstad, Sweden

S T Holgate

Senior Lecturer in Medicine, Medicine I, University of Southampton, Southampton General Hospital, Tremona Road, Southampton, SO9 4XY, United Kingdom

Y Iikura

Director, Department of Allergy, National Children's Hospital, Tokyo, Japan

O Inbar

Head, Exercise Physiology Section, The Department of Research and Sports Medicine, Wingate Institute, Netanya, Israel

M Kendall

Senior Physiotherapist, Voksentoppen Children's Asthma and Allergy Institute, Oslo, Norway

T H Lee

Clinical Lecturer, Department of Allergy and Clinical Immunology, Cardiothoracic Institute, Brompton Hospital, Fulham Road, London, SW3 6HP, United Kingdom

D Lindsay

Staff Specialist in Thoracic Medicine, Royal Prince Alfred Hospital, Missenden Road, Camperdown, 2050 NSW, Australia

O Löwhagen

Section of Allergology, Medical Department I, Sahlgren's Hospital, University of Göteborg, Göteborg, Sweden

B M Mallinson
Superintendent Physiotherapist, Booth Hall Children's Hospital, Manchester, United Kingdom

I Morisbak
The Norwegian College of Physical Education and Sports, Oslo; and The Beitostølen Health Sports Center, Beitostølen, Norway

I Neuman
Head, Department of Paediatric Allergy and Clinical Immunology, Hasharon Hospital, Petach-Tikva, Israel

W Nystad Lid
Health Sport Educator, Children's Asthma and Allergy Institute, Voksentoppen, Oslo, Norway

S Oseid
Associate Professor, The Norwegian College of Physical Education and Sport, Sognsveien 220, Oslo 8; and Children's Asthma and Allergy Institute, Voksentoppen, Oslo, Norway

P Aa Østergaard
The Children's Allergy Unit, Aalborg Hospital North, Denmark

K R Patel
Consultant Physician, Department of Respiratory Medicine, Western Infirmary, Glasgow, United Kingdom

P D Phelan
Director, Department of Thoracic Medicine, Royal Children's Hospital, Melbourne, Australia

W E Pierson
University of Washington, Seattle, Washington, USA

H E Refsum
Associate Professor, University of Oslo; and Head of Laboratory of Clinical Physiology, Ullevål Hospital, Oslo, Norway

E A Stemmann
Staedtische Kinderkliniken, Westerholter Strasse 142, 4660 Gelsenkirchen-Buer, FRG

R C Strunk
Associate Professor, Department of Pediatrics, National Jewish Hospital and Research Center/ National Asthma Center, 3800 E Colfax Avenue, Denver, Colorado 80206, USA

E Sundstén   Physiotherapist, Habilitation Unit, Box 7033, S-300 07 Halmstad, Sweden

I L Swann   Consultant Paediatrician, Burnley General Hospital, Casterton Avenue, Burnley, Lancashire, BB10 2PQ, United Kingdom

N C Thomson   Consultant Physician, Department of Respiratory Medicine, Western Infirmary, Glasgow, United Kingdom

R Verrier Jones   Consultant Paediatrician, University Hospital of Wales, Cardiff, United Kingdom

CONTENTS

PART I

INTRODUCTORY LECTURE

Chapter 1

THE PLACE OF PHYSICAL ACTIVITY IN THE LIFE OF CHILDREN AND ADOLESCENTS WITH ASTHMA

K Aas

Children's Asthma and Allergy Institute, Voksentoppen and Pediatric Research Institute, Rikshospitalet, Oslo, Norway

SUMMARY

A child with asthma is, above all, a child, and a child has a body, a mind and a soul. The concept of health encompasses them all and holistic approaches to the prophylaxis and therapy of bronchial asthma are therefore demanded. Our goals are the control of symptoms and the child's ability to cope with the disease. Both the physical and the psychosocial complications of asthma can be avoided, or at least reduced, if the problems are anticipated early enough. The problems that can be predicted depend partly on the kind of difficulties that tend to arise in any child (and adolescent) at certain times and in different personalities, and partly on the difficulties specific to bronchial asthma and the sub-population to which the individual belongs.

Children with asthma should be guided into their own natural society since this is essential for a normal personal and social development and for a balanced emotional maturation. Physical activity is one important means by which this can be achieved. Much effort should be put into stimulating enjoyable, balanced physical activities to build up fitness and self-confidence in the child's own environment. This should start at an earlier stage than usual since it is at the toddler and preschool age that the talents and techniques for play and movement, and the motivation for physical activities are founded. The training for improved physical fitness, improved health and increased exercise tolerance should be accompanied by the teaching of behavioural techniques and the vocabulary of communication appropriate to the child's background.

Participation in physical activities and play which demand a good physical condition is a prerequisite for the child to cope with the disease, to be accepted by his peers and to accept himself. In the child's own world it is the physical component of the personality that counts. As Freud said, our sense of identity is rooted in our physical being.

INTRODUCTION

Bronchial asthma is a disease or group of diseases characterised by dyspnoea of varying degree and duration due to a widespread but more or less reversible obstruction of the bronchi and bronchioles. The bronchial tissues are, to a varying extent, hyperreactive or hypersensitive to physical, chemical, pharmacological and/or immunological stimuli [1]. However, the impairment of lung function of asthma in childhood is not the sole handicap. Frequently other malfunctions and handicaps are preciptated by the respiratory disease or are determined by the life-style imposed upon the child. The disease affects the whole child.

A child with asthma is, above all, just a child − and a child is a body, a mind and a soul (Figure 1), all of which may be affected by the asthma.

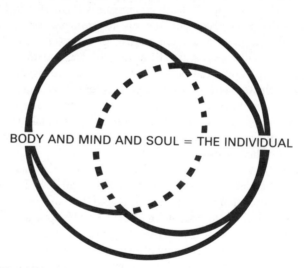

BODY AND MIND AND SOUL = THE INDIVIDUAL

Figure 1. The child with asthma is, above all, just a child with a body, a mind and a soul. The body comprises anatomy, physiology, physics, chemistry, immunology, sensations. The mind comprises intelligence, knowledge, memory, sensitivity, concentration, discipline, suggestibility. The soul comprises the emotions, religious feeling, faith

There are many components and many variables in each compartment and sometimes it may be difficult to define the borders between them. Moreover, the child belongs to, and is an essential part of, the family. Thus a chronic disease such as asthma in a child affects the whole family. The approach to prevention and therapy must therefore be based on a holistic concept of medicine.

THE HOLISTIC CONCEPT

What does a holistic concept mean in this context? In its broadest sense it could encompass all approaches from the humanitarian, the economical and the socially orientated political ones through materialistic biomedical science and active surgery to mysticism, magic and healing by prayer [2]. We have to keep an open mind on the value of mysticism and faith in our culture. As do music and poetry, for example, they may add to the quality of life and can be used deliberately to help children and families cope with difficult situations in their lives. Although I reject mysticism, magic and prayer as instruments for the treatment of the disease as such, I am sceptical of medical approaches that are strictly limited to physiology, immunology, biochemistry, pharmacology and the like. The reduction or elimination of the bronchial abnormality in asthma is important and the materialistic biomedical sciences have contributed enormously in this regard. Indeed, they may perhaps suffice in some of the mildest cases of asthma, but in most cases something more is needed.

Our objectives should be realistic. Complete cure is not a realistic objective for most children, and even the fortunate ones in whom the disease resolves are affected during their formative years. The objectives in a child with chronic asthma should be the control of symptoms with reasonable medication and other means, and the ability to cope with the disease [3]. These call for a holistic medical approach, which views the child as a functioning whole in a family which is also a functioning whole in a society which, too, is a functioning whole (Figure 2). The approach should, however, have a sound scientific foundation. This applies also to physical activity, play and sport in the life of asthmatic children and adolescents.

MOVEMENT AND PLAY

Life is movement. Movement starts *in utero* and is an expression of that life. Thus the quality of life is reduced as the capacity to move is reduced. To move feels good. For all young mammals movement in play is used as a preparation for the challenges of life to come. Human beings play from birth to death, although the character of the play changes and becomes less active as the body grows older [4]. Play for the young person most often means physical activity. The more vigorous the play, the greater the enjoyment. Human play is closely associated with creativity and fosters

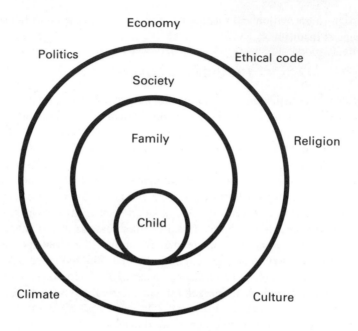

Figure 2. Holistic (comprehensive) medicine views the child as a functioning whole in a family which is a functioning whole in a society which also is a functioning whole

new ways of thinking and behaviour.

Physical activity in play and sport is part of our culture and deserves attention as such [4]. With music, poetry and faith it gives quality of life for many and may act as a valuable aid to coping. So, we have to ask, does it contribute to the health of children and adolescents with asthma? Can we use physical activity in play and sport to treat any particular aspect of the disease, perhaps replacing other less physiological methods? Can we use physical activity to prevent complications, be they physical, emotional, social or educational? Many feel that the answers are in the affirmative, but I must admit that I have had difficulty in finding convincing documentation. There is, to my knowledge, only fragmentary evidence in favour. Nevertheless there is no evidence against.

Movement in play seems to be essential in the life of all young primates [5], and physical activity seems to be a necessity for most children to become fit and happy. This is most naturally accomplished through physical activities that range from more or less vigorous play to the most competitive of sport. Many of the most enjoyable games are so vigorous that the child needs good mobility and to be in good physical condition to keep pace. It calls for breath, the more so when the child is laughing and shouting. Thus the child with asthma is from time to time or all of the time at a disadvantage and must stop playing or his asthma gets worse. To avoid this possibility he must be in good physical condition, which is a product of physical activity.

PHYSICAL ACTIVITY AND MENTAL HEALTH

There is sufficient documentation showing that physical activity makes the body stronger, fitter and healthier. But what about the mind and soul in this respect?

It is extremely difficult to elucidate scientifically the possible associations between physical activity and mental health. With the important place that play and sport occupy in our culture, research of this nature should be given high priority, not least because many forms of physical activity are inexpensive. But although documentation is scarce, some indications can be derived by extrapolation from sociological and psychological research.

Social habilitation in the child's own world is essential for normal personal and social development — and in this world it is the physical component of the personality that counts the most. As Freud expressed it: "The ego is originally a body ego. Our sense of identity is rooted in our physical being." Much of the needs of the mind and soul of the child can be satisfied through play, particularly games in which the physical activity is of many types. Play comprises activity and stimulation. It creates the feeling of togetherness and develops talents for social life. It is an ideal way of learning how to live with other people, to adapt to society and to the patterns of cultural and everyday life.

Play gives the child happy moments, but it also teaches tolerance, adjustment to others and endurance of pain and disappointment. It teaches the child how to lose as well as how to win. Through play with his peers he is enabled to test his own abilities and to adjust his self image. He learns in a playful way some of the realities of life with which he will have to cope. As far as sport is play, this applies also to sport. The ability to tolerate strenuous exercise and play gives the child (and his parents) much more latitude to act and develop according to his needs. More attention should be paid to increasing the tolerance for physical activity in the kindergarten child, since it is at the toddler age that the talent and motivation for the use of the body are developed. Physical activity may be established as a need and a desire at this age, and when integrated with play it becomes habilitation and therapy.

Children with physical handicaps may lose much. Although they may develop into wonderful people, it takes more talent, adaptation and conscious effort to develop emotionally and socially.

Some studies point to the fact that indicators of mental health such as anxiety, a feeling of depression, sleeplessness, emotional instability, social adaptability and stress can be influenced in a positive direction by physical activity [6,7]. Data are lacking, however, which would help to identify those individuals who would profit the most, and those physical activities which would be best for different personalities and different sub-sets of children with asthma. However, physical activity in play and sport tends to decrease anxiety [8].

The degree of fear and anxiety experienced during an asthmatic attack is an important psychological determinant of the course of the disease [9]. In addition to a feeling of fear/panic during the attack (situation anxiety) a rather vague and diffuse anxiety may also persist between attacks in some individuals (state anxiety). The fear never eases its grip on the patient. The trend then is to more severe attacks and more frequent admissions to hospital. Thus a vicious circle is set in motion. There is reason to believe that both these types of anxiety are decreased with the right sort of physical activity [8].

THE NEED TO LOOK INTO THE FUTURE

Physicians treating children with asthma need to be farsighted. Besides our engagement with the present, we have to look far ahead into the future. The child needs reserves of body, mind and soul to withstand the destructive forces associated with acute attacks and with the burden of a chronic disease. Reserves are particularly needed during critical and difficult periods.

The most difficult period for many is that of adolescence. Many of the problems associated with adolescence itself and of suffering from asthma at that age, are predictable and probably preventable if the reserves and preventive measures have been established from early childhood. Difficult problems associated with asthma in adolescence are failure to comply with advice about not smoking, failure to respect restrictions, and failure to comply over the use of drugs. One reason for this is that good health has a lower priority than good company. It may be that certain physical activities – in particular team activities – could help to prevent these problems, at least through peer indoctrination that good health and good physical condition are at a premium.

One must, however, accept that a few children are simply not fond of physical activity. One may speculate that this is a result of the attitude of one or both parents, or that efforts at motivation have been wrong, too strong or too late. Insistence on physical activity and sport cannot be forced on these children. Nevertheless it is usually possible to find other ways to make them take part in stimulating social activities with their peers, although it may demand more imagination, effort and resources. They may be inspired to take up archery, jazz ballet or modern dance, karate, wild-life photography or bird-watching. Clubs for these pursuits may represent excellent starting points for this purpose.

CONCLUSION

Although the means available are rather scarce, The Children's Asthma and Allergy Institute at Voksentoppen puts considerable effort into programmes of physical activity and active play. This forms an essential part of a holistic paediatric philosophy focusing on the habilitation and re-habilitation of children with chronic asthma. We believe similar approaches would be as beneficial (or more so) to all handicapped children and adolescents as they would be to healthy individuals.

References

1   Aas K.
     Heterogeneity of bronchial asthma. Subpopulations or different stages of the disease. *Allergy 1981; 36:* 3–14.

2   Frank JD.
     Holistic medicine: a view from the fence.
     Johns Hopkins Med J 1981; 149: 222–227

3   Aas K.
     To Win (Cope) with a Wheeze.
     Stuttgart and New York:G Thieme (in press)

4   Norbeck E.
     The biological and cultural significance of human play: an anthropological view.
     J Phys Educ Recr 1979; 50: 33–36

5   Loizos C.
     Play behavior in higher primates. A review. In Morris D, ed.
     Primate Ethology 1967: 176–218.
     Chicago: Aldine Publ Co

6   McCloy Layman E.
     Contributions of exercise and sports to mental health and social adjustment.
     In Johnson WR, ed. *Science and Medicine of Exercise and Sports 1980:*
     560–599. New York: Harper and Row

7   Folkins CH.
     Effects of physical training on mood.
     J Clin Psychol 1976; 32: 385–388

8   Wood DT.
     The relationship between state anxiety and acute physical activity.
     Am Correct Ther J 1977; 31: 67–69

9   Dirks JF, Kinsman RA, Horton DJ et al.
     Panic-fear in asthma. Rehospitalization following intensive long-term treatment.
     Psychosom Med 1978; 40: 5–13

PART II

THE MECHANISMS OF EXERCISE-INDUCED ASTHMA AND THE SITE OF CONSTRICTION

Chairman: Professor S Oseid, Norway

Chapter 2

HETEROGENEITY OF BRONCHIAL ASTHMA WITH RESPECT TO PHYSIOLOGICAL AND BIOCHEMICAL ASPECTS OF EXERCISE-INDUCED BRONCHOCONSTRICTION

K Aas

Children's Asthma and Allergy Institute, Voksentoppen and Pediatric Research Institute, Rikshospitalet, Oslo, Norway

SUMMARY

Bronchial asthma is a multifactorial and protean disease with many distinct clinical forms. We may be dealing with a number of diseases that are similar in many ways but have different basic mechanisms. Alternatively, we may be dealing with the different stages and degrees of one disease in which the basic mechanism expresses itself in a variety of ways. But, whatever the case, patients with asthma can be divided into distinct subpopulations according to clinical presentation, lung function tests, immunological responsiveness and hypersensitivity, non-specific hyperreactivity of different tissue components, biochemistry and pharmacochemistry, psychology and response to physical exercise.

It is important to distinguish between 'true' exercise-induced asthma and exacerbations of asthma after exercise and due to the dynamics of increased airflow during established obstruction, be it clinical or subclinical.

Exercise-induced asthma may depend on peculiar neurophysiological, neurohormonal, and/or biochemical characteristics of the patient, normal (common) consequences of exercise acting in biological systems with abnormal reactivity, or on various combinations of both.

Different sets of biochemical mediators may be released, activated or modified metabolically as a consequence of various occurrences at different levels of physical load during exercise. To the degree that exercise-induced asthma depends on non-specific hyperreactivity of the bronchial tissues, subdivision may be relevant with respect to site and nature of the hyperreactivity (autonomic innervation, receptors, smooth muscle biochemistry) and the total biochemical load on the effector cells.

The distinction may be made by means of standardised quantification of dose-response phenomena and reaction patterns within several systems supported by standardised pharmacodiagnostic approaches. It is likely that more information about exercise-induced asthma could be compiled if research was concentrated upon certain well-defined subsets of patients.

INTRODUCTION

Bronchial asthma is a multifactorial and protean disease presenting in many distinct clinical forms. This heterogeneity makes definition difficult, but for all its imperfection the definition that it is 'a disease or group of diseases characterised by dyspnoea of varying degree and duration due to a widespread but more or less reversible obstruction of the bronchi and bronchioles' may serve our present purpose.

Asthma may be subdivided in many ways – for example, by presentation and tests of lung function (Figure 1), by immunological hypersensitivity

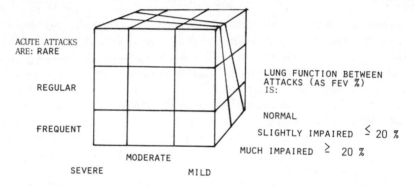

Figure 1. Asthma can be subdivided with reference to clinical presentation and lung function between acute attacks (FEV – forced expiratory volume)

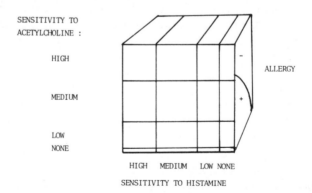

Figure 2. Asthma can be subdivided with reference to non-specific hyperreactivity and immunological hypersensitivity (allergy)

and non-specific hyperreactivity (Figure 2), by biochemistry, by psychology, by response to physical exercise and by much else besides. These distinctions may imply the existence of subgroups of patients or they may simply represent different degrees and stages of the disease. In many patients it is not a question of the presence or absence of the given traits, but of differences in intensity and significance [1—4].

In investigating these problems we must rely on information gathered from objective studies. There are, unfortunately, only three suitable models: (1) standardised work-load tests, (2) controlled induction of acute asthma by means of bronchial challenges with biochemical agents, and (3) challenges with appropriate allergens. When these tests are carried out with use of different medications and with appropriate lung function tests, they may give some indication of the type of response at the tissue level — it is, however, mandatory that the test and test conditions are standardised, and that the precision and reproducibility of the test are established.

As a result of investigations of this nature, our patients may be classified into different subsets. Nevertheless the conclusions arrived at for one subset do not allow the making of generalisations. This discussion is restricted to the heterogeneity of exercise-induced asthma, with particular emphasis on possible distinctions and differences in the underlying physiology and/or biochemistry.

True or genuine exercise-induced asthma is precipitated by a given work load even when the lung function is apparently normal at the beginning of the exercise. After a standardised exercise test 60—80 per cent of children with asthma react with bronchial obstruction [5]. In the other 20—40 per cent of patients exercise-induced asthma does not occur after the standard procedure; however, if the work load is increased, some may develop obstruction, particularly if the air inhaled is dry and cold. The distinction can, nevertheless, easily be made between those with high, medium, low or nil reactivity to a standard test.

PHYSIOLOGY

Acute bronchial obstruction may be provoked in a large number of patients by strenuous exercise. It is, therefore, important to distinguish between genuine exercise-induced asthma and episodes of subclinical obstruction becoming clinically apparent due to the dynamics of increased airflow in slightly obstructed air passages. This distinction draws attention to the relevance of the various methods and criteria adopted for defining normal base-line lung function. One pertinent question concerns the role played by existing but undetected disease of the small airways. Special tests should therefore be undertaken to distinguish between the influence of the large central and the small peripheral airways on base-line lung function.

A number of different tests of lung function are available for studying bronchial asthma during both spontaneous and experimentally-induced obstruction and symptom-free intervals. A distinction should be made between patients whose lung function is normal between attacks and those who constantly have some residual obstruction and depend on continuous use of bronchodilators. These latter are unsuitable for conventional work-load tests, but may still respond in different ways to exercise and different types of premedication.

Differences in the site of the airway response to exercise is another possible cause of heterogeneity, similar to that found in bronchial provocation tests with biochemical agents and allergens [6–8]. Mixed types of obstruction are probably the most frequent finding, but one or other type may predominate. With the use of the pharmacodiagnostic approach to exercise-induced asthma, and analysis of airway function, subgrouping may also be achieved with respect to reversibility. This may, at least partly, be associated with the site of the dominant airway response to the provocation.

Interesting features as regards heterogeneity and lung function are differences in closing volume in individuals of the same age and in static and dynamic compliance. Any differences found may be attributed, for example, to the tissue involved (spasm and/or oedema), to the dominant site of airway response, to the site of mediator action or to the localisation of the effects of various drugs. They may also depend on anatomical characteristics at the cellular level with implications for the biochemical pathways activated by exercise.

ANATOMY

Unknown, or at least undefined, properties of bronchial mast cells, amino-precursor uptake and decarboxylation (APUD) cells, tight junctions, irritant and other receptors, and other anatomical elements, may be decisive in so far as bronchial reactivity and type and degree of the disease in asthma in general is concerned, as well as being instrumental in the response to exercise.

Among the most important anatomical components involved are smooth muscle cells, small vessels, epithelium with tight epithelial junctions, vagal as opposed to adrenergic and non-adrenergic inhibitor elements, clusters of mast cells beneath the tight epithelial junctions, and the number of viable mast cells in the bronchial lumen (Figure 3). The role of APUD cells is uncertain.

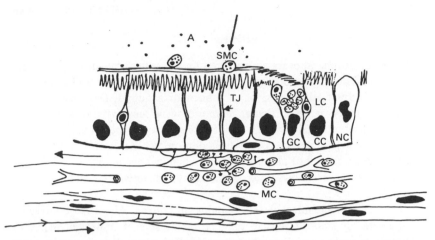

Figure 3. Longitudinal section of bronchial tissue showing some of the tissue components of particular significance for bronchial asthma. Sensitised mast cell (SMC) in lumen releases histamine on challenge and opens tight junction (TC) for allergens (A) to enter (GC = goblet cell; CC = ciliated cell; (NC = non-ciliated cell; LC = lymphocyte; MC = mast cell)

Experimental studies in monkeys and dogs have shown that mast cells can either be superficially located or be found in the lumen [10]. The same seems to apply in man. Individual variability in the number of superficial mast cells may be important in determining who will respond to inhaled allergens and maybe also who will respond to exercise. An initial release of mediators from mast cells in the lumen is likely to open the tight epithelial junctions and allow irritants or allergens access to the submucosal clusters of mast cells, receptors and effector cells. There may also be differences in the ease with which the mast cells are released. In theory, these factors may be decisive for the activity and usefulness of sodium cromoglycate in exercise-induced asthma and bronchial allergy.

The so-called APUD cells are found in the mucosa of the bronchial system and are concentrated at the bifurcations. In the intrapulmonary airways they are grouped in organ-like structures, the 'neuro-epithelial bodies'. The cells contain granules which are generally recognised as having a neurosecretory function (dense core vesicles) and contain amines and polypeptide hormones. The neuro-epithelial bodies have a cholinergic innervation and possibly afferent and efferent fibres. A sympathetic innervation cannot be ruled out. The normal function of these cells is obscure, but it is possible that they produce amines which influence the pulmonary circulation and the bronchial tone [11]. To suggest any role for APUD cells in exercise-induced asthma would be pure speculation, but might they, for example, be influenced by rapid transmucosal heat loss in some individuals?

BIOCHEMISTRY

Bronchial asthma appears above all to be a biochemical disease with imbalance of the regulatory mechanisms for bronchial tone and hyperreactivity of bronchial tissues, be it inborn or acquired. Demonstration of hyperreactivity or, in particular, immunological sensitivity, or both on the part of the bronchial tissues is almost obligatory for the diagnosis of bronchial asthma [12]. Hyperreactivity is demonstrable not only to histamine and acetylcholine, but also to other biochemical agents. One subgroup of patients, however, shows no biochemical hyperreactivity (to standard tests) [13].

The basic biochemical defect remains an enigma. Abnormal contractile behaviour of smooth muscle may be the result of abnormal mediator stimuli, defective handling of normal mediator stimuli, or a combination of both.

A malfunction somewhere in the biochemical pathway from the point of beta-adrenergic (or similar) stimulation to the metabolism of intracellular cyclic adenosine monophosphate/cyclic guanosine monophosphate (cyclic AMP/cyclic GMP) can explain many of the prominent features of bronchial asthma in a number of patients, but not in all. Other reasons for hyperirritability have been sought in vagal imbalance [11,14]. What is true for one subset of patients may be irrelevant for another.

It is possible to demonstrate a marked disparity in response between different trigger stimuli, be it between histamine and methacholine/acetylcholine [15,16], or between histamine and prostaglandin $F_{2\alpha}$ [17]. Histamine may act directly on the smooth muscles in the bronchi as well as being a trigger for parasympathetic irritant receptors in the bronchi. A subdivision may, for instance, be made between patients with high, medium, low or normal bronchial sensitivity to various mediators such as histamine and acetylcholine (Figure 2). This particular topic, however, raises many questions as to methodology and size and type of patient material.

The possible role of leukotrienes in exercise-induced asthma is particularly intriguing. Among them PGE acts as a bronchodilator and $PGF_{2\alpha}$ and slow-reacting substance as potent bronchoconstrictors. They are metabolised in the lung and the resulting $PGE/PGF_{2\alpha}$ balance depends on many variables including pH, tissue oxygenation and enzyme activities. Many of these variables may be influenced by exercise. The biochemistry acting on the effector instrument of asthma, the smooth-muscle cell, is extremely complex, and inborn or acquired differences in enzyme activities may theoretically be fundamental for the type of response to exercise – similar, for example, to the differences in response to acetylsalicylic acid found between subgroups of patients with asthma. There is much room for speculation when our knowledge is limited and the appropriate investigations have yet to be carried out.

CONCLUSION

The literature on the pharmacological prevention of exercise-induced asthma must appear confusing to those who are unaware of the heterogeneity of the asthmatic population. Differences in the prophylactic effect of various drugs are most likely to be due to subset characteristics as discussed above. There is also one subgroup of patients in whom the usual premedication has very little or no detectable effect. It might be worthwhile investigating just this one group in a search for special asthmatic pathophysiological, biochemical or other traits that are significant to them.

For investigational purposes we should select subsets of individuals who are as homogeneous as possible. Too many conclusions have obviously been drawn from studies of undifferentiated groups of patients and too many generalisations have been made from observations on small groups of patients. Conclusions have been drawn that may be correct for some subgroups, but may be wrong and harmful to others. There is a risk that the truth may be concealed as a statistically non-significant finding if an investigation is carried out in a heterogeneous population of patients suffering from a protean and multifactorial disease such as asthma. A given drug could, for example, be ineffective in the majority of patients but highly effective in an identifiable subgroup.

Heterogeneity calls for tolerance of diverging ideas, and even of conflicting reports. Might it perhaps be possible to find a subpopulation of individuals with exercise-induced asthma fitting each hypothesis?

References

1 Aas K.
Heterogeneity of bronchial asthma. Sub-populations — or different stages of the disease. *Allergy 1981; 36:* 3—14

2 Laros KD.
Diagnosis, definition and classification in chronic generalised respiratory disorder. *Respiration 1977; 34:* 250—255

3 Purcell K, Turnbull JW, Bernstein L.
Distinctions between subgroups of asthmatic children: psychological test and behaviour rating comparisons. *J Psychosom Res 1962; 6:* 283—291

4 Rackemann FM.
A working classification of asthma.
Am J Med 1947; 3: 601—606

5   Godfrey S.
    Exercise-induced asthma.
    Allergy 1978; 33: 229–237

6   Aas K.
    The Bronchial Provocation Test
    Springfield: Thomas 1975

7   Cade JF, Pain MCF.
    Pulmonary function during clinical remission of asthma. How reversible is
    asthma? *Aust NZ J Med 1973; 3:* 545–551

8   Olive JT, Hyatt RE.
    Maximal expiratory flow and total respiratory resistance during induced
    bronchoconstriction in asthmatic subjects.
    Am Rev Respir Dis 1972; 106: 366–376

9   Ingram RH Jr, McFadden ER Jr.
    Localization and mechanisms of airways responses.
    N Engl J Med 1977; 297: 596–600

10 Hogg JC, Paré PD, Boucher R et al.
    Pathologic abnoramlities in asthma. In Lichtenstein LM, Austen KF, eds.
    Asthma. Physiology, Immunopharmacology and Treatment 1977: 1–14.
    New York: Academic Press

11 Boushey HA, Holtzman J, Sheller JR, Nadel JA.
    Bronchial hyperreactivity.
    Am Rev Respir Dis 1980; 121: 389–413

12 Szentivanyi A, Flachel CW.
    The beta adrenergic theory and cyclic AMP-mediated control mechanisms in
    human asthma. In Weiss EB, Segal MS, eds.
    Bronchial Asthma: Mechanisms and Therapeutics 1976: 137–154.
    Boston: Little, Brown

13 Orehek J.
    Asthma without airway hyperreactivity: fact or artifact?
    Eur J Respir Dis 1982; 63: 1–4

14 Aas K.
    The Biochemical and Immunological Basis of Bronchial Asthma.
    Springfield: Thomas 1972

15 Spector SL, Farr RS.
    A comparison of metacholine and histamine inhalations in asthmatics.
    J Allergy Clin Immunol 1975; 56: 308–316

16 Mathé AA, Hedqvist P, Holmgren A, Svanborg N.
    Bronchial hyperreactivity to prostaglandin F2α and histamine in patients with
    asthma. *Br Med J 1973; 1:* 193–196

17 Szczeklik A, Nizankowska E, Nizankowski R.
    Bronchial reactivity to prostaglandins F2α, E2 and histamine in different types
    of asthma. *Respiration 1977; 34:* 323–331

Chapter 3

PHYSIOLOGICAL ASPECTS OF EXERCISE-INDUCED ASTHMA

Sandra D Anderson, Robin E Schoeffel, PTP Bye

Royal Prince Alfred Hospital, Camperdown, NSW, Australia

SUMMARY

Exercise induces an increase in ventilation, oxygen consumption, cardiac output and skeletal-muscle blood flow. Catecholamines are released and a variety of adrenergic effects relevant to asthma may be observed. For example, levels of adenosine $3':5'$-cyclic monophosphate (cyclic AMP) increase in response to the release of catecholamines and bronchodilatation occurs in the first few minutes of exercise. Symptomatic asthmatic patients characteristically show an improvement in flow rates and expired volumes. Ventilation perfusion inequality frequently observed at rest is improved during exercise and this is reflected by an increase in arterial oxygen tensions. Towards the end of 6—8 min of strenuous exercise there is an increase in production of lactic acid which can be measured either directly or by demonstrating a metabolic acidosis. These changes are characteristic of exercise challenge and are not usually seen in other challenges which increase ventilation alone.

However, increase in ventilation, by whatever means (exercise or hyperventilation), induces an abnormal loss of heat and water from the airways. Under ambient laboratory conditions (20—25°C, 10—60% relative humidity) most of the heat loss (approximately 80%) is due to the evaporation of water. The effect of this water loss (which may be as much as 20ml in some subjects) on the osmolarity of the respiratory tract fluid or the biochemical environment surrounding lung irritant receptors has not been elucidated. A change in osmolarity in the airways may have important physiological consequences in patients with asthma. Towards the end of a 6—8 min exercise test, children frequently show a fall in flow rates. On the cessation of exercise the increase in airways resistance becomes more marked and usually reaches a maximum within 5—7 min. This increase in airways resistance is accompanied by hyperinflation and arterial hypoxaemia. At this time the levels of catecholamines and cyclic AMP fall rapidly towards pre-exercise levels and in some adult patients a significant increase in arterial levels of histamine has been observed.

When exercise-induced asthma is prevented by prior administration of drugs many of the physiological changes are modified. The increase in airways resistance and hypoxaemia seen after the exercise are abolished, and though further increases are observed in levels of cyclic AMP, there is no increase in the levels of histamine.

INTRODUCTION

The quality of life of patients suffering from exercise-induced asthma has dramatically improved in the past 10 years as a result of our understanding of the physiological changes that occur during asthma and the development of pharmacological agents that modify these changes.

The primary physiological changes during exercise-induced asthma are hyperinflation and hypoxaemia brought about by an increase in airways resistance. This explains why many asthmatic patients find it difficult to continue or resume exercise, and why many are discouraged from taking part in sporting activities. Consequently, an understanding of the prevention and treatment of exercise-induced asthma with pharmacological agents is essential.

RESPIRATORY HEAT AND WATER LOSS DURING EXERCISE

As ventilation increases in response to exercise the amount of heat and water lost from the airways also increases. This loss is linearly related to the level of ventilation at constant inspired air conditions and for this reason is much lower in children compared with adults [1].

Under ambient laboratory conditions ($20-26°C$, $2-14mgH_2O/L$) approximately $80-90$ per cent of the heat is lost by vaporisation of water from the respiratory mucosa as a consequence of the humidification of the inspired air to $44mgH_2O/L$. It is this loss of heat and water that is thought to be the initiating stimulus in exercise-induced asthma [2]. By measuring ventilation and the temperature of inspired and expired air throughout exercise it is possible to quantitate the heat lost during exercise and to relate this to changes in flow rates.

Sensitivity to heat and water loss within the asthmatic population varies widely [1]. However, for a given individual the asthmatic response to exercise is enhanced when cooler drier air is inhaled [3] and lessened when

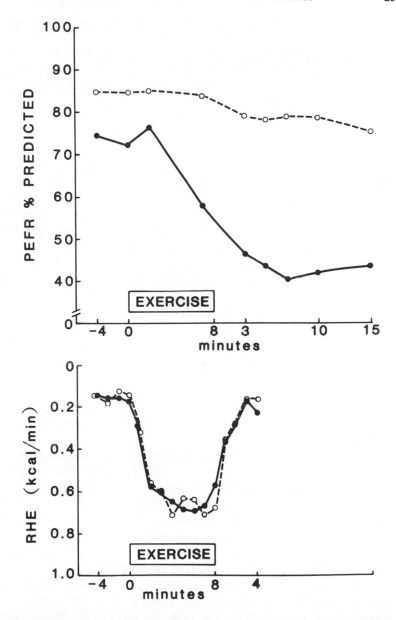

Figure 1. Mean values for peak expiratory flow rate (PEFR) and respiratory heat exchange (RHE − 1kcal = 4.2kJ) at rest and during and after exercise in eight asthmatic children who cycled after receiving salbutamol aerosol (o——o) and its placebo (•——•)

the air is conditioned to body temperature and fully saturated with water vapour [1, 4].

The respiratory heat loss in normal subjects does not differ from that in asthmatics [5] and no modifying effect is demonstrable when exercise-induced asthma is prevented with aerosols such as salbutamol [6] (Figure 1) or sodium cromoglycate [7].

FLOW RATES AND VOLUMES

Patients with asthma respond to exercise with a characteristic biphasic change in airways resistance, the magnitude of which is far greater than that observed in the normal non-asthmatic population [8].

In the symptomatic asthmatic patient exercise of a short duration (two minutes) may induce significant bronchodilatation resulting in increased flow rates and in the forced expiratory volume in one second (FEV_1). The reason for the bronchodilatation is not known. It may be due to a withdrawal of parasympathetic tone during exercise but is more likely to be due to the effects of circulating catecholamines and cyclic adenosine monophosphate (cyclic AMP) which are increased in response to exercise (see below). In children the increase in peak expiratory flow rate (PEFR), when expressed as a percentage of the pre-exercise level, is inversely correlated with the pre-existing level of airways obstruction (per cent rise in PEFR = -0.45 (resting PEFR per cent predicted) + 51.6; n = 79, r = 0.64). The more symptomatic the patient the greater the rise in PEFR in response to exercise. In some patients, exercise alone may reverse the airways obstruction that is present at rest; however, this bronchodilatation is not maintained [9].

Towards the end of six to eight minutes of vigorous exercise or within a few minutes after exercise, the flow rates fall. In children we have observed the lowest values within three to five minutes of the cessation of exercise. Exercise-induced asthma has been defined as a fall in flow rates or FEV_1 greater than 10 per cent of the pre-exercise level [10]. This increased airways resistance as measured by a reduction of either PEFR or FEV_1 is accompanied by significant increases in functional residual capacity and in some patients by an increase in total lung capacity [11, 12].

Figure 2 illustrates the changes in lung volumes and flow rates in four asthmatic children who exercised by running for six minutes on two occasions, one after receiving a placebo the other after receiving 20mg of sodium cromoglycate. Their values are compared with those observed in nine normal children. The changes in flow rates and volumes which

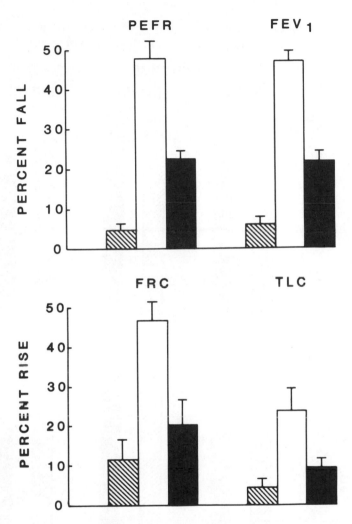

Figure 2. Mean values ± 1 SEM for the per cent fall after exercise of peak expiratory flow rate (PEFR) and forced expiratory volume in one second (FEV$_1$) and the per cent rise after exercise in functional residual capacity (FRC) and total lung capacity (TLC) in nine normal children (hatched columns) and four asthmatic children who exercised after placebo (open columns) and sodium cromoglycate (solid columns)

were observed after placebo were modified when the exercise was performed after taking sodium cromoglycate. When the airways obstruction induced by exercise was reversed with salbutamol the hyperinflation was also reversed. Many studies have reported the efficacy of bronchodilator

aerosols in exercise-induced asthma [13] – when exercise-induced asthma
is prevented by pharmacotherapy hyperinflation does not occur.

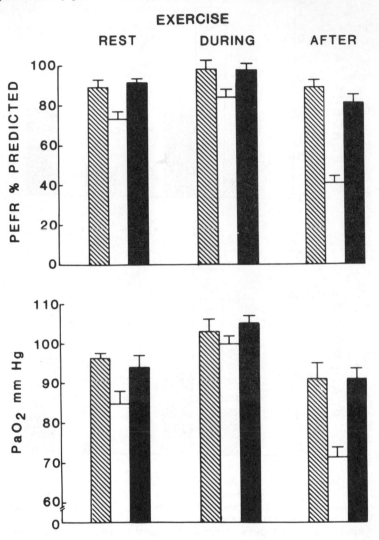

Figure 3. Mean values ± 1 SEM for peak expiratory flow rate (PEFR) expressed as a
percentage of predicted and arterial oxygen tensions (PaO$_2$) at rest and during and
after exercise in 14 asthmatics who exercised after placebo (open columns) and
terbutaline aerosol (solid columns). The data are compared with those obtained
from nine asthmatic men performing the same intensity of exercise after placebo
aerosol (hatched columns)

ARTERIAL BLOOD GAS TENSIONS AND pH

Mild arterial hypoxaemia is frequently observed at rest in adult patients with asthma who have not received medication for six hours or more and whose flow rates are 75 per cent of predicted normal or less.

During the first few minutes of exercise when bronchodilatation occurs there is a more equal distribution of ventilation in relation to perfusion in the lung [14]. At this time the arterial oxygen tensions increase towards values observed in normal subjects [15] (Figure 3). Carbon-dioxide levels, however, may be lower in asthmatics than in normal subjects and this probably reflects the relative hyperventilation compared to oxygen consumption that occurs in asthmatics in response to exercise.

When, after exercise, there is a reduction in flow rates severe hypoxaemia can occur — oxygen tensions of 50—60mmHg have been recorded in our laboratory. In children oxygen desaturation may be measured easily using an earoximeter. Hypercapnia is rare and usually only occurs in patients whose flow rates fall to less than 30 per cent of predicted normal. Values for pH in the post-exercise period may be lower in asthmatics compared with normal subjects exercising at the same work intensity.

When exercise-induced asthma is inhibited or prevented by drugs such as terbutaline sulphate oxygen tensions and saturation remain within the normal range during and after exercise (Figure 3). Lower values for carbon dioxide and higher values for pH in asthmatics compared with normal subjects have been recorded when terbutaline has been taken, implying that equivalent levels of ventilation are maintained in the post-exercise period whether bronchoconstriction is present or not. As a result, the rate of recovery from the metabolic acidosis induced by exercise is more rapid in asthmatic patients who have taken terbutaline.

CATECHOLAMINES

Endogenous noradrenaline and adrenaline are released by strenuous exercise. Levels of noradrenaline measured during and after exercise in adult asthmatics with exercise-induced asthma have been reported to be similar to those in normal subjects [16—18] though there is some evidence that they are decreased in asthmatic children [19]. Figure 4 illustrates the plasma noradrenaline levels at rest and during and after 6—10 minutes of treadmill running in 10 adult male asthmatics. The levels are highest at the end of strenuous exercise and it is important that measurements are made at that time. The levels rapidly fall with the cessation of exercise and are near pre-exercise levels within 15 minutes.

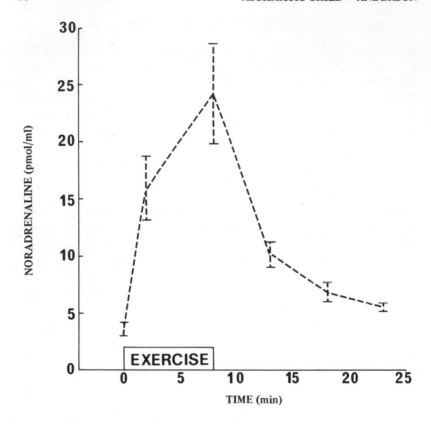

Figure 4. Mean values ± 1 SEM for arterial plasma noradrenaline at rest and during and after running exercise in 10 adult asthmatic men

The bronchodilatation that occurs during exercise is thought to be brought about by the increased levels of circulating catecholamines.

ARTERIAL PLASMA CYCLIC ADENOSINE MONOPHOSPHATE

Cyclic adenosine monophosphate (cyclic AMP) is generated by activation of adenylate cyclase in response to circulating catecholamines and beta-sympathomimetic agents; it produces a variety of adrenergic effects including relaxation of smooth muscle and inhibition of the release of mediators. Documenting increases in cyclic AMP in response to the release of endogenous catecholamines, as in exercise, and to the administration of bronchodilator drugs provides a useful index of preserved adrenergic responsiveness in asthmatic patients.

We have measured (by radioimmunoassay) plasma cyclic AMP at rest and during and after exercise in nine asthmatic and seven normal adult men. The asthmatic patients were taking six to eight puffs of a beta-sympathomimetic aerosol daily for control of their symptoms which had varied in duration from six months to 40 years [20]. Exercise was performed on a treadmill for 6–10 minutes and maximum heart rates were reached in the last few minutes of exercise. The exercise was followed by a severe attack of asthma in all the patients (mean ± 1 SEM per cent fall in PEFR = 45.4 ± 4.6; range, 23–69%) but not in the normal subjects. Terbutaline sulphate aerosol (1.25mg) was given to aid recovery and 90 minutes later an equivalent dose was given immediately before a second exercise test. Terbutaline inhibited exercise-induced asthma in all the asthmatics (mean ± 1 SEM per cent fall in PEFR = 9.2 ± 2.3; range, 1.0–20.7%). Figure 5 illustrates the levels of cyclic AMP observed at rest and during and after exercise in the nine asthmatic patients who exercised with and without terbutaline. Signi-

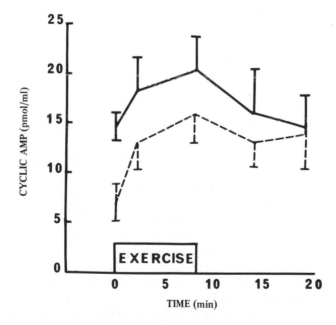

Figure 5. Mean values ± 1 SEM for arterial plasma cyclic adenosine monophosphate (cyclic AMP) at rest and during and after exercise in nine asthmatic men who performed running exercise after placebo (solid line) and terbutaline aerosol (broken line)

ficant increases in cyclic AMP occurred in eight of the nine patients and in all normal subjects in response to exercise after placebo and there was no significant difference between the two groups. After terbutaline, levels of cyclic AMP were higher in all patients and normal subjects with further increases taking place during the second exercise test in seven of the nine asthmatics and six of the seven normal subjects. Again there was no significant difference between the asthmatic patients and normal subjects.

An attenuated increase in cyclic AMP in response to the inhalation of isoprenaline [21] and the stress of exercise has been reported by other workers [22] for patients with asthma. Our patients may have differed in that only one was receiving an oral beta-sympathomimetic drug and no patient was taking methylxanthines or oral steroids. Further, their airways obstruction which was recorded at rest, six hours after the last medication (mean ± 1 SEM per cent predicted PEFR = 72.5 ± 5.0) was completely reversed during exercise after terbutaline (mean ± 1 SEM per cent predicted PEFR = 97.0 ± 2.0%).

Thus normal changes in cyclic AMP have been measured in response to strenuous exercise and after the administration of terbutaline aerosol in patients taking beta-sympathomimetic aerosols daily for control of symptoms.

It would appear that exercise-induced asthma can occur at a time when values for cyclic AMP are increased in response to exercise. However, a critical level of cyclic AMP may be achieved after the administration of terbutaline and this may be sufficient to modify the contraction of smooth muscle or inhibit the release of mediators from mast cells.

ARTERIAL PLASMA HISTAMINE

The release of chemical mediators such as histamine and leukotrienes from mast cells lying superficially in the airways has been considered an important mechanism of exercise-induced asthma [8]. The development of sensitive radioimmunoassays has allowed the measurement of histamine in human plasma. For this reason histamine has been used as a marker of mediator release with the reservation that it need not be the main or the only mediator involved in the contraction of airway smooth muscle.

Arterial plasma concentrations of histamine were measured at rest and during and after exercise in nine asthmatic and two normal adult subjects. The subjects exercised by running on two occasions two hours apart before and after the administration of the beta-sympathomimetic agent terbutaline sulphate [23]. The sensitivity of the assay and the reproducibility of the measurements suggested that a significant increase had occurred in response to exercise when the values for plasma histamine were greater than 9pmol/ml (1ng/ml) and more than three standard deviations from the resting level.

Applying these criteria a significant increase in histamine levels was observed in five of the nine asthmatics but in neither of the two normal

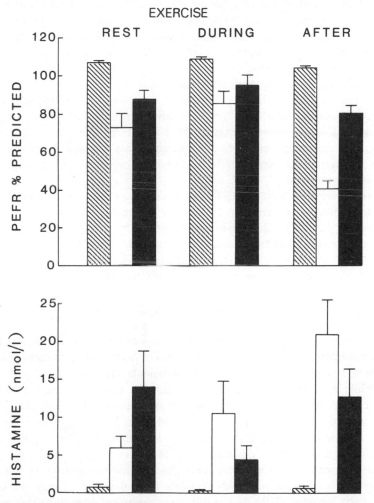

Figure 6. Mean values ± 1 SEM for peak expiratory flow rate (PEFR) and arterial plasma levels of histamine at rest and during and after exercise in five adult asthmatic men who performed exercise after placebo (open columns) and terbutaline aerosol (solid columns). The data for two non-asthmatic men who exercised after placebo are illustrated for comparison (hatched columns)

subjects. The highest levels of histamine were observed between one and 15 minutes after exercise and were associated with severe exercise-induced asthma (Figure 6). The levels of histamine returned to pre-exercise values within 30 minutes after exercise but rose again after 5mg of terbutaline was given by nebulisation. This observation implies that histamine was available locally in the lung for some considerable time after the exercise. The increase in histamine levels may have been due to the relaxant effect of terbutaline on vascular smooth muscle [24, 25]. After the drug had been given there may have been an increase in blood flow in areas of lung constricted by histamine or hypoxia. In this way histamine may have been 'flushed' out of poorly perfused areas.

A second dose of 5mg of terbutaline was given 15 minutes before the second exercise test. The levels of histamine fell during exercise and remained below resting levels in the post-exercise period which implies that the terbutaline modified any further release of histamine in response to exercise. Mild exercise-induced asthma occurred in one patient after repeated exercise.

There are now several studies in which the release of histamine into arterial plasma in some patients with exercise-induced asthma has been reported [26, 27]. Changes in venous plasma levels of histamine have also been reported in exercise-induced asthma [28], but they are smaller and may not truly reflect the release of histamine from the lung owing to deactivation of histamine in the peripheral circulation.

CONCLUSION

The physiological changes that accompany exercise-induced asthma may be modified by pharmacological agents. This advance in treatment permits the normal performance of exercise by patients with asthma.

While the loss of heat and water from the airways is the most likely initiating stimulus for exercise-induced asthma, its role in the mechanism of asthma is not clear. Loss of heat and water induce significant cooling of the airways [29]. However, water loss alone may be important by inducing a change in the osmolarity of the respiratory tract fluid [1]. Patients with asthma are sensitive to the inhalation of both hypotonic and hypertonic aerosols and loss of water from the airways may act as an osmotic stimulus [30]. As a result the environment of both irritant receptors and mast cells may be altered so that bronchoconstriction occurs either reflexly or by a direct action of mast cell mediators on airway smooth muscle.

The increase in circulating levels of catecholamines and cyclic AMP which occurs during strenuous exercise does not appear to provide a protective effect — at least in the absence of beta-sympathomimetic aerosols [20]. This may be due to the fact that intracellular events in the airways are not reflected in changes in catecholamines and cyclic AMP in plasma. Thus physiological studies have not elucidated the mechanism of exercise-induced asthma. Further studies on the release of chemical mediators during and after exercise and the possible inhibition of this release by pharmacological agents are required.

SUMMING UP

In patients with asthma, exercise induces physiological changes that are not observed in non-asthmatic subjects — they include an increase in airways resistance, hyperinflation and arterial hypoxaemia, all of which can be inhibited or completely prevented when drugs such as the beta-sympathomimetic amines or sodium cromoglycate are administered as aerosols prior to exercise. Thus premedication can restore to normal the physiological changes observed in asthmatics with exercise-induced asthma.

In both asthmatic and normal subjects exercise increases the loss of heat and water from the airways and this loss is not modified by the administration of drugs.

During exercise the circulatory levels of catecholamines and cyclic AMP are significantly increased, which may account for the bronchodilatation observed in the first few minutes of exercise in the symptomatic asthmatic patient. Further increases in cyclic AMP take place after the use of bronchodilator aerosols but the changes that occur in asthmatics are similar to those in normal subjects.

In some patients with asthma a significant increase in arterial plasma histamine has been demonstrated at a time when exercise has induced asthma. This release of histamine in response to exercise has been modified by terbutaline sulphate administered before exercise but only a small number of patients has been studied.

References

1   Anderson SD, Schoeffel RE, Follet R et al.
    Sensitivity to heat and water loss at rest and during exercise in asthmatic patients.
    Eur J Respir Dis 1982. In press
2   Deal EC, McFadden ER, Ingram RH, Jaeger JJ.
    Hyperpnea and heat flux:initial reaction sequence in exercise-induced asthma.
    J Appl Physiol 1979; 46: 476–483

34 ASTHMATIC CHILD – ANDERSON

3   Strauss RH, McFadden ER, Ingram RH, Jaeger JJ.
    Enhancement of exercise-induced asthma by cold air.
    N Engl J Med 1977; 297: 743–747

4   Strauss RH, McFadden ER, Ingram RH et al.
    Influence of heat and humidity on the airway obstruction induced by exercise
    in asthma. *J Clin Invest 1978; 61:* 433–440

5   O'Cain CF, Dowling NB, Slutsky AS et al.
    Airway effects of respiratory heat loss in normal subjects.
    J Appl Physiol 1980; 49: 875–880

6   Anderson SD, Schoeffel RE.
    Respiratory heat and water loss during exercise in patients with asthma. The
    effect of repeated exercise challenge. *Eur J Respir Dis 1982.* In press

7   Breslin FJ, McFadden ER, Ingram RH.
    The effects of cromolyn sodium on the airway response to hyperpnea and cold
    air in asthma. *Am Rev Respir Dis 1980; 122:* 11–16

8   Anderson SD, Silverman M, Konig P, Godfrey S.
    Exercise-induced asthma. A review.
    Br J Dis Chest 1975; 69: 1–39

9   Joseph J, Bandler L, Anderson SD.
    Exercise as a bronchodilator.
    Aust J Physiother 1976; 12: 47–50

10 Mellis CM, Kattan M, Keens TG, Levison H.
    Comparative study of histamine and exercise challenges in asthmatic children.
    Am Rev Respir Dis 1978; 117: 911–915

11 Anderson SD, McEvoy JD, Bianco S.
    Changes in lung volumes and airway resistance after exercise in asthmatic
    subjects. *Am Rev Respir Dis 1972; 106:* 30–37

12 Freedman S, Tattersfield AE, Pride NB.
    Changes in lung mechanics during asthma induced by exercise.
    J Appl Physiol 1975; 38: 974–982

13 Anderson SD, Seale JP, Ferris L, Schoeffel RE.
    An evaluation of pharmacotherapy for exercise-induced asthma.
    J Allergy Clin Immunol 1979; 64, part 2: 612–624

14 Young IH, Corte P, Schoeffel RE.
    Pattern and time course of ventilation perfusion inequality in exercise induced
    asthma. *Am Rev Respir Dis 1982; 125:* 304–311

15 Anderson SD, Silverman M, Walker SR.
    Metabolic and ventilatory changes in asthmatic patients during and after exercise.
    Thorax 1972; 27: 718–725

16 Anderson SD, Pojer R, Smith ID, Temple D.
    Exercise-related changes in plasma levels of 15-keto-13, 14-dihydro-prostaglandin
    $F_{2\alpha}$ and noradrenaline in asthmatic and normal subjects. *Scand J Respir Dis
    1976; 57:* 41–48

17 Zielinski J, Chodosowska E, Radomysk A et al.
    Plasma catecholamines during exercise induced bronchoconstriction in bronchial
    asthma. *Thorax 1980; 35:* 823–827

18   Chryssanthopoulos MD, Barboriak JJ, Fink JN et al.
     Adrenergic responses of asthmatic and normal subjects to submaximal and
     maximal work levels. *J Allergy Clin Immunol 1978; 61:* 17–22

19   Barnes PJ, Brown MJ, Silverman M, Dollery CT.
     Circulating catecholamines in exercise and hyperventilation induced asthma.
     Thorax 1981; 36: 435–440

20   Bye PTP, Anderson SD, Daviskas E et al.
     Plasma cyclic AMP levels in response to exercise and terbutaline sulphate aerosol
     in normal and asthmatic subjects. *Eur J Respir Dis 1980; 61:* 287–297

21   Trembath PW, Shaw J.
     Adrenoceptor responsiveness in bronchial asthma. Effect of isoprenaline inha-
     lation on plasma cyclic 3'5' AMP levels. *Br J Clin Pharmacol 1976; 3:* 1001–1005

22   Hartley JPR, Davies CJ, Charles TJ et al.
     Plasma cyclic nucleotide levels in exercise-induced asthma.
     Thorax 1981; 36: 823–827

23   Anderson SD, Bye PTP, Schoeffel RE et al.
     Arterial plasma histamine levels at rest, and during and after exercise in patients
     with asthma:effects of terbutaline aerosol. *Thorax 1981; 36:* 259–267

24   Stockley RA, Finnegan P, Bishop JM.
     Effect of intravenous terbutaline on arterial blood gas tensions, ventilation and
     pulmonary circulation in patients with chronic bronchitis and cor pulmonale.
     Thorax 1977; 32: 601–605

25   Persson CGA, Ekman M, Efjefült I.
     Terbutaline preventing permeability effects of histamine in the lung.
     Acta Pharmacol Toxicol (Copenh) 1978; 42: 395–397

26   Karr RM, Brach BB, Wilson MR et al.
     Change in levels of arterial blood histamine during exercise induced asthma.
     J Allergy Clin Immunol 1979; 63: 153

27   Hartley JP, Charles TJ, Monie RD et al.
     Arterial plasma histamine after exercise in normal individuals and in patients
     with exercise-induced asthma. *Clin Sci 1981; 61:* 151–157

28   Barnes PJ, Brown MJ.
     Venous plasma histamine in exercise- and hyperventilation induced asthma in
     man. *Clin Sci 1981; 61:* 159–162

29   Deal EC, McFadden ER, Ingram RH, Jaeger JJ.
     Esophageal temperature during exercise in asthmatic and non-asthmatic subjects.
     J Appl Physiol 1979; 46: 484–490

30   Schoeffel RE, Anderson SD, Altounyan REC.
     Bronchial hyperreactivity in response to inhalation of ultrasonically nebulised
     solutions of distilled water and saline. *Br Med J 1981; 283:* 1285

Chapter 4

THE ROLE OF THE MAST CELL IN EXERCISE-INDUCED ASTHMA

P H Howarth, S T Holgate

University of Southampton, United Kingdom

SUMMARY

Considerable controversy exists over the role of the release of mediators from mast cells as a causative factor in the exercise-induced bronchoconstriction of asthma. We have examined the changes in histamine levels in whole blood and plasma, in white blood-cell counts and in the calibre of the airways in nine normal and nine atopic mild asthmatic subjects after exercise. Subjects were exercised at room temperature on a treadmill set at a $10°$ slope for five minutes. The speed of the treadmill varied for any one individual from 4–6kph. Minute ventilation was recorded during exercise and, on a separate day matched during isocapnic hyperventilation in the asthmatic subjects, to reproduce the respiratory heat exchange.

The airway response was recorded as specific airway conductance (sGaw), before and at 2, 5, 10, 15, 30 and 60 minutes after bronchial provocation. After each recording venous blood was withdrawn from an indwelling cannula for the analysis of histamine levels and white blood-cell counts.

A fall in sGaw was noted in both normal and asthmatic subjects after exercise amounting to 8 ± 3 per cent (1 SEM) and 60.5 ± 5 per cent respectively. A comparable fall was achieved with isocapnic hyperventilation in the asthmatics.

Resting plasma histamine levels measured by a sensitive rat kidney HMT assay were significantly higher in the asthmatic (5.23 ± 0.58nmol/L) than normal subjects (3.15 ± 0.63nmol/L). No change in the plasma histamine level was detected after exercise in either group, nor was there any change in the asthmatics with isocapnic hyperventilation. Exercise in all subjects produced a biphasic increase in the white blood-cell count, with peaks at 2–15 minutes and 60 minutes. There was no early peak after isocapnic hyperventilation, but the late peak persisted.

By using sGaw as a sensitive index of airway calibre it is apparent that both asthmatic and normal subjects respond to exercise with bronchoconstriction, but differ in the magnitude of their response. Isocapnic hyperventilation, which is dependent upon airway cooling alone, was sufficient to reproduce the same degree of bronchoconstriction as with exercise. The elevated plasma histamine levels encountered in asthma may reflect increased release of mediators associated with the basal mast cell which, in turn, could be responsible for the observed increased responsiveness of the airways. It is possible that .the increase in plasma histamine after exercise recorded by some workers might relate to the early increase in blood basophil count and this would explain why a similar increase in plasma histamine has not been reported after isocapnic hyperventilation.

INTRODUCTION

Exercise may induce bronchoconstriction in asthmatic subjects and this is a reflection of their non-specific airway hyperreactivity. The response has been recognised for a long time and since it is physiological and can easily be studied in the laboratory, it has been used as a model of asthma to gain insight into the mechanism of the bronchoconstriction. Two major functions of the upper air passages are to humidify fully and to heat to body temperature the inspired air; as a consequence the mucosal lining is cooled. It is now accepted that the airway cooling resulting from the respiratory heat exchange is the initial event in the bronchoconstriction that follows exercise [1]. Modifying the respiratory heat exchange by altering minute ventilation, humidity or temperature of the inspired air influences the degree of bronchoconstriction [2–5]. Isocapnic hyperventilation with matched respiratory heat exchange is able to produce identical bronchoconstriction to that produced by exercise [1].

Bronchoconstriction and moderate airway cooling

It is uncertain how moderate airway cooling induces bronchoconstriction although there are two main schools of thought: one supports a central role for the vagus nerve; the other favours local mast-cell degranulation with release of mediators.

Vagal reflex mechanisms

Vagal irritant receptors are found under the mucosal surface in the oropharynx and large airways. In animals, stimulation of these receptors at both sites induces bronchoconstriction which can be abolished by cutting or cooling the cervical vagosympathetic nerves [6]. Indirect evidence of a role for the vagus in exercise-induced asthma in man has come from *in-vivo* experiments with oropharyngeal anaesthesia [7] and pretreatment with muscarinic cholinergic antagonists [8]. Oropharyngeal anaesthesia is, however, non-specific and variable in its effect.

Antimuscarinic agents are most effective at blocking exercise-induced asthma in those patients with a predominant large-airway response to exercise as assessed by helium-oxygen expiratory flow-volume curves [9], which is consistent with the anatomy of the vagal innervation of the airways. The large doses of antimuscarinic agents, however, that are required to block exercise-induced asthma – 4–6mg inhaled atropine sulphate or 1–2mg ipratropium bromide – produce maximal bronchodilatation [8,10] which makes interpretation difficult as it may alter reactivity of the airways and non-specifically modulate exercise-induced asthma [11]. Yet, even with these doses, little or no effect on exercise-induced asthma is found in 30–50 per cent of asthmatic patients.

Secretion of inflammatory mediators

Since the role of vagal reflex mechanisms in exercise-induced asthma is controversial it follows that other mechanisms may be involved. One possibility is that inflammatory mediators may be secreted from the mast cells in response to airway cooling after exercise since cold degranulates mast cells in cold urticaria [12].

In the lung, mast cells are found in the lumen, beneath the basement membrane of the airways, near blood vessels in the submucosa, adjacent to submucous glands, scattered throughout the muscle bundles and in the alveolar septa. Human peripheral lung fragments contain approximately 10^6 mast cells/g and constitute 0.01–0.1 per cent of the total lung cell population [13]. Preformed mediators associated with the human pulmonary mast cell include histamine, exoglycosidases, tryptase, carboxypeptidase B, chemotactic factors and heparin proteoglycan [14]. These mediators are packaged in modified lysosomal granules which are capable of being secreted in response to specific stimulation of the mast cell. In addition, activation of the mast cell results in the *de-novo* synthesis and release of prostaglandin (PG) D_2 by the cyclooxygenase pathway of arachidonic acid metabolism. Slow-reacting substance of anaphylaxis – now recognised to be the lipoxygenase products leukotrienes (LT), C_4, D_4 and E_4 – together with LTB_4, $PGF_{2\alpha}$, PGE_2 and platelet-activating factor are secondary mediators whose formation requires, in addition to mast cells, the participation of other cells in the microenvironment [15].

While many of the pathophysiological features of asthma can be related to inflammation in the airways, secondary to the release of inflammatory mediators [13], evidence that mast cells degranulate with exercise is largely indirect. It has been suggested that the fact that sodium cromoglycate, a 'mast-cell stabilising drug', prevents exercise-induced asthma provides support for involvement of the mast cells [8]. Evidence is now available, however, to suggest that sodium cromoglycate may have alternative actions, such as blocking afferent 'C' fibres which may be involved in vagal reflex mechanisms [16]. Exercise is followed by a refractory period during which another similar exercise task results in less bronchoconstriction [17]. It has been suggested that the refractory period represents depletion of mast-cell mediators, but an alternative explanation is that it is a delayed inhibitory effect produced by such agents as catecholamines and steroids released during exercise. Bronchial provocation with antigen in some patients is associated with late bronchoconstriction occurring after 6–24 hours [18], which may be secondary to release of mediators by the mast cells and recruitment of other effector cells such as neutrophilic leucocytes [19]. No similar late reaction follows exercise-induced asthma.

Measurement of circulating inflammatory mediators

To approach the problem more directly, attempts have been made to measure the levels of circulating inflammatory mediators in the plasma, before and after exercise, as an index of intrapulmonary mast-cell degranulation. Plasma histamine has been commonly used as a marker of mast-cell degranulation, since it is one of the major granule-associated mediators [20–22]. Unfortunately, biological and fluorometric assays for histamine have proven either too insensitive or too non-specific to detect low levels of histamine in biological fluids. The development of a radioenzymatic assay involving the methylation of histamine greatly improved the sensitivity [23]. This assay most frequently employed guinea-pig brain histamine methyltransferase which contains other methyltransferase activities, thereby giving poor specificity and high blank values. Predictably, studies of plasma histamine before and after exercise employing this assay gave variable results [22,24,25]. Moreover, up to 30-fold differences in plasma histamine levels between different groups were reported in a quality control study [26]. Two methods have been successfully used to improve the specificity of this assay: in one the more specific rat kidney histamine methyltransferase is substituted for the guinea-pig enzyme [27], and in the other a thin layer chromatographic step is incorporated to separate methylated histamine from contaminants [28]. Using this latter method, Barnes and his colleagues [29] found an increase in plasma histamine after exercise in asthmatic subjects, but not in normal subjects, which led them to suggest that pulmonary mast-cell degranulation occurred in exercise-induced asthma. However, basophilia is a normal response to exercise and some histamine from the basophils may leak into the plasma without necessarily implying that the intrapulmonary mast cells have degranulated [30].

MATERIALS AND METHODS

Bearing this problem in mind, we have investigated the changes in histamine levels in whole blood and plasma, the white blood-cell count and airway calibre in both normal and mild atopic asthmatic subjects, after a standard treadmill exercise test, and on a separate day after matched isocapnic hyperventilation in the asthmatic subjects. Before and at regular intervals from two to 60 minutes after bronchial provocation, airway resistance was measured in a constant-volume whole body plethysmograph, on line to a microprocessor, and the results expressed as specific airways conductance (sGaw). After each recording, blood was taken for measurement of plasma and total blood histamine levels and white blood-cell count. The blood was taken into chilled EDTA to inhibit diamine oxidase activity, and the plasma separated by centrifugation at 2000g for 10 minutes. Only the top 1ml of plasma was used for measuring histamine levels. Both plasma histamine and whole-blood histamine were assayed using a rat kidney histamine methyltransferase radioenzyme assay with a sensitivity of 0.45nmol/L linearity over a histamine range of 0–90.09nmol/L (r = 0.998) and an intra-assay coefficient of variation of seven per cent [31].

RESULTS

In both the normal and the asthmatic subjects exercise produced a fall in sGaw amounting to 8 ± 3 per cent (1 SEM) and 60.5 ± 5 per cent, respectively. Isocapnic hyperventilation produced a 57 ± 6 per cent fall in sGaw in the asthmatics which was not significantly different from that produced by exercise. The mean minute ventilation was 49.19L/min during exercise and 48.95L/min during isocapnic hyperventilation.

Resting plasma histamine levels were significantly higher in the asthmatic subjects, 5.23 ± 0.58nmol/L, than in the normal subjects, 3.15 ± 0.63nmol/L ($p<0.01$). The total blood histamine levels in the two groups were respectively, 847 ± 143 and 643 ± 74.3nmol/L, which are not significantly different. It was found that histamine levels in plasma and whole blood correlated in both normal and asthmatic subjects ($p < 0.01$), suggesting that most of the plasma histamine is derived from the basophil. The regression slopes were different for normal subjects compared to asthmatics — 121 and 64, respectively.

In a separate experiment, details of which are not presented here, it was found that the basophils of the asthmatics had a higher spontaneous histamine leak (13.40 ± 2.0 per cent), compared to those of the normal subjects (6.46 ± 0.71 per cent), which would explain the higher plasma histamine level and the different regression slopes.

There was no significant change in the plasma histamine levels after exercise but there was an immediate increase in the white blood-cell counts and total blood histamine levels in all subjects that was not accounted for by haemoconcentration. A comparable increase in the white blood-cell counts and whole-blood histamine levels did not occur with isocapnic hyperventilation.

DISCUSSION

Thus, by using a sensitive radioenzymatic assay for histamine we have shown that there is no significant increase in the plasma histamine levels after either exercise or isocapnic hyperventilation. We have also confirmed the finding, consistent with reports in the literature, that asthmatics have higher resting levels of plasma histamine than normal subjects [22,29]. The discrepancies between our findings and those of studies in which an increase in plasma histamine levels has been found after exercise [24,29] may relate to the handling of the blood samples and in particular to the release of histamine into plasma from circulating basophils. We have clearly demonstrated a close correlation between plasma levels and whole-blood levels of histamine, both in normal and asthmatic subjects. As histamine in whole blood is derived from basophils, these cells may be more relevant than tissue mast cells when considering changes in plasma histamine levels. And since basophilia occurs with exercise, changes in plasma histamine levels could arise either from contamination with basophils of the plasma during sampling or from spontaneous release from increased numbers of basophils. If either were the case, the absence of change in the plasma histamine levels after isocapnic hyperventilation might be predicted as we have shown that there is no subsequent leucocytosis (Figure 1). The rise in plasma histamine levels reported with exercise occurs only in asthmatics and not in normal subjects [29]. For our hypothesis to stand, the basophilia after exercise must either be greater in asthmatic than in normal

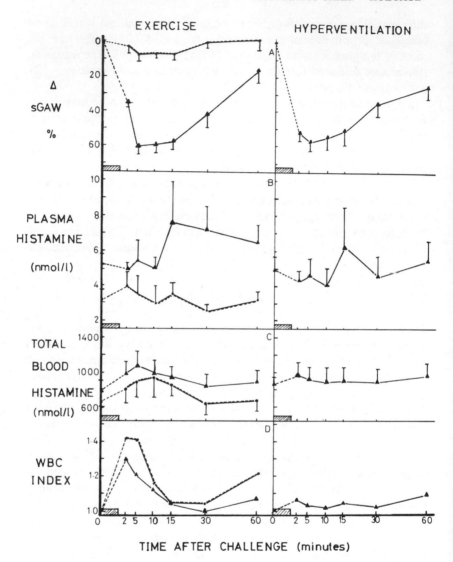

Figure 1. Time-dependent changes in specific airways conductance, sGaw, plasma histamine, total blood histamine and white blood cell (WBC) index after five minutes' treadmill exercise (left panels) and matched isocapnic hyperventilation (right panels) in adult normal (●- - -●) and allergic asthmatic (▲——▲) subjects. (WBC index = $\frac{\text{WBC/PCV at time x}}{\text{WBC/PCV at time 0}}$ where PCV = packed cell volume)

subjects or the basophils of asthmatics should show a greater spontaneous release of histamine. Reference to Figure 1 shows clearly that there is no greater basophilia after exercise in asthmatics. We have, however, shown in the same group of subjects that the spontaneous release of histamine from the basophils of asthmatics is up to two times greater than that which occurs from the basophils of normal subjects. This finding would also explain the higher resting plasma histamine levels encountered in asthmatic compared with normal subjects.

Of great interest is the recent demonstration that exercise, but not hyperventilation, causes an increase in serum high molecular weight neutrophil chemotactic activity [Nagakura et al, unpublished observations]. Neutrophil chemotactic activity is reported to be a mediator released in association with preformed mast-cell mediators − ECF-A and histamine − in cold urticaria [12]. Neutrophil chemotactic activity has also been putatively identified, however, in human basophils [32]. It is not clear how specific is the rise in neutrophil chemotactic activity after exercise for human mast-cell degranulation.

As histamine is an unreliable index of mast-cell degranulation and no rise in $PGF_{2\alpha}$ or its 15 keto 13,14-dihydro metabolite has been detected after exercise [33,34], direct evidence for mast-cell degranulation is lacking. However, plasma levels of mediators may not be a reflection of their release within the lungs as the release may be local and the half-life of the mediator short. It is likely that mast-cell associated mediators are an important contributory factor in exercise-induced asthma, but it is not essential to invoke their release on exercise. The response of the smooth muscle of guinea-pig trachea to cooling *in vitro* is greatly enhanced by prior exposure to histamine [35].

We have demonstrated that both normal and asthmatic subjects show a similar time-related bronchoconstriction to exercise, but differ in the magnitude of their response. McFadden and his co-workers have reported similar findings with isocapnic hyperventilation [36]. The difference in reactivity of normal and asthmatic airways could be explained by chronic release of mast-cell associated mediators around the airways causing inflammation and influencing the threshold at which the airways of asthmatic subjects react to stimuli. Mast-cell mediators might open up bronchial epithelial tight junctions transmitting stimuli to afferent mucosal vagal nerve endings. The interlinking of mast-cell degranulation with access to afferent vagal nerve endings and thus bronchoconstriction would be an attractive hypothesis. It could explain the non-specific airway hyperreactivity of asthmatics and their response to sodium cromoglycate both immediately before challenge and in the long term in modulating their airway hyperreactivity.

References

1 Deal EC, McFadden ER, Ingram RH, Haeger JJ.
Hyperpnea and heat flux: initial reaction sequence in exercise-induced asthma.
J Appl Physiol 1979; 46: 476–483

2 Kivity S, Souhrada JF, Melzer E.
A dose-response-like relationship between minute ventilation and exercise-induced bronchoconstriction in young asthmatic patients.
Eur J Respir Dis 1980; 61: 342–346

3 Weinstein PE, Anderson JA, Kvale PK, Sweet LC.
Effect of humidifcation on exercise-induced asthma (EIA).
J Allergy Clin Immunol 1976; 57: 250–251

4 Bar-Or O, Neuman I, Dotan R.
Effects of dry and humid climates on exercise-induced asthma in children and preadolescents. *J Allergy Clin Immunol 1977; 60:* 163–168

5 Deal EC, McFadden ER, Ingram RH et al.
Role of respiratory heat exchange in production of exercise-induced asthma.
J Appl Physiol 1979; 46: 467–475

6 Widdicombe JG, Sterling GM.
The autonomic nervous system and breathing.
Arch Intern Med 1970; 126: 311–329

7 McNally JF, Enright P, Souhrada JF.
The role of the oropharynx in exercise-induced bronchoconstriction.
Am Rev Respir Dis 1978; 117: 372A

8 Thomson NC, Patel KR, Kerr JW.
Sodium cromoglycate and ipratropium bromide in exercise-induced asthma.
Thorax 1978; 33: 694–699

9 McFadden ER, Ingram RH, Haynes RL, Wellman JJ.
Predominant site of flow limitation and mechanisms of post exertional asthma.
J Appl Physiol 1977; 42: 746–752

10 Deal EC, McFadden ER, Ingram RH, Jaeger JJ.
Effects of atropine on potentiation of exercise-induced bronchospasm by cold air.
J Appl Physiol 1978; 45: 238–243

11 Tattersfield AE.
Measurement of bronchial reactivity: a question of interpretation.
Thorax 1981; 36: 561–565

12 Soter NA, Wasserman SI, Austen KF.
Cold urticaria: release into the circulation of histamine and eosinophil chemo-tactic factor of anaphylaxis. *N Engl J Med 1976; 294:* 687–690

13 Kaliner MA.
Mast cell derived mediators and bronchial asthma. In Hargreave FE, ed.
Airway Reactivity 1979. Ontario, Canada: Astra Pharmaceuticals Ltd

14 Schwartz LB, Austen KF.
Enzymes of the mast cell granule.
J Invest Dermatol 1980; 74: 349–353

15 Lewis RA, Holgate ST, Jackson Roberts L II et al.
    Preferential generation of prostaglandin D_2 by rat and human mast cells.
    In Becker EL, Simon AS, Austen KF, eds. *Biochemistry of the Acute Allergic
    Reactions* (in press). New York: Alan R Liss

16 Dixon M, Jackson DM, Richards IM.
    The action of sodium cromoglycate on 'C' fibre endings in the dog lung.
    Br J Pharmacol 1980; 70: 11–13

17 Edmunds AT, Tooley M, Godfrey S.
    The refractory period after exercise-induced asthma: its duration and relation to
    the severity of exercise. *Am Rev Respir Dis 1978; 117:* 247–254

18 Pepys J, Hargreave FE, Chan M, McCarthy DS.
    Inhibitory effects of disodium cromoglycate on allergen-inhalation tests.
    Lancet 1968; ii: 134–137

19 Nagy L, Lee TH, Kay AB.
    Neutrophil chemotactic activity in antigen-induced late asthmatic reactions.
    N Engl J Med 1982; 306: 497–501

20 Bhat KN, Arroyave CM, Marney SR et al.
    Plasma histamine changes during provoked bronchospasm in asthmatic patients.
    J Allergy Clin Immunol 1976; 58: 647–656

21 Harries MG, Burge PS, O'Brien et al.
    Blood histamine levels after exercise testing.
    Clin Allergy 1979; 9: 437–441

22 Hartley JPR, Charles TJ, Seaton A et al.
    Arterial plasma histamine after exercise in normal individuals and in patients
    with exercise-induced asthma. *Clin Sci 1981; 61:* 151–157

23 Snyder SH, Baldessarini R, Axelrod J.
    A sensitive and specific enzymatic isotopic assay for tissue histamine.
    J Pharmacol Exp Ther 1966; 153: 544–549

24 Ferris L, Anderson SD, Temple DM.
    Histamine release in exercise-induced asthma.
    Br Med J 1978; 2: 1697

25 Simon RA, Ginsberg M, Timms RM, Stevenson DD.
    Exercise-induced bronchospasm: a study of plasma mediators.
    J Allergy Clin Immunol 1979; 63: 153

26 Gleich GJ, Hull WM.
    Measurement of histamine: a quality control study.
    J Allergy Clin Immunol 1980; 66: 295–298

27 Shaff RE, Beaven MA.
    Increased sensitivity of the enzymatic isotopic assay of histamine: measurement
    of histamine in plasma and serum. *Anal Biochem 1979; 94:* 425–430

28 Brown MJ, Ind PW, Barnes PJ et al.
    A sensitive and specific radiometric method for the measurement of plasma
    histamine in normal individuals. *Anal Biochem 1980; 109:* 142–146

29 Barnes PJ, Brown MJ.
    Venous plasma histamine in exercise and hyperventilation-induced asthma in
    man. *Clin Sci 1981; 61:* 159–162

30   Durer H, Pernow B.
     Histamine and leucocytes in blood during muscular work in man.
     Scand J Clin Lab Invest 1958; 10: 394–396

31   Church MK, Pao GJK, Holgate ST.
     Characterisation of histamine secretion from human lung dispersed mast cells:
     effects of anti-IgE, calcium ionophore A23187, compound 48/80 and basic
     polypeptides. *J Immunol* (in press)

32   Austen KF.
     *Biological Implications of the Structural and Functional Characteristics of the
     Chemical Mediators of Immediate Hypersensitivity. The Harvey Lectures,
     Series 73:* 93–161. New York: Academic Press

33   Anderson SD, Pojer R, Smith ID, Temple D.
     Exercise-related changes in plasma levels of 15-keto 13,14-dihydro-prostaglandin
     $F_{2\alpha}$ and noradrenaline in asthmatic and normal subjects.
     Scand J Respir Dis 1976; 57: 41–48

34   Field J, Allegra J, Trautlein J et al.
     Measurement of plasma prostaglandins during exercise-induced bronchospasm.
     J Allergy Clin Immunol 1976; 58: 581–585

35   Souhrada M, Souhrada JF.
     The direct effect of temperature on airway smooth muscle.
     Respir Physiol 1981; 44: 311–323

36   Deal EC, McFadden ER, Ingram RH et al.
     Airway responsiveness to cold air and hyperpnea in normal subjects and those
     with hay fever and asthma. *Am Rev Respir Dis 1980; 121:* 621–628

Chapter 5

MAST-CELL MEDIATORS IN EXERCISE-INDUCED ASTHMA

T H Lee, A B Kay

Brompton Hospital, London, United Kingdom

SUMMARY

Concentrations of plasma histamine and a heat stable serum neutrophil chemotactic factor have been measured in atopic asthmatics who developed exercise-induced asthma after a treadmill task. Plasma histamine was measured with a novel double isotope radioenzymatic assay and neutrophil chemotactic factor was identified by its elution in the void volume fractions of Sephadex G-200.

There was a significant increase in neutrophil chemotactic factor and plasma histamine in the asthmatics after exercise. The time course of their appearance accompanied the development of exercise-induced asthma and their elaboration could be inhibited by the prior administration of sodium cromoglycate. There was no significant rise in neutrophil chemotactic factor after histamine bronchoprovocation or in the concentrations of plasma histamine after methacholine inhalation challenge, which produced a similar fall in the forced expiratory volume in one second (FEV_1).

The physicochemical characterisation of the neutrophil chemotactic factor released during exercise-induced asthma showed that (1) it was a macromolecule with an estimated size $>500,000$ daltons, (2) it eluted at approximately $0.15mol/L$ NaCl from DEAE-Sephacel (pH 7.8), (3) it had an isoelectric point between 6.0 and 6.5 and (4) it was susceptible to inhibition by trypsin and chymotrypsin. Since these features have also been identified as characteristic of the neutrophil chemotactic factor released after antigen bronchial challenge, our results suggest that these neutrophil chemotactic factors may be identical substances.

INTRODUCTION

Exercise-induced asthma refers to the increase in airflow obstruction which, in many asthmatics, follows physical exertion. It is not a 'disease' but rather a manifestation of bronchial hyperreactivity. The typical pattern of response consists in a phase of bronchodilatation during the first few minutes of exercise; this is followed by a lag period before the maximal limitation of airflow develops between five and 10 minutes after exercise [1]. The airways obstruction usually recovers over the next 60 minutes [1, 2]. Although this clinical association has been recognised at least since the time of Aretaeus in the second century AD, the pathogenesis of exercise-induced asthma is still not understood.

MEDIATOR HYPOTHESIS

In 1966 McNeill and his colleagues [3] suggested that chemical mediators, such as histamine and slow-reacting substance of anaphylaxis (SRS-A), may be released in asthmatics after exercise and contribute towards the bronchoconstriction. The demonstration of a refractory period (during which the post-exercise increase in airways resistance is reduced) should exercise be repeated within two [4] to four hours [5] would be compatible with the view that a mediator had been depleted and that time was required for its regeneration. The observation that some drugs that inhibit the degranulation of mast cells *in vitro* – such as sodium cromoglycate [6], beta-adrenergic receptor agonists [7, 8] and diethylcarbamazine [9] – could prevent exercise-induced asthma has also supported the view that activation of the mast cells plays a role in exercise-induced asthma. However, there are other drugs that have potent mast-cell stabilising properties which have no effect on exercise-induced asthma [10]. It has been suggested, therefore, that sodium cromoglycate exerts its effect *in vivo* by other mechanisms, such as the inhibition of phosphodiesterase inhibition [11] or a direct action on a neurological reflex [12]. However, the concentration of the drug necessary to inhibit phosphodiesterase *in vitro* was much higher than that attainable *in vivo*, so it would seem unlikely that this is the site of action of sodium cromoglycate.

Histamine

Other evidence for the possible involvement of mediators in the pathogenesis of exercise-induced asthma has depended on the demonstration of their release into the circulation [13–16]. Unfortunately histamine is rapidly metabolised in the blood and is very labile *in vitro*. Assays hitherto used for its measurement have been insensitive and, for the fluorometric assay, also non-specific. A further difficulty is that basophilia is a normal response to exercise and may contribute to an increased concentration of histamine in the plasma, despite the careful collection of samples and separation of the plasma [17]. These factors have contributed to conflicting results in the literature [18–22], so making it desirable to search for another marker of mast-cell activation.

Neutrophil chemotactic factor

In 1977 Atkins and his co-workers [23] detected a high molecular weight, heat stable neutrophil chemotactic factor (NCF) in the circulation of asthmatic patients after the inhalation of a specific antigen. Similar neutrophil chemotactic factors have also been identified in patients suffering from physical urticarias after the appropriate challenge [24–26]. The evidence suggests that neutrophil chemotactic factor might be associated with the mast cell. For instance, the release of neutrophil chemotactic factor closely paralleled the appearance of recognised mast-cell mediators such as histamine and eosinophil chemotactic factor of anaphylaxis (ECF-A) [24–27]. Bronchial challenge in asthmatics with methacholine [23] was not associated with the release of neutrophil chemotactic factor, whereas the prior administration of sodium cromoglycate to asthmatics challenged with specific antigen inhibited the wheezing and the appearance of circulating neutrophil chemotactic factor [28]. The *in-vitro* release of neutrophil chemotactic factor from lung fragments or dispersed mast cells is poorly documented, although it has been shown that the release of similar neutrophil chemotactic factor from rat peritoneal mast cells can be detected after challenge with rabbit anti-rat antisera [29], giving some direct evidence of the mast-cell origin of this substance. Although the origin of the high molecular weight neutrophil chemotactic factor is not definitely established, these previous observations suggest that its appearance may be a useful marker for mast-cell degranulation.

Neutrophil chemotactic factor in exercise-induced asthma

We have recently been studying the circulating activity of neutrophil chemotactic factor during exercise-induced asthma in atopic asthmatics in order to ascertain whether there was any evidence for the release of mediators associated with the mast cell [30].

A heat stable neutrophil chemotactic factor has been identified in the serum of atopic asthmatic subjects after treadmill exercise. The peak activity was detected at 10 minutes and returned to prechallenge values by one hour [30]. Neutrophil chemotactic factor activity was not detected in the sera of seven non-asthmatic individuals performing the same task. The appearance of neutrophil chemotactic factor was exercise-dose dependent [31] and accompanied the development of airflow obstruction. Furthermore, its release could be inhibited by the prior administration of sodium cromoglycate [30]. In contrast, histamine challenge in atopic asthmatics, at concentrations giving a comparable change in forced expiratory volume at one second (FEV_1) to that evoked by exercise was not associated with the appearance of circulating neutrophil chemotactic factor [30]. Therefore the release of neutrophil chemotactic factor was not due to the bronchoconstriction alone.

The physicochemical properties of the exercise-induced neutrophil chemotactic factor were similar to those of the neutrophil chemotactic factor released in response to antigen challenge [30] : (1) they both eluted as macromolecules with an estimated molecular size greater than 500,000 daltons, when subjected to Sephadex G-200 chromatography; (2) the neutrophil chemotactic factors, partially purified by gel filtration, eluted as a single peak of activity after anion exchange chromatography on DEAE-Sephacel; (3) they had an isoelectric point between 6.0 and 6.5, as determined by chromatofocusing on Polybuffer Exchanges 94; and (4) their activities were substantially reduced after incubation with trypsin and chymotrypsin. This suggested that peptide bonds were important for the expression of their chemotactic activity.

Since the appearance of neutrophil chemotactic factor is believed to reflect activation of the mast cells, our results support the view that mediators of hypersensitivity are released in exercise-induced asthma.

Neutrophil chemotactic factor and basophils

Earlier work has suggested that the increases in mediator concentrations induced by exercise may originate from 'leaky' basophils, since a basophilia occurs after exercise [17]. However, the release of neutrophil chemotactic factor in asthmatics who had exercise-induced asthma was significantly greater than in those subjects who did not have exercise-induced asthma [31] despite a similar post-exercise basophilia [T Nagakura et al, unpublished observations]. This suggests that the release of neutrophil chemotactic factor could not be explained simply by the increase in basophils alone.

EXERCISE-INDUCED ASTHMA AND
ISOCAPNIC HYPERVENTILATION WITH COLD AIR

It is well recognised that swimming is the form of exercise least likely to limit airflow and that asthmatics often complain of a deterioration of their asthma in the cold weather. These clinical observations have been explained over the past few years by studies which have suggested that respiratory heat exchange is the likely initiating stimulus for the exercise-induced asthma.

It has been shown that cold air could potentiate exercise-induced asthma [32, 33] and that the severity of the airways obstruction, when breathing air of ambient temperature, was inversely proportional to the water content of the inspired gas [34—37]. Increasing the humidity at ambient temperatures reduced the incidence of exercise-induced asthma and inhaling fully saturated air at body temperature completely prevented its occurrence. Deal and his colleagues [33] postulated that exercise-induced asthma was due to the heat exchange that occurred at the bronchial mucosa which, in turn, was due to the vaporisation of water necessary for the conditioning of the inspired gas by the airways. They developed quantitative expressions which suggested that respiratory heat loss was directly proportional to the minute ventilation. They further reasoned that, since the level of ventilation was an important determinant of the quantity of heat transferred from the mucosa, it should be possible to reproduce the extent of the obstruction to airflow on exercise by performing isocapnic hyperventilation [38]. To test this hypothesis, they subjected asthmatic patients to isocapnic hyperventilation through a heat exchanger [38]. Hyperventilation with fully saturated air (heat flux 0) did not result in bronchoconstriction. However, as the water content and temperature of the inspired gas were decreased — thereby increasing the thermal burden on the airways — bronchoconstriction occurred.

Despite these elegant experiments it is still not understood how respiratory heat exchange obstructs the airflow. It is tempting to speculate that a situation analogous to cold urticaria exists in the airways and that cold air degranulates mast cells in the bronchial mucosa [39]. However, in a recent study, using isocapnic hyperventilation with air at $-11°C$ to provoke asthma, no significant release of mediators into the circulation was detected. We have compared treadmill exercise and a matched isocapnic hyperventilation procedure with cold air in the same asthmatic subjects [T Nagakura et al, unpublished observations]: despite similar falls in FEV_1, exercise, but not isocapnic hyperventilation, was followed by the release of neutrophil chemotactic factor and by a basophilia. This observation is supported by the work of Barnes and Brown [16] who demonstrated an increase in histamine concentrations during exercise-induced asthma, but not after isocapnic hyperventilation.

These findings suggest that there is a difference between true exercise-induced asthma and the bronchoconstriction produced by isocapnic hyperventilation. There are other recognised differences, too: there is a phase of bronchoconstriction during exercise [1], a lag period before the development of airways obstruction [1] and a refractory period after exercise [1], all features which are reported to be absent in isocapnic hyperventilation [40]. These differences emphasise that although respiratory heat exchange may initiate exercise-induced asthma, other factors may modulate and sustain this initial stimulus.

NEUTROPHIL CHEMOTACTIC FACTOR AND HISTAMINE

As we have already discussed, previous work on changes in the concentrations of histamine during exercise-induced asthma have given inconclusive results partly due to the technical difficulties of collecting the samples and assay methodology. A sensitive double-isotope radioenzymatic method has recently been developed by Brown and his colleagues [41], in which the specificity has been increased by the incorporation of a thin-layer chromatography step. Using this technique, small but significant increases of plasma histamine have been detected during exercise-induced asthma [31]. The time course of its appearance was similar to that of neutrophil chemotactic factor, as previously reported for the appearance of these two mediators in the physical urticarias [24–27]. In contrast, methacholine challenge which gave a fall in FEV_1 similar to that in the treadmill task released neither histamine nor neutrophil chemotactic factor [31].

CONCLUSIONS

The pathogenesis of exercise-induced asthma is likely to be multifactorial. There is good evidence that respiratory heat exchange is the initiating event, but the mechanism by which heat loss causes exercise-induced asthma is unknown. There are differences between isocapnic hyperventilation and exercise-induced asthma and it seems possible that the initiating stimulus is maintained by other mechanisms. We believe that the release of mediators is probably important in this respect, but other factors may also play a part. The reason why mediators are released by exercise is not known, but the reported disturbances in the secretion of catecholamines [42–44] in exercise-induced asthma may have an important modulating influence on mast-cell activation.

References

1   Anderson SD, Silverman M, König P, Godfrey S.
     Exercise-induced asthma.
     Br J Dis Chest 1975; 69: 1–39

2   Jones RS, Buston MH, Wharton MJ.
     The effect of exercise on ventilatory function in the child with asthma.
     Br J Dis Chest 1962; 56: 78–86

3   McNeill RS, Nairn JR, Millar JS, Ingram CG.
     Exercise-induced asthma.
     Q J Med 1966; 35: 55–67

4   Haynes RL, Ingram RH Jr, McFadden ER Jr.
     As assessment of the pulmonary responses to exercise in asthma and an analysis
     of the factors influencing it. *Am Rev Respir Dis 1976; 114:* 739–752

5   Edmunds AT, Tooley M, Godfrey S.
     The refractory period after exercise-induced asthma: its duration and relation to
     the severity of exercise. *Am Rev Respir Dis 1978; 117:* 247–254

6   Davies SE.
     Effect of disodium cromoglycate on exercise-induced asthma.
     Br Med J 1968; 3: 593–594

7   Poppius H, Salorinne Y.
     Comparative trial of salbutamol and an anticholinergic drug SCH 1000, in pre-
     vention of exercise-induced asthma. *Scand J Respir Dis 1973; 54:* 142–147

8   Jones RS, Wharton MJ, Buston MH.
     The place of physical exercise and bronchodilator drugs in the assessment of
     the asthmatic child. *Arch Dis Child 1963; 38:* 539–545

9   Sly RM.
     Effect of diethylcarbamazine pamoate upon exercise-induced bronchospasm.
     J Allergy Clin Immunol 1974; 53: 82

10   Stokes TC, Morley J.
     Prospects for an oral Intal.
     Br J Dis Chest 1981; 75: 1–14

11   Roy AL, Warren BT.
     Inhibition of cyclic AMP phosphodiesterase by DSCG.
     Biochem Pharmacol 1974; 23: 917–920

12   Woenne R, Kottan M, Levinson H.
     Sodium cromoglycate-induced changes in the dose response curves of inhaled
     methacholine and histamine in asthmatic children.
     Am Rev Respir Dis 1979; 119: 927–932

13   Ferris L, Anderson SD, Temple DM.
     Histamine release in exercise-induced asthma.
     Br Med J 1978; 1: 1967

14   Simon RA, Ginsberg M, Timms RM, Stevenson DD.
     Exercise-induced bronchospasm: a study of plasma mediators.
     J Allergy Clin Immunol 1979; 63: 153

15   Karr RM, Brach BB, Wilson MR et al.
     Change in levels of arterial blood histamine during exercise-induced asthma.
     J Allergy Clin Immunol 1979; 63: 153

16   Barnes PJ, Brown MJ.
     Venous plasma histamine in exercise- and hyperventilation-induced asthma in
     man. *Clin Sci 1981; 61:* 159–162

17   Duner M, Pernow B.
     Histamine and leucocytes in blood during muscular work in man.
     Scand J Clin Lab Invest 1958; 10: 394–396

18   Deal EC, Wasserman SI, Soter NA et al.
     Evaluation of role played by mediators of immediate hypersensitivity in exercise-
     induced asthma. *J Clin Invest 1980; 15:* 659–665

19   Granerus G, Simonsson BG, Skoogh BE, Wetterqvist H.
     Exercise-induced bronchoconstriction and histamine release.
     Scand J Respir Dis 1971; 52: 131

20   Harries MG, Burge PS, O'Brien I et al.
     Blood histamine levels after exercise testing.
     Clin Allergy 1979; 9: 437–441

21   McFadden ER, Soter NA.
     A search for chemical mediators of immediate hypersensitivity and humoral
     factors in the pathogenesis of exercise-induced asthma.
     In Austen KF, Lichtenstein LM, eds. *Asthma, Immunology, Immunopharma-
     cology and Treatment 1977;* 337.
     New York: Academic Press

22   Sherman NA, Morris HG, Arroyave CM, Selner JC.
     Changes in plasma cyclic adenosine monophosphate, cyclic guanosine mono-
     phosphate, histamine and prostaglandins during exercise-induced asthma.
     J Allergy Clin Immunol 1979; 63: 154

23   Atkins PC, Norman M, Weiner H, Zweiman B.
     Release of neutrophil chemotactic activity during immediate hypersensitivity
     reactions in humans. *Ann Intern Med 1977; 86:* 415–418

24   Wasserman SI, Soter NA, Centre DM, Austen KF.
     Cold urticaria. Recognition and characterisation of a neutrophil chemotactic
     factor which appears in serum during experimental cold challenge.
     J Clin Invest 1977; 60: 189–196

25   Soter NA, Wasserman SI, Austen KF.
     Cold urticaria: release into the circulation of histamine and eosinophil chemo-
     tactic factor of anaphylaxis during cold challenge.
     N Engl J Med 1976; 294: 687–690

26   Soter NA, Wasserman SI, Pathak MA et al.
     Solar urticaria: release of mast cell mediators into the circulation after
     experimental challenge. *J Invest Dermatol 1979; 72:* 282

27   Soter NA, Wasserman SI, Austen KF, McFadden ER.
     Release of mast cell mediators and alterations in lung function in patients with
     cholinergic urticaria. *N Engl J Med 1980; 302:* 604–608

28 Atkins PC, Norman M, Zweiman B.
Antigen-induced chemotactic activity in man, correlation with bronchospasm
and inhibition by DSCG. *J Allergy Clin Immunol 1978; 62:* 149–155

29 Centre DM, Soter NA, Wasserman ST, Austen KF.
Characterisation of neutrophil specific chemotactic activity from rat mast cells.
Am Rev Respir Dis 1980; 121: Suppl 61

30 Lee TH, Nagy L, Nagakura T et al.
Identification and partial characterisation of an exercise-induced chemotactic
factor in bronchial asthma. *Clin Invest 1982; 69:* 889–899

31 Lee TH, Brown MJ, Nagy L et al.
Exercise-induced release of histamine and neutrophil chemotactic factor in
atopic asthmatics. *J Allergy Clin Immunol 1982.* In press

32 Strauss RH, McFadden ER, Ingram RH, Jaeger JJ.
Enhancement of exercise-induced asthma by cold air.
N Engl J Med 1977; 297: 743–747

33 Deal EC, McFadden ER, Ingram RH et al.
Role of respiratory heat exchange in production of exercise-induced asthma.
J Appl Physiol 1979; 46: 467–475

34 Strauss RH, McFadden ER, Ingram RH et al.
Influence of heat and humidity on the airway obstruction induced by exercise
in asthma. *Clin Invest 1978; 61:* 433–440

35 Bar-Or, Neuman I, Dotan R.
Effects of dry and humid climates on exercise-induced asthma in children and
preadolescents. *J Allergy Clin Immunol 1977; 60:* 163–168

36 Chen WY, Horton DJ.
Heat and water loss from the airways and exercise-induced asthma.
Respiration 1977; 34: 305–313

37 Weinstein PE, Anderson JA, Kvale PK, Sweet LC.
Effects of humidifcation on exercise-induced asthma (EIA).
J Allergy Clin Immunol 1976; 57: 250–251

38 Deal EC, McFadden ER, Ingram RH, Jaeger JJ.
Hyperpnea and heat flux: initial reaction sequence in exercise-induced asthma.
J Appl Physiol 1979; 46: 476–483

39 Deal EC, McFadden ER, Ingram RH, Jaeger JJ.
Effects of atropine on the potentiation of exercise-induced bronchospasm by
cold air. *J Appl Physiol 1978; 45:* 238–243

40 Stearns DR, McFadden ER Jr, Brestin FJ, Ingram RH Jr.
Reanalysis of the refractory period in exertional asthma.
J Appl Physiol 1981; 50: 503–508

41 Brown MJ, Ind PW, Causon R, Lee TH.
A novel double-isotope technique for the enzymatic assay of plasma histamine:
application to estimation of mast cell activation assessed by antigen challenge
in asthmatics. *J Allergy Clin Immunol 1982; 69:* 20–24

42 Barnes PJ, Brown MJ, Silverman M, Dollery CT.
Circulating catecholamines in exercise- and hyperventilation-induced asthma.
Thorax 1981; 36: 435–440

43   Warren JB, Keynes RJ, Brown MJ et al.
     Blunted sympatho-adrenal response to exercise in asthmatic subjects.
     Br J Dis Chest 1982; 76: 147–150

44   Nagakura T, Iikura Y, Miyakawa T.
     Serum dopamine β-hydroxylase and free fatty acids in exercise-induced asthma.
     Clin Allergy. In press

DISCUSSION

HAIDER (Bury, UK)	One of the problems of exercise testing is the standardisation of exercise itself. I find a significant number of children do not show the abnormalities of clinical or pulmonary airways function on conventional testing in hospital surroundings. Nevertheless they become evident when the tests are performed by the parents at home. The duration of exercise is probably less important in terms of time but more important in terms of breathlessness.
ANDERSON	Perhaps the children have a high level of catecholamines in a hospital environment. Certainly we have experience of people who, when they first come to the laboratory, do not have exercise-induced asthma but who develop it subsequently.
	However, we have found that even vigorous treadmill exercise for eight minutes at heart rates of 175 beats/min will not induce an attack of asthma in 23 per cent of children. Exercise-induced asthma is not a consistent occurrence: some children may only have exercise-induced asthma when they have infections or in unusually dry weather.
PIERSON (Seattle, USA)	Does arterial hypoxaemia correlate with the severity of exercise-induced bronchospasm?
ANDERSON	I have not actually done the necessary calculations — the changes in flow rates were changes in oxygen tension. What distinguishes our tests from those of anybody else is that we really do get severe exercise-induced asthma — our falls in lung function measurements are around 45—50 per cent. In fact, we would not ask a patient to volunteer for a blood study unless we knew he or she would have severe exercise-induced asthma. Obviously, therefore, all the patients in whom we introduced arterial lines had hypoxaemia.

However, only three of the 20 patients we have studied had values for arterial oxygen tension less than 60mmHg (7.8 kPa).

We have seen reductions in oxygen saturation down to 70 per cent in children who have had, say a 70 per cent fall in peak flow or FEV_1. So, yes, I think there is a correlation. Probably the most severe asthmatic reaction is associated with the most severe hypoxaemia.

WINSNES
(Drammen,
Norway)

What are the effects (if any) of alpha- and beta-receptor blocking agents on exercise-induced asthma? The answer might elucidate the possible role of noradrenaline in exercise-induced asthma.

ANDERSON

The effects of drugs on exercise-induced asthma depend entirely on the route of administration. The alpha-blockers — thymoxamine, phentolamine and prazosin — have all been shown to block exercise-induced asthma when given by aerosol. However, we have found little use for these agents when they are given orally.

With respect to the beta-blocking drugs, the only studies I know of have all used the oral form and I think that the effect of these agents is to increase the resting level of airways resistance rather than enhance exercise-induced asthma.

CAMPBELL
(Penarth, UK)

How do 'mediators' make the airways hyperreactive?

HOLGATE

Some elegant studies have been carried out in the USA on tracheal smooth muscle from the cat demonstrating that when the muscle is sensitised in the active state its pattern of work changes from that of multiple units to that of a single unit. It behaves more as a single muscle contracting, rather than as many individual muscle fibres contracting. It is this electrophysiological change in the muscle brought about by the presence of inflammatory mediators that I believe underlies hyperreactivity.

ANDERSON   I wonder if the intensity and duration of exercise and
                        the degree of obstruction induced in the studies of
                        Drs Holgate and Lee were all too small for histamine
                        to be released?

HOLGATE   The exercise task that produced a 60 per cent fall in
                        specific airways conductance was associated with a 30
                        per cent fall in the forced expiratory volume in one
                        second and I would suggest that this is a reasonable
                        exercise task. It may not be the maximum exercise-
                        induced bronchoconstriction that could be produced
                        but it makes the patient sufficiently uncomfortable
                        for us to hesitate to provoke them any further.

JENSSEN (Trond-   Do you have any idea of the purity of chemotactic
heim, Norway)   factor that you elute from your column?

LEE   That is a question to which we are devoting a great
                        deal of time. One of the most difficult problems facing
                        us in characterising the precise nature of this chemo-
                        tactic factor is starting material. There is only so
                        much blood that you can take from an asthmatic
                        after a challenge test, and the difficulty of having
                        small amounts of starting material is that it is not
                        possible to raise lines on any conventional gels to
                        determine the purity of our preparation.

HOLGATE   If isocapnic hyperventilation causes the same broncho-
                        constriction as occurs in exercise but without the
                        release of neutrophil chemotactic factor, how is it
                        that mediators released with exercise contribute to
                        this bronchoconstriction?

LEE   That is a difficult question. I think that the broncho-
                        constriction of exercise-induced asthma is likely to be
                        caused by many factors — and the release of a media-
                        tor is just one of them. There are differences between
                        a true exercise task and hyperventilation. For instance,
                        there is the refractory period. There is also the bron-
                        chodilatation that occurs during exercise but not
                        during isocapnic hyperventilation. In certain indivi-

duals there is a long period after exercise before the development of maximal airflow obstruction. In our experience isocapnic hyperventilation produces maximal airflow obstruction earlier than exercise and I would suggest that although respiratory heat loss initiates the obstruction to airflow, mediators probably have a modulating influence on this.

THOMSON (Glasgow, UK)   Some asthmatics develop late asthmatic responses three to eight hours after allergen inhalation tests. Have you observed similar late responses after exercise? If so, was this associated with changes in neutrophil chemotactic factor?

LEE   We have observed late asthmatic reactions after exercise in a study carried out in collaboration with Dr Iikura. However, our results are preliminary and detailed analysis of the data is still required.

Chapter 6

CLIMATIC CONDITIONS AND THEIR EFFECT ON EXERCISE-INDUCED ASTHMA

O Bar-Or

Children's Therapeutic Exercise and Fitness Centre, McMaster University, Hamilton, Ontario, Canada

SUMMARY

Exercise-induced asthma does not occur consistently in any given asthmatic patient, even when exertion and medication are standardised. A major reason for this inconsistency is the fluctuation in climatic conditions. Specifically, it is the temperature and humidity of inspired air that determines airway response to exercise: while dry or cold air increases the risk of exercise-induced asthma humid or warm air has a protective influence.

Evaporative and convective respiratory heat loss, which are dependent on the water content and temperature of inspired air and on ventilation, have been implicated as the main trigger for exercise-induced asthma. The mechanism has, however, not yet been elucidated, nor is it clear why respiratory heat loss is less important in swimming than in running.

Natural humidification and warming of inspired air by nasal breathing has been shown to prevent exercise-induced asthma in asthmatics who exert themselves at mild or moderate intensities. No data, however, are available on the feasibility for the asthmatic of nasal breathing during high intensity exertion or spontaneous play.

Some of the still unresolved questions about climatic effects on exercise-induced asthma are: (1) Is it only the direct effect on the bronchial mucosa that determines bronchial response to exercise or is the exposure of other parts of the skin (for example, the face) to thermal influence also of importance? (2) Can asthmatic individuals 'acclimatise' to cold/dry air stress? (3) Will exposure to *extremely* dry/hot weather be detrimental to the exercising asthmatic because of the marked hyperpnoea and resultant evaporative loss? (4) How do climatic conditions interact with other weather conditions (for example, ionisation) in their effect on exercise-induced asthma?

INTRODUCTION

In spite of its high prevalence exercise-induced asthma is an inconsistent occurrence in any given asthmatic. Even when the type, duration and intensity of exercise, as well as medication, are standardised an asthmatic may respond to exercise with bronchoconstriction on one day but not on another. A number of factors have been implicated as responsible for this inconsistency, and amongst them is fluctuation in climatic conditions.

In a broad sense 'climatic conditions' encompass such variables as ambient temperature, humidity of the atmosphere, wind velocity, solar and other thermal radiation, barometric pressure and ionisation of the air. Since our knowledge of the relationship between climate and exercise-induced asthma is at present limited to the effects of air temperature and humidity, I shall review the data on these two components only.

Although I shall focus on the exercising asthmatic, I shall also mention the effects of climate on the incidence of asthmatic attacks in the resting patient. Artificial conditioning of the inspired air is of the utmost importance to the genesis or prevention of exercise-induced asthma – which is not to deny the value of our built-in air conditioner, the nose.

CLIMATE AND THE RESTING ASTHMATIC

Epidemiological studies [for example, 1–5] and anecdotal observations [6, 7] have indicated that a decrease in ambient temperature, especially during autumn and winter, is associated with, or followed by, a greater incidence of asthmatic attacks. For example, Greenburg and his colleagues [2, 3] found that the number of emergency visits to the clinic on account of asthma in three New York hospitals drastically increased with the onset of cold weather. The increase did not coincide with any rise in moulds, pollen counts or air pollutants. Tromp and Bouma [4] monitored complaints such as cough, wheeziness, breathlessness and asthmatic attacks among children living in an asthma clinic in Holland. In a three-year follow-up they found a definite increase in incidence of these complaints during periods of cool weather in winter and spring, but not during summer. Unfortunately, epidemiological data of this nature are inherently difficult to interpret because changes cannot be looked at in isolation from other climatic components [see, for example, 1] or air-borne pathogens.

In the laboratory, various protocols have been used to monitor climatic effects on the asthmatic. Inhalation of cold air reduced the forced expiratory volume in one second (FEV_1) and specific air conductance (sGaw) among asthmatics [8, 9]. A one-minute cold shower (15°C) followed by sitting in front of a fan for one minute induced a 21 per cent drop in FEV_1 and a 98 per cent rise in airway resistance (Raw) among asthmatics, but not among healthy controls [10]. Inhalation of warm humid air (37°C, 100 per cent relative humidity) during the cold shower virtually reversed the effect on respiratory function of body cooling [11] (Figure 1).

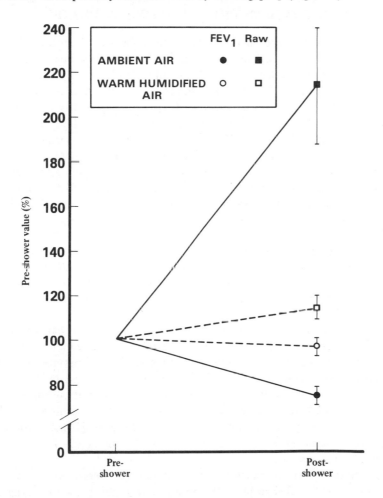

Figure 1. Cold shower and inhalation of warm humid air in the resting asthmatic. Pulmonary functions of eight adult patients were tested before and after a shower at 15°C. Comparison between inhalation of 37°C, 100 per cent relative humidity (warm, humid) and 23°C, 30 per cent relative humidity (ambient) air (FEV_1 = forced expiratory volume in one second; Raw = airway resistance) (Data of Horton and Chen [11])

Unlike cooling, drying or humidifying the air without changing its temperature does not seem to affect airway resistance of the resting asthmatic [12, 13]. Introduction of mist particles of various size was found beneficial to some asthmatic children but detrimental to others [14].

CLIMATE AND THE EXERCISING ASTHMATIC

Research into the combined effects on the asthmatic of climate and exercise is of quite recent origin. In the mid-1970s four laboratories (in Detroit, Colorado, Boston and the Wingate Institute) simultaneously, but independently, started studying this issue. In three, the temperature- or humidity-controlled inspired air was introduced by a mask [15, 16] or through a mouthpiece [17]. In the fourth, subjects were free-breathing in a climate-controlled chamber [13]. The results indicated that, during exercise: (1) dry inspired air was more asthmagenic in neutral ambient temperature than humidified air [13, 15], (2) cold inspired air was more asthmagenic than air at neutral ambient temperature [17], (3) inspired air warmed to 37°C and saturated with water vapour virtually prevented exercise-induced asthma [16], and (4) raising the temperature of the inspired air to about 37°C, but keeping the water vapour content at low values reduced, but did not entirely abolish, bronchoconstriction [16]. Similar results were later obtained by others [18–24]. In only two asthmatic adults [25] did warming of the inspired air (30–34°C) and its humidification (water vapour content not stated) not reduce the degree of exercise-induced asthma.

The common denominator of the above experiments is that increase in airway cooling brings about a greater degree of exercise-induced asthma, whereas its reduction has the opposite effect. The first to show this relationship in a quantitative manner were Chen and Horton [16]. As summarised in Figure 2, they found a fairly consistent relationship between the fall in FEV_1 and the respiratory heat loss. Analysis of this relationship was subsequently refined by Deal and his colleagues [20, 21] for wide ranges of temperature (–10 to +80°C) and humidity (0–100% relative humidity) of inspired air.

Respiratory heat exchange has two components – convection and evaporation. Heat exchange by radiation in the respiratory tract is negligible. Heat loss by convection can be calculated from equation (1):

$$HL_C = \dot{V}_E \cdot HC(T_E - T_I) \tag{1}$$

where HL_C is the heat loss by convection in kJ/min; $\dot{V}_E$, the minute ventilation (BTPS) in L/min; HC, the thermal capacity – the product of

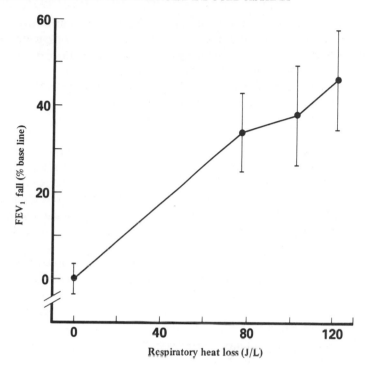

Figure 2. Respiratory heat loss and airway resistance. Eight asthmatic adolescents and young adults underwent treadmill walks at four combinations of humidity and temperature of inspired air (FEV$_1$ fall = per cent decrease of forced expiratory volume in one second after exercise. Values are mean ± 1 SE) (Adapted from Chen and Horton [16])

specific heat and density — of air (= 1.27 × 10^{-3} kJ/L/°C); and T$_E$ and T$_I$, the temperature of the expired and inspired air, respectively, in °C, both measured at the mouth. It is apparent from equation (1) that in most prevailing climates, in which T$_E$ exceeds T$_I$, heat will be *lost* by convection. Inversely, during hot weather (about 35°C or more) the air inspired may be warmer than the air expired and the net result will be convective heat *gain*.

Heat loss by evaporation is calculated from equation (2):

$$HL_e = \dot{V}_E \cdot HV(WC_E - WC_I) \tag{2}$$

where HL$_e$ is the heat loss by evaporation in kJ/min; HV, the latent heat loss of vaporisation of water (= 2.43 kJ/g); and WC$_E$ and WC$_I$, the vapour content of the expired and inspired air, respectively, in g per litre of air.

Because expired air is usually saturated at $37°C$ WC_I is lower than WC_E. The exception is when the inspired air is warmer than body temperature and is saturated. In this very unlikely climatic condition there will be a net heat *gain* by condensation, rather than loss by evaporation.

The overall respiratory heat loss (RHL) is obtained by combining the losses by convection and evaporation, as in equation (3):

$$RHL = \dot{V}_E \left[HC \left(T_E - T_I\right) + HC \left(WC_E - WC_I\right) \right] \tag{3}$$

One should realise that out of the two components of the total respiratory heat loss, it is the loss by evaporation that usually dominates. For example, drying the inspired air at $37°C$ from 100 per cent to 50 per cent relative humidity (which is by no means a dry climate) would induce an evaporative loss of $0.06\,kJ$ per litre of air. To obtain a similar degree of cooling by convection the ambient temperature would have to be lowered from $37°C$ to $-10°C$.

Exertion affects respiratory cooling primarily by the marked increase in $\dot{V}_E$, which in moderate exercise can be $8-10$ times that at rest. During exhausting exercise, it can be $15-20$ times the resting values. Another effect is on T_E (and therefore WC_E), as core body temperature can rise by $2-3°C$ in moderate or severe exercise. Airway cooling, however, which results from increase in T_E is negligible in comparison with the marked changes induced by hyperpnoea.

The importance of airway cooling in triggering exercise-induced asthma is now universally accepted. There still is, however, no agreement as to whether airway cooling can offer a *unifying* explanation of the variety of phenomena related to exercise-induced asthma. Proponents of the unifying approach have stated that 'the role of exercise can be viewed as only the means to increase respiratory heat exchange through hyperpnea' [21] and that the non-ventilatory events which take place during exercise are tangential to the genesis of exercise-induced asthma. Indeed, in the study of Deal and his colleagues [20], hyperventilation at rest induced broncho-constriction to a degree predictable from their previously constructed FEV_1-respiratory heat loss relationship during exericse.

Others agree about the importance of respiratory heat loss but hold that the unifying approach may be an oversimplification. Firstly, the FEV_1-respiratory heat loss regression line and correlation coefficient constructed by Deal and his colleagues [20] are based on repeated measurements on the same group of individuals rather than on independent individual values [24, 26]. Thus, the predictive strength of the regression line underestimates inter-individual variability. A specific conceptual weakness of such a regression line is that it is invalid for people who differ in body size from those studied by Deal. Children, for example, have smaller $\dot{V}_E$ than adults and cannot reach some of the absolute levels of respiratory heat loss found by Deal. Still, their per cent fall in FEV_1 is as marked as is that of adults. A case in point is shown in Figure 3 in which Deal's data for adults is compared with data reported by Bar-Yishay and his colleagues [24] for 13-year-old asthmatic boys. For these boys to reach a degree of respiratory heat loss such as is found in adults they would have to increase their $\dot{V}_E$ to levels beyond their $\dot{V}_{E\ max}$. To reconcile the above discrepancy the FEV_1-respiratory heat loss equation should be modified to take account of differences in body size. One approach is to define relative heat loss in *relative*

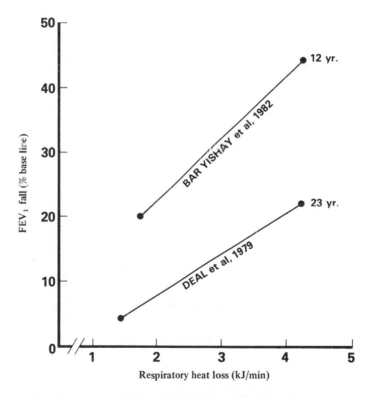

Figure 3. Effect of age on the relationship between exercise-induced asthma and respiratory heat loss. A comparison of post-exertional fall in forced expiratory volume in one second (FEV_1) between children and adults (Data from Bar-Yishay et al [24] and Deal et al [20])

terms, using per cent $\dot{V}_{E\,max}$ or per cent $\dot{V}_E$ at rest instead of absolute $\dot{V}_E$. Another, and conceptually more correct, approach is to equate the respiratory heat loss of individuals according to body size (height, skin surface area or height[3]), as has recently been attempted [24]. Another phenomenon that cannot be explained in full by respiratory heat loss is the low asthmagenicity of swimming, as discussed below.

The mechanism by which airway cooling triggers exercise-induced asthma is not clear. Discussion of the chain of events that may take place after a cold stimulus overlaps discussion of mechanisms that underlie the genesis of exercise-induced asthma in general. This topic is covered in detail elsewhere in these proceedings.

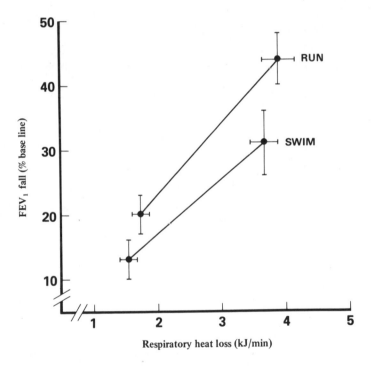

Figure 4.   The protective nature of swimming against exercise-induced asthma as related to respiratory heat loss. Thirteen adolescent asthmatics ran and swam while inhaling dry or humid air (FEV$_1$ fall = per cent decrease of forced expiratory volume in one second after exercise. Mean ± 1SE) (Adapted from Bar-Yishay et al [24])

SWIMMING AND EXERCISE-INDUCED ASTHMA –
THE CLIMATE ANGLE

The protective nature of air of high humidity on the one hand and the low asthmagenicity of swimming on the other raises the hypothesis that the highly humid air at water level is the reason why swimming seldom induces bronchoconstriction. This hypothesis was tested at my laboratory in the Wingate Institute [27]. The pulmonary response to swimming was measured in asthmatic children with documented running-induced asthma. Unbeknown to the children they inhaled dried air (6–7mg H_2O/L air). Contrary to our expectations this treatment did *not* induce bronchoconstriction, suggesting that the protective nature of swimming was due to factors other than low respiratory heat loss. In a subsequent study [24], drying of inspired air was more thorough (approximately 2mg H_2O/L air). Bronchoconstriction was induced but, as shown in Figure 4, to a lesser extent than after a run, even though the respiratory heat loss was equated in both modes of exercise.

These data strongly suggest that the low respiratory heat loss during swimming is just one factor, among others, which protects the asthmatic against exercise-induced asthma.

NASAL VERSUS ORAL BREATHING
AND EXERCISE-INDUCED ASTHMA

The preceding discussion has focused on extraneous modifications of inspired air and their effect on the exercising asthmatic. One should realise, however, that the temperature and humidity of air reaching the lower airways are to a great extent determined by whether it passes through the mouth or through the in-built air conditioner, the nose. Nasal air conditioning is so efficient that even during extremes of ambient temperature and humidity the air reaching the nasopharynx is 32–37°C and nearly always 100 per cent humid [see, for example, 28]. It is thus expected that climatic provocation of exercise-induced asthma will be attenuated, or even prevented, if subjects are made to inhale through their noses. Indeed, this was the finding in two studies from Denver: 7–14-year old asthmatics walked on a treadmill at 75–80 per cent of their aerobic capacity. Air temperature was 20–22°C and relative humidity 25–30 per cent. When breathing spontaneously, bronchoconstriction was apparent after exertion. It was more severe when oral breathing was enforced, and practically abolished with nasal breathing [29]. Thus, even though ventilation was identical in both, nasal breathing was apparently efficient in preventing airway cooling. In another report by the same group [30] nasal breathing was also effective in reducing bronchoconstriction after isocapnic hyperventilation at rest. Benefit to asthmatics of nasal breathing was recently confirmed during free running [31].

Is it practicable to breathe through the nose during exercise? While no data are available on the feasibility for asthmatics of nasal breathing during spontaneous activity the following information is of relevance: most people inhale through their nose while at rest and switch to oronasal breathing during exercise [for example, 32]. The stage at which oronasal breathing starts depends on nasal airway resistance [33], nasal work of breathing and the rating of perceived exertion of breathing [32] of each individual. The breathing pattern also depends on previous experience and training. Exercise was found to increase the cross section of the nasal airway and thus to decrease the airway resistance of healthy adults exercising in a neutral [34] or in a dry [35] environment. The same was shown for patients suffering from allergic rhinitis [36]. This increase in nasal patency is probably due to sympathetic discharge and vasoconstriction. In contrast, exposure to cold has been found to *increase* the resistance of the nasal airway at rest [28, 37]. It is therefore of extreme practical importance to conduct a definitive study with asthmatics, assessing their ability to inhale through the nose during high intensity exertion, expecially on cold and dry days.

PRACTICAL IMPLICATIONS OF CLIMATIC EFFECTS ON EXERCISE-INDUCED ASTHMA

To the clinician, scientist, educator, parent or patient a number of practical lessons can be derived from the above information:

1) asthmatics should be instructed to reduce their physical activities on cold or dry days, tailoring the nature and extent of the reduction to the individual;

2) nasal breathing during exertion should be taught and encouraged;

3) for outdoor activities in extremely cold weather face masks (some are available commercially) can be used. These trap warm and humid expired air and induce partial conditioning of inspired air;

4) standardisation of temperature and especially humidity is important in any clinical environment (physician's office or a hospital laboratory) where exercise-induced asthma is to be assessed;

5) scientists planning research on exercise-induced asthma must consider respiratory heat loss to be a major independent variable in any future study [for example, 38]. It is safe to assume that much of the inconsistency in previous findings (for example, on the effects of hyperventilation or of different exercise stimuli) could have been avoided had climate been taken into consideration;

6) cold-induced asthma is a reproducible and quantifiable phenomenon. It can be used (at rest or during exercise) to evaluate efficacy of drugs [for example, 39] or for further understanding of the mechanisms that underlie exercise-induced asthma [19, 40].

References

1   Derrick EH.
    The seasonal variation of asthma in Brisbane: its relation to temperature and humidity. *Int J Biometeorol 1965; 9:* 239–251

2   Greenburg L, Field F, Reed JI, Erhardt CL.
    Asthma and temperature change.
    Arch Environ Health 1964; 8: 642–647

3   Greenburg L, Field F, Reed JI, Erhardt CL.
    Asthma and temperature change. II – 1964 and 1965 epidemiological studies of emergency clinic visits for asthma in three large New York City Hospitals.
    Arch Environ Health 1966; 12: 561–563

4   Tromp SW, Bouma J.
    Effect of weather on asthmatic children in the eastern part of the Netherlands.
    Int J Biometeorol 1965; 9: 233–238

5   Hobday JD, Stewart AJ.
    The relationship between daily asthma attendance, weather parameters, spore count and pollen count. *Aust NZ J Med 1973; 3:* 552–556

6   Bury JD.
    Climate and chest disorders.
    Br Med J 1972; 4: 613

7   Steer RG.
    Asthma and the weather.
    Med J Aust 1976; 7: 38

8   Millar JS, Nairn JR, Unkles RD, McNeill RS.
    Cold air and ventilatory function.
    Br J Dis Chest 1965; 59: 23–27

9   Simonsson BG, Jacobs FM, Nadel JA.
    Role of autonomic nervous system and the cough reflex in the increased responsiveness of airways in patients with obstructive airway disease.
    J Clin Invest 1967; 46: 1812–1818

10 Chen WY, Horton DJ.
    Airways obstruction in asthmatics induced by body cooling.
    Scand J Respir Dis 1978; 59: 13–20

11   Horton DJ, Chen WY.
     Effects of breathing warm humidified air on bronchoconstriction induced by
     body cooling and by inhalation of metacholine. *Chest 1979; 75:* 24–28

12   Fontana VJ, Fost A, Rappaport I.
     Effects of rapid change in humidity on pulmonary function studies in normal
     and asthmatic children in a controlled environment. *J Allergy 1969; 43:* 16–21

13   Bar-Or O, Neuman I, Dotan R.
     Effects of dry and humid climate on exercise-induced asthma in children and
     preadolescents. *J Allergy Clin Immunol 1977; 60:* 160–168

14   Rodriguez GE, Branch JB, Cotton EK.
     The use of humidity in asthmatic children.
     J Allergy Clin Immunol 1975; 56: 133–140

15   Weinstein RE, Anderson JA, Kvale P, Sweet LC.
     Effects of humidification on exercise-induced asthma (EIA).
     J Allergy Clin Immunol 1976; 57: 250–251

16   Chen WY, Horton DJ.
     Heat and water loss from the airways and exercise-induced asthma.
     Respiration 1977; 34: 305–313

17   Strauss RH, McFadden ER, Ingram RH, Jaeger JJ.
     Enhancement of exercise-induced asthma by cold air.
     N Engl J Med 1977; 297: 743–747

18   Strauss RH, McFadden ER, Ingram RH et al.
     Influence of heat and humidity on the airway obstruction induced by exercise
     in asthma. *J Clin Invest 1978; 61:* 433–440

19   Deal EC, McFadden ER, Ingram RH, Jaeger JJ.
     Effects of atropine on the potentiation of exercise-induced bronchospasm by
     cold air. *J Appl Physiol 1978; 45:* 238–243

20   Deal EC, McFadden ER, Ingram RH et al.
     Role of respiratory heat exchange in production of exercise-induced asthma.
     J Appl Physiol 1979; 46: 467–475

21   Deal EC, McFadden ER, Ingram RH, Jaeger JJ.
     Hyperpnea and heat flux: initial reaction sequence in exercise-induced asthma.
     J Appl Physiol 1979; 46: 476–483

22   Anderson SD, Daviskas E, Schoeffel RE, Unger SF.
     Prevention of severe exercise-induced asthma with hot humid air.
     Lancet 1979; ii: 629

23   Malo JL, Filiatrault S, Martin RR.
     Combined effects of exercise and exposure to outside cold air on lung functions
     of asthmatics. *Bull Eur Physiopathol Respir 1980; 16:* 623–635

24   Bar-Yishay E, Gur I, Inbar I et al.
     Differences between swimming and running as stimuli for exercise-induced
     asthma. *Eur J Appl Physiol.* In press

25   Lefcoe NM, Carter RP, Ahmad D.
     Exercise bronchoconstriction in normal subjects and asthmatics.
     Am Rev Respir Dis 1971; 104: 562–567

26   Anderson SD.
     Exercise-induced asthma – new ideas about an old problem – response.
     In Hargreave FE, ed. *Airway Reactivity 1980; 30.*
     Mississauga: Astra

27 Inbar O, Dotan R, Dlin RA et al.
Breathing dry or humid air and exercise-induced asthma during swimming.
Eur J Appl Physiol 1980; 44: 43–50

28 Proctor DF, Andersen I, Lundqvist GP.
Human nasal mucosal function at controlled temperatures.
Respir Physiol 1977; 30: 109–124

29 Shturman-Ellstein R, Zeballos RJ, Buckley JM, Souhrada JF.
The beneficial effect of nasal breathing on exercise-induced bronchoconstriction.
Am Rev Respir Dis 1978; 118: 65–73

30 Zeballos RJ, Shturman-Ellstein R, McNally JF et al.
The role of hyperventilation in exercise-induced bronchoconstriction.
Am Rev Respir Dis 1978; 118: 877–884

31 Mangla PK, Menon MPS.
Effect of nasal and oral breathing on exercise-induced asthma.
Clin Allergy 1981; 11: 433–439

32 Niinimaa V, Cole P, Mintz S, Shephard RJ.
The switching point from nasal to oronasal breathing.
Respir Physiol 1980; 42: 61–71

33 Patrick GA, Sharp GR.
Oronasal distribution of inspiratory flow during various activities.
J Physiol 1970; 206: 22p–23p

34 Niinimaa V, Cole P, Shephard RJ.
Nasal work of breathing at rest and during exercise.
Med Sci Sports Exerc 1980; 12: 126

35 Andersen I, Lundqvist GR, Jensen PL, Proctor DF.
Human response to 78-hour exposure to dry air.
Arch Environ Health 1974; 29: 319–324

36 Richerson HB, Seebohm PM.
Nasal airway response to exercise.
J Allergy 1968; 41: 269–284

37 Takagi Y, Proctor DF, Salman S, Evering S.
Effects of cold air and carbon dioxide on nasal air flow resistance.
Ann Otol Rhinol Laryngol 1969; 78: 40–48

38 Kilham H, Tooley M, Silverman M.
Running, walking and hyperventilation causing asthma in children.
Thorax 1979; 34: 582–586

39 Breslin FJ, McFadden EA, Ingram RH.
The effects of cromolyn sodium on the airway response to hyperpnea and cold air in asthma. *Am Rev Respir Dis 1980; 122:* 11–16

40 O'Byrne PM, Ryan G, Morris M et al.
Asthma induced by cold air and its relation to nonspecific bronchial responsiveness to metacholine. *Am Rev Respir Dis 1982; 125:* 281–285

Chapter 7

THE EFFECT OF BREATHING DRY OR HUMID AIR ON EXERCISE-INDUCED ASTHMA CAUSED BY RUNNING OR SWIMMING

I Neuman

Hasharon Hospital, Petach-Tikva, Israel

SUMMARY

Among the factors that possibly influence the responses of asthmatic children to exercise, atmospheric conditions have so far received little attention. This study was performed to determine whether the humidity of the air in conjunction with the type of exercise should be considered.

Twenty extrinsic perennial asthmatic children with histories of exercise-induced asthma showed no changes in pulmonary function whether sitting in dry or humid conditions. However, five or 10 minutes after running on the treadmill, bronchoconstriction was distinctly more pronounced in the dry rather than the humid atmospheres. Nine of the asthmatic children undertook eight-minute exercise challenge tests of 'tethered-swimming' at constant metabolic rates. No reduction in pulmonary function was found five or 10 minutes after the swimming exercise whether they were inspiring dry air (25–35% relative humidity) or humid air (80–90% relative humidity). A further 13 children exercised for six minutes by running on a treadmill followed by tethered-swimming while breathing air to 80–90% relative humidity. Metabolic rates were closely matched. The falls in forced expiratory volume in one second (FEV_1) after exercise were again significantly greater after running compared with swimming and were unaltered whether humid or dry air was breathed.

The changes in FEV_1 were also related to respiratory heat loss calculated from measurements of inspired and expired gas temperatures and humidity. At a standardised respiratory heat loss, the differences between running and swimming were highly significant.

These experiments suggest that exercise-induced asthma is more likely to occur in dry rather than humid air possibly due to heat loss from the airway mucosa caused by evaporation. They also suggest that the type of exercise appears to influence the severity of exercise-induced asthma even under the same metabolic stress and respiratory heat loss. Finally these experiments show that swimming does not readily lead to exercise-induced asthma.

INTRODUCTION

All the climatic studies reported here were carried out at the Department of Research and Sports Medicine at the Wingate Institute and the Hasharon Hospital in Israel.

Although extrinsic asthma is by definition dependent on the environment, only little attention has so far been given to the possibility that climatic conditions may determine the variability in exercise-induced asthma and that some climates may be less favourable to the exercising asthmatic than others. Yet the occurrence of exercise-induced asthma has been shown to vary with the seasons [1].

While it has been a common clinical practice to advise some asthmatics to change their climatic environment by moving to a dry geographical region, no systematic studies were available until our work in 1977, to show whether it was the dryness *per se* or the lack of allergens that was beneficial. As Dr Anderson has shown the bronchial lability typical of exercise-induced asthma in a child can be seen after six minutes of running. During the early part, there is a small but definite degree of bronchodilatation. After about four minutes of running, this gives way to constriction and once the exercise is stopped there is a profound fall in the peak expiratory flow rate (PEFR) as the full exercise-induced asthma develops three to four minutes later [2].

STUDY OF THE EFFECT OF HUMIDITY ON RUNNING

Twenty children with extrinsic perennial asthma, allergic rhinitis and exercise-induced asthma were included in our climatic study in 1977 [3] which was carried out during winter months in order to reduce the chance that seasonal allergens might affect the results.

Each child underwent two testing sessions in a climatic chamber. For both, similar protocols were used, the only difference being that in one of the sessions the relative humidity was set at 90 per cent (humid) while in the other it was set at 25 per cent (dry). The air temperature in both sessions was kept constant at $25-26°C$.

The two sessions were randomly assigned to each child and were separated by one to three weeks. After a rest period in a neutral environment and then in the assigned environment, treadmill running was carried out for six minutes at sub-maximal heart rates.

This study showed that the level of humidity affected the bronchial resistance only during exercise and not at rest. Dryness proved less favourable to the free-breathing exercising asthmatic child than did high ambient humidity. In this study the trigger for the exercise-induced asthma could have been loss of respiratory heat and water due to breathing dry air [3].

STUDY OF THE EFFECT OF HUMIDITY ON SWIMMING

In another study performed in our laboratory an attempt was made to clarify the role played by the humidity of the inspired air in preventing or reducing asthmatic reactions after swimming [4]. This time nine children with extrinsic perennial asthma, allergic rhinitis and proven exercise-induced asthma were included. Test sessions were carried out during the dry Israeli summer months, again to minimise the influence of seasonal allergens. After a rest period and passive immersion, the children underwent a swimming challenge consisting of an eight-minute tethered breast-stroke swim. They breathed through a low resistance valve either connected to a Douglas bag containing dry air or placed just above the surface of the water. Pulmonary function tests were carried out before the exercise and five and 10 minutes afterwards. Although a trend toward lower values was apparent in the 'dry' swimming conditions none of the differences between the 'dry' and 'humid' swimming conditions was statistically significant. However, neither 'humid' nor 'dry' swimming caused significant decreases in pulmonary function compared with 'dry' running which had produced significant changes in the same children.

COMPARISON BETWEEN RUNNING AND SWIMMING

In the third study, a more rigorous comparison was made between running and swimming as stimuli for exercise-induced asthma [5]. On two occasions 13 asthmatic children were given six minutes of either treadmill running or tethered breast-stroke swimming while breathing either dry or humid air. A high-speed thermistor was used to measure the temperature of the inspired and expired gases during the exercise periods.

This study showed once again that running provoked more exercise-induced asthma than swimming. During the humid air studies, the children did not develop as much exercise-induced asthma as in the dry air periods although their forced expiratory volumes in one second (FEV_1) before exercise were similar in both cases. There were no significant differences in the temperatures and humidities of the gases used in the two types of exercise and the only differences noted between the tests were that the temperatures of the expired gases after inhalation of humid air were significantly higher ($p < 0.0001$). Presumably this is a reflection of the reduced cooling of the airways.

CONCLUSION

We have shown that there are significant differences in the asthmagenicity between humid and dry climates and also between swimming and running exercises that are unrelated to the respiratory heat loss of these two types of exercises.

On the strength of these studies we have decided to control and describe the climatic conditions in our future work on exercise-induced asthma.

In a recent study the presence of vasoactive materials was checked in 10 children before and after asthma induced by six minutes of free-range running in dry climatic conditions with a relative humidity below 30 per cent [Neuman et al, unpublished observations]. In one group of children, significant changes in blood kallikrein levels were found after the provocation perhaps indicating an involvement of this vasoactive material in exercise-induced asthma. In one child kallikrein levels in the blood were high before provocation of the exercise-induced asthma and the levels did not significantly increase after the provocation. Perhaps in this child the level of kallikrein in the blood was already sufficient to provide an additional trigger for the asthmatic symptoms.

Since no change was found in humoral immunoglobulins or in the complement system, kallikrein activation of exercise-induced asthma is probably not an immune-dependent mechanism. Thus, in some cases, there is an actual enhancement of kallikrein in exercise-induced asthma while in others there is no further enhancement when the levels are already pathologically high before the onset of exercise-induced asthma.

References

1   Eggleston PA.
     Exercise-induced asthma in children with intrinsic and extrinsic asthma.
     Pediatrics 1975; 56: 1

2   Godfrey S, Silverman M, Anderson SD.
     Problems of interpreting exercise-induced asthma.
     J Allergy Clin Immunol 1973; 52: 199

3   Bar-Or O, Neuman I, Dotan R.
     Effects of dry and humid climates on exercise-induced asthma in children and
     preadolescents. *J Allergy Clin Immunol 1977; 60:* 163–168

4   Inbar O, Dotan R, Dlin RA, Neuman I, Bar-Or O.
     Breathing dry or humid air and exercise-induced asthma during swimming.
     Eur J Appl Physiol 1980; 44: 43–50

5   Bar-Yishay E, Gur I, Inbar O, Neuman I, Dlin RA, Godfrey S.
     Eur J Appl Physiol 1982; in press

DISCUSSION

JENSSEN (Trondheim, Norway)	Evaporation from the airways is dramatically increased during hyperventilation, which can be compensated for by hypersecretion. The loss of water will lead to contraction of macromolecules in the secretion and thereby changes in its visco-elastic properties. Is there any evidence that the obstruction to the airways after exercise is caused not merely by bronchospasm, but also possibly by the secretions?
BAR-OR	I am not aware of any information from either the cooling or the drying point of view which could corroborate this possibility. However, Dr Anderson tells me that she is now conducting some studies into the possible relationship between changes in osmolality and bronchoconstriction. Changes in osmolality are likely to result from drying of the airways, so maybe there is something relevant here, but, as I say, I am not familiar with any direct evidence.
BURGE (Birmingham, UK)	In my experience, exercise on foggy days causes even more asthma than on cold days. Could the asthma provoked by cold showers be more dependent on the water aerosol inhaled than on the inspiration of cold air — indeed was the air inspired during cold showering actually cold?
BAR-OR	This is a possibility. Rodriguez and his colleagues [reference 14 in my paper] have investigated the size of droplets and the triggering of bronchoconstriction at rest. They found that some asthmatic children respond with bronchoconstriction and others with bronchodilatation. As far as I know Chen and Horton [reference 10 in my paper] did not measure the temperature of the inhaled air during their cold shower study. The statement regarding foggy days in England raises an important issue since other climatic factors, such as the level of pollutants or pollens in the air, could very well mask or unmask effects of temperature

and humidity. Unfortunately our information is still mainly based on laboratory rather than real-life data in this respect.

OSEID
(Chairman)

Do you have any experience with face masks of different kinds for the prevention of exercise-induced asthma?

BAR-OR

We have no first-hand experience but there is definitely a theoretical benefit to such masks if they can increase the dead space — that is, if they can trap some of the warm, humid expired air. With such a device there is a trade-off whereby, although the dead space during exercise is increased, a sort of counter-current effect is induced by means of which inhaled air is warmed and humidified before entering the respiratory tract. I think that certainly such masks can be of benefit.

LINDSAY
(Camperdown,
Australia)

Is it true that *no* heat loss is *always* (that is, in all subjects) associated with *no asthma* (as indicated by your own data and that of Deal and his colleagues in adults and children)?

BAR-OR

I do not think so. There are occasionally individuals who do respond with bronchoconstriction even if both humidity and temperature are brought close to body conditions (BTPS). This is another example of the heterogeneity of exercise-induced asthma — in some asthmatics, whether children or adults, factors other than respiratory heat loss play a role.

FITZGERALD
(Ardkeen,
Ireland)

Does permanent relocation to a more suitable' climate have a *proven* long-term role in the treatment of asthmatics?

BAR-OR

Not to my knowledge. All the studies on climate and exercise-induced asthma are of a few minutes' duration only — or at the most an hour or so. From the practical point of view, the effect of long-term exposure is very definitely a key question.

LITTLEWOOD (Leeds, UK)	Does diet affect the response to exercise? Are the bronchi ever sensitised by food allergens which increase the severity of subsequent exercise-induced broncho-constriction?
NEUMAN	We showed that tartrazine and other food allergens may enhance the activation of the same body kinin system that we showed in exercise-induced asthma. So if the patient takes both food additives and exercise at the same time it may enhance exercise-induced asthma — it is bad to take candy and run.
HAIDER (Bury, UK)	We all know that swimming is the exercise that asth-matic children can do best. Asthma is expiratory dyspnoea. Could it be that the compression of the chest by the water helps with expiration? Has the airway resistance been measured with the chest in and out of the water? Did Dr Neuman make measure-ments before and after passive immersion?
NEUMAN	We did not make these measurements, but it could be that the compression of the chest by the water may help the asthmatic swimmer.
HOLGATE (Southampton, UK)	Do you think the higher borderline levels of kallikrein in patients with asthma reflects chronic mast-cell stimulation?
NEUMAN	The kallikrein of the body kinin system is only one active material that is interwoven with so many other vasoactive materials, such as prostaglandins, C3A and C5A, which are active in the complement system and we are looking for their presence. We have thus far only particles of information and those we have presented here. We found no enhancement of C3A or C5A in exercise-induced asthma. When in the future we are able to measure the slow reacting substance of anaphylaxis (SRS-A) we may find one more vasoactive material that participates in the enhancement of exercise-induced asthma. There is probably more

than one vasoactive material that influences exercise-induced asthma and one vasoactive hormone may activate other vasoactive pathways.

LEE
(London, UK)

How do you measure kallikrein and how specific is the assay?

NEUMAN

It is very specific — it is an immunoassay.

RICHARDSON
(Bromley, UK)

Dr Neuman's technique of tethered swimming ignores the exhalation against the resistance of water that is part of natural swimming. This would seem to introduce an element of artificiality and perhaps even problems of standardisation. Would Dr Neuman please comment?

NEUMAN

Dr Richardson is right and our work with swimmers is only the beginning. We showed that swimming is less asthmagenic than running, and that was the purpose of our work. In the future we could introduce a higher resistance valve for exhalation and then we would know its influence.

BUNDGAARD
(Copenhagen,
Denmark)

All asthmatics can be made to show exercise-induced asthma. If the variations in ventilatory capacity during or after exercise at the first challenge are not great, they will probably become so at the second or third challenge. If exercise-induced asthma is still not in evidence, the ventilation or the work load should be increased and the humidity of the inhaled air decreased. The asthmatic patients who do not respond with large variations in ventilatory capacity after an appropriate challenge have not yet been described in the literature. When normal people perform the same exercise challenge as asthmatics, similar variations in ventilatory capacity are observed — they are simply much smaller. A fall in $\dot{V}_{25}$ of up to 20 per cent may be observed in normal people after exercise, whereas the fall in asthmatics is greater than 30—40 per cent. Asthmatics show changes in forced expiratory volume in one second (FEV_1) greater than 15–20 per cent during and after exercise whereas in normal people the changes are no greater than 5–10 per cent. These facts demonstrate that the changes in ventilatory capacity during and after exercise in asthmatics and non-asthmatics are similar – the only difference is that in asthmatics they are greater.

Might one or more mediators be responsible for exercise-induced asthma? Maybe in part. But it must be remembered that hyperventilation alone is as good as exercise for inducing asthma. Therefore only mediators that are located in the bronchial tree can be expected to take part in the pathogenesis of exercise-induced asthma. The possible mediator(s) must be located in the region of nerves or muscle since inhibition of these components inhibits exercise-induced asthma.

It is well known that all biochemical processes are highly dependent of temperature and concentration. During exercise much heat is lost from the respiratory tract, the temperature decreasing down to about 26°C in the sub-sub-segments of the lung. At the same time a great deal of water is lost from the surface of the lung – a loss that must change the concentrations of some of the substances on the surface of the respiratory tract. Therefore both temperature and concentrations change greatly during exercise. As soon as the exercise is stopped, ventilation is reduced and the temperature and the relative humidity in the respiratory tract return to normal. The changes in the lung volumes and in the ventilatory capacity, however, continue to increase until the maximal response is observed at about 5–10 min after the exercise has ceased. Thus, at the time when the response to exercise is at its maximum in the asthmatic, the temperature and relative humidity in the lungs have returned to normal. These observations together with the fact that inhaled drugs more effectively inhibit exercise-induced asthma than orally given drugs, point to the conclusion that there must be some slow-reacting, adrenergic-sensitive receptors in the lungs which are essential for producing cold- and exercise-induced asthma.

Chapter 8

INFLUENCE OF DIFFERENT DEGREES OF BRONCHO-CONSTRICTION ON REFRACTORINESS IN EXERCISE-INDUCED ASTHMA

J M Henriksen, R Dahl, G R Lundqvist*

Aarhus Kommunehospital, and *University of Aarhus, Denmark

SUMMARY

Increasing the water content of inhaled air has recently been shown to decrease the bronchospastic response to exercise. However, the mechanism underlying this phenomenon is still not understood. Few studies have been designed to evaluate the refractory period that follows an episode of exercise-induced asthma.

The results of our study support the hypothesis that cooling of the bronchial mucosa during exercise is the initiating stimulus for exercise-induced bronchoconstriction. Our finding that the refractory period after an episode of exercise-induced bronchoconstriction is unrelated to the severity of previous bronchoconstriction suggests that exercise-induced bronchoconstriction is not due to mast-cell derived mediators.

INTRODUCTION

Several studies have demonstrated a decreasing bronchospastic response to exercise with increasing water content of inhaled air [1, 2]. Despite this advance in the understanding of exercise-induced asthma, the fundamental mechanism underlying this phenomenon is still not clearly defined. It has been suggested that exercise-induced asthma is the result of the release of mediators derived from the mast cells. For instance, the relative refractoriness seen after an episode of exercise-induced asthma has been considered to be due to depletion of stored mediators, which take time to regenerate [3]. However, few studies have been designed to evaluate the refractory period, and the effect of exercise as such in repeated exercise-induced asthma is not known.

In order to investigate the relationship between previous exercise-induced asthma of different intensities and the pulmonary response to exercise one hour later we carried out a study in a clean air climatic chamber [4]. In paired exercise tests, humidity was used to produce different degrees of bronchoconstriction in three first tests. Room temperature was held constant at 23°C.

MATERIAL AND METHODS

Patients

Eleven asthmatic children, between 9 and 15 years of age, with a history of exercise-induced asthma were studied with the approval of their parents. The selection criterion was a fall in peak expiratory flow rate (PEFR) of at least 15 per cent from base line after submaximal exercise. They were all considered atopic as demonstrated by clinical histories and skin prick tests with common allergens.

Medication (terbutaline, salbutamol or sodium cromoglycate) was withheld for at least 12 hours before all experiments.

Study design

After one hour's rest in the climate chamber each subject performed two exercise tests daily on three consecutive days. The first test of each pair was carried out, in random order, in 15 per cent, 50 per cent and 85 per cent relative humidity, respectively, at 23°C, corresponding to 2.6g, 8.5g and 14.6g water per kg dry air. After one hour's rest the test was repeated in a relative humidity of 50 per cent.

Exercise testing

The exercise tests were performed on a bicycle ergometer. Work loads were held constant for five to six minutes and were adjusted to 80 to 85 per cent of the maximum working capacity. The load for each individual was also kept constant throughout the studies. The children were provided with a nose clip during exercise to ensure identical respiration in the separate tests. Heart rate was monitored by radiotelemetry.

Pulmonary function

PEFR was measured with a Wright Peak Flowmeter on entry to the chamber, immediately before exercise, after 2, 4 and 6 minutes of exercise and 3, 5, 10, 15 and 20 minutes after exercise. Forced expiratory volume in one second (FEV_1, BTPS) was measured with a Vitalograph before and 5, 10 and 20 minutes after exercise. The best of three efforts was used in the calculations. Values were calculated as a percentage of expected normal values. The results were expressed in terms of resting values (base line) and lowest values after exercise.

The data were analysed by two factor analysis of variance, and Student's t test for paired comparisons. Correlation coefficients (r) between parameters were calculated from the individual values by the method of linear least squares.

RESULTS

Resting PEFR (per cent expected) during the study ranged from 75 ± 10 per cent (mean ± SD) to 79 ± 10 per cent before acclimatisation ($F = 1.04$, 3.20 df, NS) and from 76 ± 13 per cent to 81 ± 9 per cent before exercise ($F = 0.66$, 5.50 df, NS). No significant changes in resting PEFR were found during acclimatisation (t test).

Figure 1 illustrates the mean changes in per cent expected PEFR during the exercise experiments. The PEFR increased during exercise and decreased to a minimum three to five minutes after cessation of work. In the first tests with variable humidity, the degree of bronchoconstriction was highly dependent on relative humidity (85 per cent relative humidity vs 50 per cent relative humidity, $p < 0.05$; 85 per cent relative humidity vs 15 per cent relative humidity, $p < 0.001$ and 50 per cent relative humidity vs 15 per cent relative humidity, $p < 0.01$). In the second tests, which were all performed in 50 per cent relative humidity, the bronchoconstrictive responses did not differ statistically according to the t tests. However,

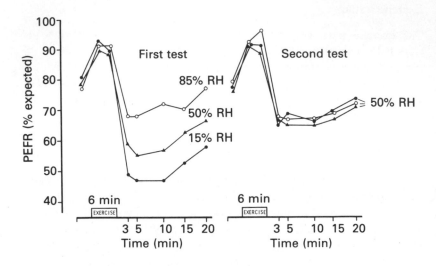

Figure 1. Mean changes in peak expiratory flow rates (PEFR per cent expected) during and after exercise challenges in 11 asthmatic children. The first tests were performed in variable relative humidity (RH) on three consecutive days. The corresponding second test was performed in 50 per cent relative humidity one hour after the first test

when both the first and the second tests were performed under the same conditions (50 per cent relative humidity), the second test caused significantly less exercise-induced bronchoconstriction than did the first test (p < 0.02).

Figure 2 shows base-line and lowest post-exercise FEV_1 values (mean ± SE) during the study. No significant within or between day changes in resting values were found (F = 0.57, 5.50 df, NS). However, a positive linear correlation between the degree of bronchoconstriction in the first test and the difference in base-line FEV_1 between the two tests was found (r = 0.68, p < 0.001) (Figure 3).

The exercise-induced changes in FEV_1 paralleled those in PEFR.

Maximum heart rates during the study ranged from 186 ± 8 (mean ± SD) to 189 ± 8 beats/min (F = 2.21, 5.50 df, NS).

DISCUSSION

The heat lost by evaporation from the bronchial mucosa during exercise is directly related to the minute ventilation and the water content of the inhaled air [1, 2]. The present study has confirmed the central role of

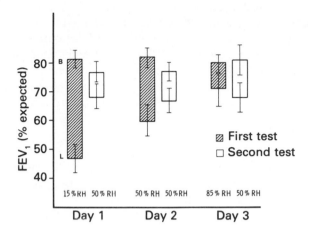

Figure 2. Base-line (B) and lowest (L) post-exercise FEV$_1$ values (mean ± SE) in paired exercise tests on three consecutive days. Room temperature, 23° C. Relative humidity (RH) 15 per cent, 50 per cent and 85 per cent, respectively, in the first tests and 50 per cent in the three second tests

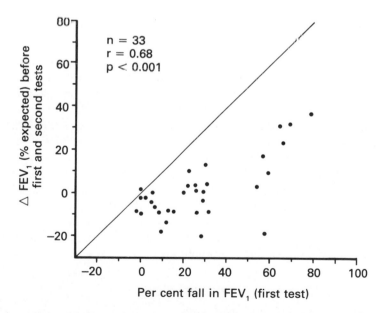

Figure 3. The rationship between per cent fall in FEV$_1$ (first tests) and the difference in resting per cent of expected FEV$_1$ before the first and the second tests. The line of identity is shown

respiratory heat loss in exercise-induced asthma.

The lack of a relationship between the severity of exercise-induced bronchoconstriction in the first and second tests is in contrast to the findings of Edmunds and his colleagues [3]. In a comparable study they found that there was an inverse relationship between the severity of exercise-induced bronchoconstriction in the first and second tests and suggested that this was due to consumption of stored mediators. The discrepancy between the results of the two studies might partly be explained by different protocols. Edmunds and his colleagues used varying work loads to produce different amounts of exercise-induced bronchoconstriction in the first tests, and the paired tests were performed at 30-minute intervals. In addition, they based their conclusions on responses calculated as per cent fall from base line – which, in fact, had not been reached again before the second tests when the first tests had been followed by vigorous bronchoconstriction.

When we expressed our data in terms of per cent fall from base line no significant difference between the responses in the three second tests was found (not presented in the results section above), but there was a tendency to an inverse relationship between the responses in the first and second tests. However, this trend could be explained by the method of calculation and was not found when the results were expressed in terms of lowest values after exercise. Moreover, on analysing the data of Edmunds and his colleagues in terms of lowest post-exercise values, we found no significant difference between the responses in their second tests. So, from this point of view their results are consistent with ours and it seems likely that refractoriness in repeated exercise at short intervals is independent of the magnitude of the previous exercise. These results emphasise that the methods of calculation must be taken into account when refractoriness in exercise-induced asthma is evaluated.

We find that these results are in disagreement with the hypothesis that mast-cell derived mediators are implicated in exercise-induced asthma, instead they indicate that refractoriness in exercise-induced asthma is associated with exercise *per se* or with other mechanisms. Advantage of this phenomenon should be taken in sports and physical games since it shows the beneficial effect of warming up.

CONCLUSION

We have confirmed that dry air increases and humid air decreases the bronchospastic response to exercise. Refractoriness in exercise-induced asthma is independent of the degree of the previous bronchoconstriction.

The degree of refractoriness in exercise-induced asthma is overestimated if the pulmonary responses are expressed in terms of per cent fall from base line. Refractoriness in exercise-induced asthma can be related to previous exercise as such. It is suggested that exercise-induced bronchoconstriction is due to factors other than mediators derived from the mast cells.

References

1   Chen WY, Horton DJ.
     Heat and water loss from the airways and exercise induced asthma.
     Respiration 1977; 34: 305–313

2   Strauss RH, McFadden ER, Ingram RH et al.
     Influence of heat and humidity on the airway obstruction induced by exercise in asthma. *J Clin Invest 1978; 61:* 433–440

3   Edmunds AT, Tooley M, Godfrey S.
     The refractory period after exercise induced asthma.
     Am Rev Respir Dis 1978; 117: 247–254

4   Henriksen JM, Dahl R, Lundqvist GR.
     Influence of relative humidity and repeated exercise on exercise-induced bronchoconstriction. *Allergy 1981; 36:* 463–470

Chapter 9

THE VARIABILITY OF BRONCHOCONSTRICTION AFTER REPEATED AND PROLONGED EXERCISE TESTS IN ASTHMATICS

I Gillam, L I Landau*, P D Phelan*, Mary H D Chennells†

Victoria College, Burwood, Victoria, *Royal Children's Hospital, Melbourne, †Melbourne University, Australia

SUMMARY

In this study in young asthmatics we investigated the relationship between the reduced bronchoconstrictor response seen in the second of two exercise tests, and the predominant site of limitation of flow within the bronchial tree.

Twenty-two subjects were run twice on a treadmill for six minutes. The two exercise tests — exercise 1 and exercise 2 were run 60 minutes apart. The following measurements of pulmonary function were made before and at fixed intervals after exercise: peak expiratory flow rate (PEFR), forced expiratory volume in one second (FEV_1), forced expiratory flow between 25 per cent and 75 per cent of the vital capacity (FEF_{25-75}), lung volumes, maximum expiratory flow at 50 per cent of the total lung capacity ($\dot{V}_{50}$) and the percentage increase in maximum expiratory flow ($\dot{V}_{max}$) at 50 per cent of the vital capacity when breathing a helium-oxygen gas mixture (He responsiveness).

The degree of protection afforded by the first exercise test was determined by comparing the change in the percent fall index of exercise 2, relative to the percent fall index of exercise 1. Asthmatics who were afforded 'little or no protection' by the first exercise test, demonstrated statistically significant decreases in their He responsiveness before and after exercise 2. In these cases, the He responsiveness approached abnormal values, suggesting a predominance of small airways obstruction. In asthmatics with 'significant protection', the He responsiveness remained within normal limits throughout the paired exercise tests suggesting that the predominant site of airways obstruction was in the large central airways. These observations were supported by the fact that there was a smaller decrease in the post-exercise 2 values of those pulmonary function tests considered more representative of small airways obstruction (FEF_{25-75} and $\dot{V}_{50}$), in the group of subjects showing 'significant protection'.

These findings suggest that vagal mechanisms may predominate in asthmatics showing a significantly reduced bronchoconstrictor response in paired exercise tests. The study supports the importance of vagal mechanisms in exercise-induced asthma but there is a need for further studies.

INTRODUCTION

The degree of bronchoconstriction produced in asthmatic subjects by repeated exercise tests on a single day was first studied in four patients by McNeill and his associates [1] in 1966. It was noted that when exercised six times, 45 minutes apart, two of the four patients showed successive reductions in their exercise-induced asthma, one had only a partial reduction, and the fourth maintained the bronchoconstrictor response. The 'protective' nature of exercise on a subsequent exercise challenge has been established by others [2,3], as has the variability of the phenomenon between individuals.

Additional evidence for the heterogeneity of the asthmatic population's response to exercise has been presented by McFadden and his colleagues [4]. By examining the density dependence of expiratory flow and the response to two pharmacological agents, they defined two distinct subgroups of patients with exercise-induced asthma according to the predominant site of limitation of flow within the bronchial tree.

Few studies have investigated the extent of exercise-induced asthma elicited by prolonged exercise [5,6]. In the only comprehensive study of the effect of the duration of exercise on exercise-induced asthma, Silverman and Anderson [5] found that two of the eight subjects "ran through their asthma" [7], although there was considerable variability within the group.

The following study investigated the possibility that a relationship exists between the observed variability of exercise-induced asthma after repeated exercise testing and the predominant site of limitation of flow, as determined by the density dependence of expiratory flow. In addition, the variability between individuals of exercise-induced asthma after prolonged exercise was documented, and compared to the 'protective' effect seen with repeated exercise testing. This was of interest since both phenomena have been attributed to the depletion of bronchoconstrictor mediators [1,7].

SUBJECTS AND METHODS

Twenty-two asthmatic subjects (age range, 10–27 years) were selected on the basis of minimal to moderate airways obstruction at rest, a percent fall index of greater than 14 per cent in peak expiratory flow rate (PEFR) after the first exercise test [8], and their ability to perform the pulmonary function tests required. Subjects were instructed to avoid all medications except steroids for at least six hours before testing. Six of the 22 subjects were taking steroids by inhalation at the time of testing. Informed consent for these procedures was obtained.

PEFR was measured using a Wright peak flow meter. A water filled spirometer was used to measure vital capacity (VC), forced expiratory flow in one second (FEV_1) and forced expiratory flow between 25 and 75 per cent of the vital capacity (FEF_{25-75}).

The maximum expiratory flow-volume (MEFV) curve was recorded with the patient seated in a constant pressure integrated flow plethysmograph [9] and performing a forced vital capacity manoeuvre. The MEFV curve was analysed, by measuring the $\dot{V}_{max}$ at 50 per cent of the total lung capacity ($\dot{V}_{50}$) and expressed as TLC/sec, so that different size lungs could be compared [10].

The subject was then connected via a two-way Rudolph valve to a meteorological balloon containing a low density, 80 per cent helium–20 per cent oxygen gas mixture, and instructed to perform three slow vital capacity manoeuvres. As the subject reached total lung capacity (TLC) on the third inspiration, he was disconnected from the circuit and the MEFV curve repeated. Flows through the pneumotachograph with the He-O_2 gas mixture were corrected electrically to account for the slight increase in viscosity.

The helium and air MEFV curves were superimposed at total lung capacity and the 'He responsiveness', was calculated as shown in equation (1)

$$\text{He responsiveness (\%)} = \frac{\dot{V}_{max}\ 50\%\ VC\ (He\text{-}O_2) - \dot{V}_{max}\ 50\%\ VC\ (air) \times 100}{\dot{V}_{max}\ 50\%\ VC\ (air)} \tag{1}$$

Body plethysmography was used to determine the thoracic gas volume at functional residual capacity, by the method of Du Bois and his colleagues [11].

Normal values for PEFR, spirometry and lung volumes in children (< 16 years) were taken from Cook and Hamann [12] and Murray and Cook [13] and in adults from Cotes [14] and Bates and his colleagues [15]. A value of 0.41 TLC/sec was taken as the lower limit of normal (mean − 2SD) for $\dot{V}_{50}$ in both adults and children [16].

The standard exercise test consisted of six minutes' running on a motor-ised treadmill at 10 per cent gradient and at a speed sufficient to bring the subject's heart rate to at least 170 beats/min at the end of the exercise. Exercise was continuous, but the treadmill was slowed to walking pace in order to perform PEFR measurements at two-minute intervals during exer-cise. The test was discontinued if the subject showed signs of breathless-ness or registered a fall in PEFR of greater than 50 per cent from the pre-exercise value.

Pulmonary function testing was performed immediately prior to, during, and at up to 30 minutes after exercise.

The response to exercise was quantified according to the method of Godfrey and his colleagues [17] as shown in equation (2)

$$\text{Percent fall index} = \frac{\text{Pre-exercise value} - \text{Lowest value post exercise}}{\text{Pre-exercise value}} \times 100 \qquad (2)$$

After they had successfully completed the initial exercise test, the 22 subjects completed a second, identical exercise test, 60 minutes after the start of the first. All subjects had recovered spontaneously and were not wheezing at the start of the second test. No bronchodilators were given between the two exercise tests.

To determine the effect of the first exercise test on the second for each individual patient an index called 'percent protection', was introduced [3]. It is calculated as shown in equation (3)

$$\text{Percent protection} = \frac{\% \text{ fall after exercise 1} - \% \text{ fall after exercise 2}}{\% \text{ fall after exercise 1}} \qquad (3)$$

The data were analysed by means of a t-test for paired values in the same subject. One- and two-way analyses of variance were used to determine whether there was a difference between the means of the 'protection' groups, and before and after exercise tests, respectively. Duncan's multiple range test was applied to determine the level of significance between indi-vidual pairs of group means [18].

All 22 subjects were invited to attend the laboratory for further exercise testing on two days within a week to test the reproducibility of their exer-cise-induced asthma and to calculate the coefficient of variation for each percent fall index. Seventeen patients repeated the protocol as above. In addition, a prolonged running test was conducted. This consisted of 16 minutes' running at an identical workload to the standard six-minute test.

RESULTS

The results of the pre-exercise pulmonary function tests on the 22 subjects are shown in Table I. The mean He responsiveness was 30.7 ± 18.38 per cent (range, 0% to 62%). There were significant (p<0.002) reductions in the four mean percent fall indices of exercise period 2 when compared to exercise period 1, using a two tailed paired t-test. Significant differences were found between the pre-exercise pulmonary function of the two exercise tests (Table II).

The effect of a prior exercise test on the second bronchoconstrictor

TABLE I. The mean (±SD) results of the pre-exercise pulmonary function tests on the 22 subjects, expressed as a percentage of the predicted normal value

Test	Result
PEFR	89.1 ± 16.6%
FEV_1	86.6 ± 13.8%
FEF_{25-75}	64.2 ± 26.2%
$\hat{V}_{50}$	63.9 ± 32.8%
Total lung capacity	111 ± 10%
Residual volume	138 ± 47%

TABLE II. Mean percent fall indices and mean pre-exercise pulmonary functions for paired exercise tests one hour apart (n = 22)

Pulmonary index	PEFR Exercise period		FEV_1 Exercise period		FEF_{25-75} Exercise period		$\hat{V}_{50}$ Exercise period	
	1	2	1	2	1	2	1	2
Percent fall index	33.8	22.6	26.8	16.1	46.0	27.1	39.6	23.0
(±SD)	±12.6	±12.5	±13.9	±13.8	±18.5	±21.6	±19.0	±23.9
p	<0.002		<0.002		<0.002		<0.002	
Pre-exercise level (% predicted)	89.1	82.6	86.6	81.1	64.2	53.8	63.9	65.4
(±SD)	±16.6	±17.5	±13.8	±13.3	±26.2	±20.6	±32.8	±37.4
p	<0.002		<0.01		<0.002		NS	

NS = not significant

response showed considerable variability between individuals. In order to describe this individual variation, the percent protection index was calculated. Individuals who had a greater percent fall index in the second exercise test, were defined as having zero percent protection.

To relate the changes in He responsiveness to the percent protection, subjects were divided into groups according to their 'degree of protection' (Table III). This was defined by the coefficient of variation of the respective percent fall indices for each pulmonary parameter used to assess exercise-induced asthma. The mean coefficients of variation were 41.2, 51.6, 36.3 and 67.5 for PEFR, FEV_1, FEF_{25-75} and $\dot{V}_{50}$, respectively. These coefficients of variation are higher than those previously reported [8], because of the mild exercise-induced asthma response in this group of asthmatics.

TABLE III. Grouping of patients according to degree of protection

Group	Degree of protection
Little or no protection	Less than 10% protection
Some protection	Between 10% and one CV% protection
Appreciable protection	Between one and two CV% protection
Significant protection	Greater than two CV% protection

CV = coefficient of variation

Figures 1 and 2 illustrate the changes in the He responsiveness before and after exercise in the paired tests, for each of the protection groups, and two of the four pulmonary function indices (PEFR and FEF_{25-75}). These two graphs are representative of the changes in all four parameters monitored.

The graphs indicate that those individuals who are afforded little or no protection by a bout of exercise also show a marked decrease in their He responsiveness before and after the second exercise test which approaches abnormal values [16]. Conversely, individuals who show an appreciable degree of protection have no significant change in their He responsiveness which stays well within the normal range.

To determine if the changes in the He responsiveness for any of the percent protection groups were statistically significant at pre-exercise period 1 to post-exercise period 2, a two way ANOVA test was performed. All four indices of pulmonary function used to assess exercise-induced asthma showed statistically significant decreases in the He responsiveness in the

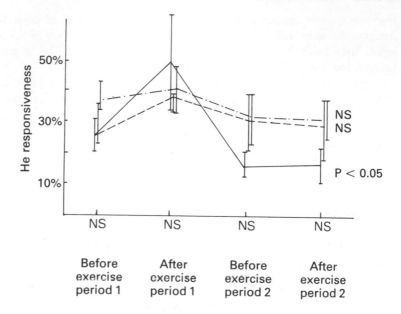

Figure 1. Relationship between the degree of protection afforded by a six-minute running test and the He responsiveness before and after exercise periods 1 and 2. Grouped according to the coefficient of variation of the percent fall index for peak expiratory flow rate (PEFR). Error bars indicate ± SE of the mean; NS = not significant. —— <10% protection (n=6); – – – 10–14% protection (n=6); – · – >41% protection (n=10)

group with little or no protection. Application of Duncan's Multirange Test revealed that, virtually without exception, the He responsiveness before and after exercise period 2, was significantly lower than the He responsiveness after exercise period 1 in the groups with the lowest degrees of protection. Furthermore, one-way ANOVA demonstrated that there were statistically significant differences between percent protection groups before exercise period 2 (Figures 1 and 2).

Seventeen of the 22 subjects successfully repeated the paired-exercise tests. On this occasion, the group with little or no protection demonstrated no tendency toward abnormal values for the He responsiveness, before or after exercise period 2.

Comparison of the percent protection indices for the 17 subjects who completed both series of tests, revealed that although the correlation coefficients were positive they were low: PEFR (0.49), FEV_1 (0.56), FEF_{25-75} (0.39) and $\dot{V}_{50}$ (0.03).

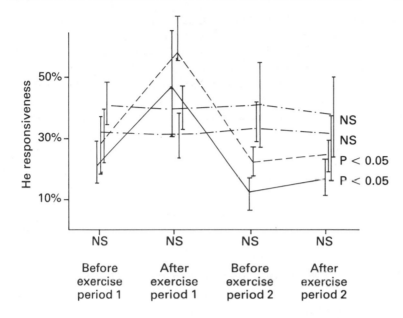

Figure 2. Relationship between the degree of protection afforded by a six-minute running test and the He responsiveness before and after exercise periods 1 and 2. Grouped according to the coefficient of variation of the percent fall index for the forced expiratory flow between 25 and 75 per cent of the vital capacity (FEF_{25-75}). Error bars indicate ±SE of the mean; NS = not significant. —— <10% protection (n=5); — — — 10–35% protection (n=5); — · — 36–70% protection (n=7); — · · — >70% protection (n=5)

TABLE IV. Mean (±SD) percent fall indices for the six-minute and 16-minute runs

Test	Six-minute run	Sixteen-minute run
PEFR	21.0 ± 10.7	25.9 ± 16.2
FEV_1	17.4 ± 10.2	18.0 ± 14.9
FEF_{25-75}	33.2 ± 18.0	31.5 ± 20.1

Thirteen subjects completed a prolonged 16-minute running test. The mean (±SD) percent fall indices for the six-minute and the 16-minute runs are shown in Table IV. There were no significant differences between the mean percent fall indices or the pre-exercise values for the six- and 16-minute exercise tests.

Considerable variability between subjects was apparent in response to the prolonged run when individual percent fall indices for the six- and 16-minute runs were compared. Five of the 17 subjects experienced significantly worse exercise-induced asthma after the 16-minute run, but four others experienced less exercise-induced asthma than after the six-minute run. The inter-subject variability was evaluated by the calculation of index, analogous to the percent protection index, used in the paired exercise tests above. The ability of an individual to 'run through his asthma' (that is, to experience less exercise-induced asthma after prolonged running than after the shorter six-minute run) was indicated by this protection index.

There were poor correlations between the 'run through' phenomenon and the percent protection afforded by paired exercise tests: PEFR (0.92), FEV_1 (0.10) and FEF_{25-75} (−0.07).

DISCUSSION

The results of the present study indicate that the degree of protection afforded by a prior exercise test varies between individuals and appears to be related to a subject's He responsiveness just before and after the second exercise test. Those individuals whose He responsiveness is reduced — indicating persisting small airways obstruction — showed minimal protection.

As in previous studies [2,3,19] a statistically significant decrease was seen in the second of the two mean percent fall indices when exercise tests were repeated.

Subjects with a normal increase in $\dot{V}_{max}$ when breathing helium can be interpreted as having predominantly large airways obstruction, although some degree of peripheral airway obstruction may be masked [16,20,21].

The innervation of the tracheobronchial tree is not homogeneous. The use of tantalum bronchography to study the changes in airway calibre in anaesthetised dogs has shown that vagal stimulation consistently resulted in constriction of all airways from the trachea to the bronchioles 0.5mm in diameter [22,23]. Sympathetic stimulation results in selective dilatation of small airways [24].

Other studies have provided support for these findings by examining the effect of cholinergic antagonists on the density dependence of expiratory flow. After the inhalation of atropine, the He responsiveness decreased in normal [25] and asthmatic subjects [26] indicating that the predominant site of action of the drug was on the large central airways, thus shifting the site of limitation of flow away from them.

The results of this study indicate also that the predominance of small airways obstruction before or after exercise period 2 is an important discriminating feature, suggesting that the individual will be afforded no protection by a prior exercise test. The protection that is seen in those asthmatics with a large airway response to paired exercise tests, and the observed effects on single exercise tests with the cholinergic antagonist ipratropium bromide [4,27], suggest that the reduced bronchoconstrictor response may be dependent on vagal mechanisms. Individuals who failed to obtain protection and lost their He responsiveness may have broncho-constriction that is not solely dependent on vagal tone.

The cause of the possible reduced vagal involvement in exercise-induced asthma after the second exercise test in some asthmatics, could be related to depletion of the pool of bronchoconstrictor mediators [1,2,19] or refractoriness of sensory receptors in the smooth muscle itself. Depletion of the mediator pool would appear to be well suited to explain the protection phenomenon, since Loring and his colleagues [28] have demonstrated in dogs that the constriction of bronchial smooth muscle is dose-dependent. The results of the present study indicate that if the depletion of mediators is to play a central role in the protection phenomenon, the mediators must induce bronchoconstriction in the large airways via a vagally dependent reflex. Gold [29] has concluded that while bronchoconstrictor mediators have a direct local effect on bronchial smooth muscle, the mediators also stimulate rapidly adapting vagal sensory receptors causing reflex potentiation of the bronchoconstriction. It is likely that the sensory receptors involved are the 'irritant receptors' found in the trachea and larger bronchi [30].

Although it is possible that the bronchial smooth muscle could become refractory to repeated stimulation by bronchoconstrictor mediators [31], this would seem to be unlikely. Schoeffel and her colleagues [3] compared repeated histamine challenges with exercise tests repeated 40 minutes apart and found no statistically significant decreases in the percent fall for the repeated histamine challenges; they did, however, find significant differences between the percent fall indices for the repeated exercise tests. They concluded that their results provided indirect evidence that depletion of bronchoconstrictor mediators was the underlying cause of the protection phenomenon seen during repeated exercise tests, rather than smooth muscle itself becoming refractory to the applied stimulus.

Some workers have produced evidence that bronchoconstrictor mediators, such as histamine, are released into arterial blood in some asthmatic individuals in response to exercise [32—34], although others [35,36] have not observed this change. Anderson and her colleagues [34] noted that, while the increase in arterial plasma histamine levels in some asthmatics coincided with the post-exercise decrease in pulmonary function, this relationship was not apparent in others – thus further emphasising the heterogeneity of exercise-induced asthma. Of considerable interest was the fact that one patient who demonstrated a significant increase in plasma histamine levels after exercise, showed a smaller increase after a second exercise test 40 minutes later which was associated with a protective effect. Other physical stimuli, including cold, have also resulted in the release of histamine in allergic subjects [37]. Previous evidence that mediators are implicated in exercise-induced asthma have been based on the observation that sodium cromoglycate inhibits the release of mediators from mast cells [38], and that it prevents exercise-induced asthma in some subjects [4].

McFadden and Ingram [39] have accumulated considerable evidence that airway cooling is of central importance in the causation of exercise-induced asthma, and that the degree of exercise-induced asthma elicited is directly related to the respiratory heat loss. Jaeger and his colleagues [40] measured the temperatures in the upper and lower oesophagus in an attempt to assess the amount of cooling that occurred in the airways and showed that while the temperature of the upper oesophagus decreased in accordance with the respiratory heat exchange, the temperature in the lower oesophagus remained fairly constant. The heterogeneity of protection could be related either to the varied cooling of the airways or to differences in the amount of histamine released.

In order to observe the protective effect after exercise or an equivalent ventilatory challenge it would appear that it is necessary to have experienced a previous attack of exercise-induced asthma, although the evidence is not conclusive [41,42].

When 17 of the 22 subjects were retested the observed relationship between a reduced He responsiveness and little or no protection was found not to be readily repeatable. This may simply be due to the inherent variability of exercise-induced asthma. All 17 subjects who were retested are included in the analysis even though four had percent fall indices of PEFR in the normal range. However, if these subjects are not considered, the numbers in each protection group become quite small and susceptible to individual fluctuation. The absence of a distinct group with small airway obstruction in the second series may account for the lack of a clearcut relationship between the He responsiveness and the degree of protection.

It was of interest to compare an individual's ability to 'run through' his exercise-induced asthma during a prolonged 16-minute exercise test with his response to repeated six-minute exercise tests. Both phenomena have been reported to show considerable variability between individuals [1,5] and, in both, the underlying mechanism has been suggested as depletion of bronchoconstrictor mediators [7].

Considerable variability between individuals was observed in this study when the percent fall indices of the six- and the 16-minute running tests were compared. There were no significant differences between the mean percent fall indices of the two tests, thus confirming the findings of an earlier report [5]. When the percent protection index '6 vs 16' was plotted against the percent protection for the paired six-minute tests, a poor correlation was found, suggesting that the mechanisms involved may be different.

References

1   McNeill RS, Nairn JR, Millar JS, Ingram CG.
    Exercise-induced asthma
    Q J Med 1966; 35: 55–67

2   Edmunds AT, Tooley M, Godfrey S.
    The refractory period after exercise-induced asthma: its duration and relation to the severity of exercise. *Am Rev Respir Dis 1973; 117:* 247–254

3   Schoeffel RE, Anderson SD, Gillam I, Lindsay DA.
    Multiple exercise and histamine challenge in asthmatic patients.
    Thorax 1980; 35: 164–170

4   McFadden ER, Ingram RH, Haynes RL, Wellman JJ.
    Predominant site of flow limitation and mechanism of post-exertional asthma.
    J Appl Physiol 1977; 42: 746–752

5   Silverman M, Anderson SD.
    Standardization of exercise tests in asthmatic children.
    Arch Dis Child 1972; 47: 882–889

6   Eggleston PA, Guerrant JL.
    A standardized method of evaluating exercise-induced asthma.
    J Allergy Clin Immunol 1976; 58: 414–425

7   Anderson SD, Silverman M, König P, Godfrey S.
    Exercise-induced asthma: a review.
    Br J Dis Chest 1975; 69: 1–39

8   Godfrey S.
    Exercise Testing in Children 1974
    Philadelphia: Saunders

9   Leith DE, Mead J.
    Principles of body plethysmograph.
    In *Procedures for Standardized Measurements of Lung Mechanics 1974*.
    Bethesda Md: Distributed by the division of Lung Diseases, National Heart and Lung Institute

10 Zapletal A, Motoyama EK, Van de Woestijne KP et al.
    Maximum expiratory flow-volume curves and airway conductance in children and adolescents. *J Appl Physiol 1969; 26:* 308–316

11 Du Bois AB, Botelho SG, Bedell GN et al.
    A rapid plethysmographic method for measuring thoracic gas volume; comparison with nitrogen washout method for measuring functional residual capacity in normal subjects. *J Clin Invest 1956; 35:* 322

12   Cook CD, Hamman L.
      Relation of lung volumes to height in healthy persons between the ages of 8 and
      38 years. *J Pediatr 1961; 59:* 710–714

13   Murray JF, Cook CD.
      Measurement of peak expiratory flow rates in 220 normal children from 4.5 to
      18.5 years of age. *J Pediatr 1963; 62:* 186–189

14   Cotes JE.
      Lung Function 3rd edition 1975.
      Oxford: Blackwell

15   Bates DV, Macklem PT, Christie RV.
      Respiratory Function in Disease 1971.
      Philadelphia: Saunders

16   Landau LI, Mellis CM, Phelan PD et al.
      'Small airways disease' in children: no test is best.
      Thorax 1979; 34: 217–223

17   Godfrey S, Silverman M, Anderson SD.
      Problems of interpreting exercise-induced asthma.
      J Allergy Clin Immunol 1973; 52: 199–209

18   Duncan DB.
      Multiple range and multiple F-tests.
      Biometrics 1955; 11: 1–42

19   James L, Facaine J, Sly RM.
      Effect of treadmill exercise on asthmatic children.
      J Allergy Clin Immunol 1976; 57: 408–416

20   Despas PJ, Leroux M, Macklem PT.
      Site of airway obstruction in asthma as determined by measuring air and helium-
      oxygen mixture. *J Clin Invest 1972; 51:* 3235–3243

21   Lavelle TF, Rotman HH, Weg JG.
      Iso-volume curves in the diagnosis of upper airway obstruction.
      Am Rev Respir Dis 1978; 117: 845–852

22   Cabezas GA, Graf PD, Nadel JA.
      Sympathetic versus parasympathetic nervous regulation of airways in dogs.
      J Appl Physiol 1971; 31: 651–655

23   Kessler GF, Austin JHM, Graf PD et al.
      Airway constriction in experimental asthma in dogs: tantalum bronchographic
      studies. *J Appl Physiol 1973; 35:* 703–709

24   Woolcock SJ, Macklem PT, Hogg JC et al.
      Effect of vagal stimulation on central and peripheral airways in dogs.
      J Appl Physiol 1969; 26: 806–813

25   Ingram RH, McFadden ER.
      Localization and mechanisms of airways responses.
      N Engl J Med 1977; 297: 596–600

26   Snow RM, Miller WC, Blair HT, Rice DL.
      Inhaled atropine in asthma.
      Ann Allergy 1979; 42: 286–289

27   Thomson NC, Patel KR, Kerr JW.
     Sodium cromoglycate and ipratropium bromide in exercise-induced asthma.
     Thorax 1978; 33: 694–699

28   Loring SH, Drazen JM, Ingram RH.
     Canine pulmonary response to aerosol histamine: direct versus vagal effects.
     J Appl Physiol 1977; 42: 946–952

29   Gold WM.
     Cholinergic pharmacology in asthma. In Austin KF, Lichtenstein LM, eds.
     Asthma: Physiology, Immunopharmacology and Treatment 1973: 169–184.
     New York: Academic Press

30   Mortola J, Sant' Ambrogio G, Clement MG.
     Localization of irritant receptors in the airways of the dog.
     Respir Physiol 1975; 24: 107–114

31   Krell RD, Chakrin LW.
     Canine airway responses to acetylcholine, prostaglandin F_2, histamine, and
     serotonin after chronic antigen exposure.
     J Allergy Clin Immunol 1976; 58: 664–675

32   Ferris L, Anderson SD, Temple DM.
     Histamine release in exercise induced asthma.
     Br Med J 1978; 1: 1967

33   Karr RM, Brach BB, Wilson MR et al.
     Change in levels of arterial blood histamine during exercise induced asthma.
     J Allergy Clin Immunol 1979; 63: 153

34   Anderson SD, Bye PTP, Schoeffel RE et al.
     Arterial histamine levels at rest, and during and after exercise in patients with
     asthma: effects of terbutaline aerosol. *Thorax 1981; 36:* 259–267

35   Harries MG, Burge PS, O'Brien I et al.
     Blood histamine levels after exercise.
     Clin Allergy 1979; 9: 437

36   McFadden ER Jr, Soter NA.
     A search for chemical mediators of immediate hypersensivitiy and humoral
     factors in the pathogenesis of exercise-induced asthma.
     In Austen KF, Lichtenstein LM, eds.
     Asthma: Immunology, Immunopharmacology and Treatment 1977: 337.
     New York: Academic Press

37   Soter NA, Wasserman SI, Austen KF.
     Cold urticaria: release into the circulation of histamine and eosinophil chemo-
     tactic factor of anaphylaxis during cold challenge.
     N Engl J Med 1976; 294: 687–690

38   Orr TSC, Pollard MC, William J, Cox JSG.
     Mode of action of disodium cromoglycate studies on immediate type hyper-
     sensitivity reactions using 'double desensitization' with two antigenically dis-
     tinct rat reagins. *Clin Exp Immunol 1970; 7:* 745–757

39   McFadden ER, Ingram RH.
     Exercise-induced asthma.
     N Engl J Med 1979; 301: 763–769

40   Jaeger JJ, Deal EC Jr, Roberts DE et al.
     Cold air inhalation and esophageal temperature in exercising humans.
     Med Sci Sports Exerc 1980; 12: 365–369

41   Anderson SD, Daviskas E, Schoeffel RE, Unger SF.
     Prevention of severe exercise-induced asthma with hot humid air.
     Lancet 1979; ii: 629

42   Stearns DR, McFadden ER Jr, Breslin FJ, Ingram RH Jr.
     Reanalysis of the refractory period in exertional asthma.
     J Appl Physiol 1981; 50: 503–508

Chapter 10

THE USE OF SHORT PERIODS OF EXERCISE IN THE PREVENTION AND REVERSAL OF EXERCISE-INDUCED ASTHMA

R Schnall, L I Landau, P D Phelan

Royal Children's Hospital, Melbourne, Australia

SUMMARY

A refractory period is a well-recognised phenomenon after an episode of exercise-induced bronchoconstriction. However, the ability of non-asthmagenic exercise to provide protection has only recently been appreciated.

The beneficial effect of 30 second sprints on the prevention and reversal of exercise-induced bronchoconstriction was investigated in adolescents and young adults with asthma. Seven sprints each 2.5 minutes apart reduced the fall in peak expiratory flow rate (PEFR) caused by a 6 minute run undertaken 30 minutes after the last sprint by 54 per cent. Two sprints and four sprints reduced the fall in PEFR by 32 per cent and 43 per cent respectively. In a separate experiment, seven sprints 30 minutes before a 6 minute run reduced the fall in PEFR by 59 per cent but if the sprints took place only 10 minutes before the run, the fall was reduced by 36 per cent.

Seven 30 second sprints immediately and 10 minutes after the completion of a bronchoconstriction-inducing 6 minute run produced partial reversal of the bronchoconstriction. Seven 30 second periods of hyperventilation of room air did not protect against exercise-induced bronchoconstriction. Seven 30 second sprints did not alter the PD_{20} for histamine-induced bronchoconstriction.

The results of these studies suggest that during and after exercise the catecholamines that are released may induce an increment in the number of available receptors on bronchial smooth muscle.

INTRODUCTION

Exercise-induced bronchoconstriction can limit the enjoyment of physical activities by children and adolescents. Although sodium cromoglycate is effective in its prevention and the inhalation of $beta_2$-adrenergic drugs is effective in both its prevention and its reversal, some patients prefer not to use medication for normal sporting activities. Observations that the initial response to exercise is bronchodilatation [1], that some people with asthma can 'run through' exercise-induced bronchoconstriction and that there is a refractory period after episodes of exercise-induced bronchoconstriction [2], suggested that short periods of more intense physical activity might effectively prevent or reverse exercise-induced bronchoconstriction [3].

In addition to their possible practical applications to sporting activities, the studies reported here were undertaken in the hope that they might provide information on the underlying mechanisms of tachyphlaxis in exercise-induced asthma.

MATERIALS AND METHODS

The studies were undertaken on groups of five adolescents and young adults with asthma. All had experienced episodes of exercise-induced bronchoconstriction. Bronchodilators and sodium cromoglycate were withheld for at least eight hours before the tests and the subjects were asked to refrain from vigorous exercise for at least two hours beforehand.

All studies were conducted in an air-conditioned room with a controlled environment. The temperature during the course of the study ranged from 22 to 24°C. Relative humidity ranged from 33 to 60 per cent. The mean heat content of the ambient air was $9.56 \pm 1.94 \times 10^{-3}$ kcal/litre. The amount of heat needed to raise the air to 37°C fully saturated was $19.78 \pm 1.11 \times 10^{-3}$ kcal/litre (1 kcal $\approx$ 4.2 kJ).

In the running tests, subjects ran on a treadmill set at a 10 per cent grade. The speed was determined from data related to heart rate recorded with exercise of varying intensity as a function of age, sex and height [4], but was modified according to the exercise and sporting habits of the individual. During sprints the speed of the treadmill was increased by 25 to 35 per cent.

The peak expiratory flow rate (PEFR) was recorded with a Wright's peak flowmeter. Forced vital capacity (FVC), forced expiratory volume in one second (FEV_1) and forced expiratory flow between 25 and 75 per cent of vital capacity (FEF_{25-75}) were measured with a water filled spirometer. Base-line results were taken as the best of three measurements — provided that the individual measurements agreed within 10 per cent. All other measurements were taken as the best of two so that the number of forced expiratory manoeuvres could be kept within reasonable limits [5]. The results were expressed as per cent predicted for height and sex [6].

Five series of experiments form the basis of this report (the tests for each individual in each series of experiments were completed within 14 days):

(1) The protective effects of 2, 4 and 7 30-sec sprints performed at 2.5-min intervals 20min before an asthmagenic 6-min run were compared.

(2) The protective effects of 7 30-sec sprints performed at 2.5-min intervals 10min, 20min and 30min before an asthmagenic 6-min run were compared.

(3) The bronchodilatory effect of 7 30-sec sprints at 2.5min intervals begun 2min and 10min after a 6-min run was observed.

(4) The hyperventilatory response to the 7 30-sec sprints was recorded on a volume-time plot on a X-Y recorder. In the fourth series of tests, the subjects performed 7 periods of hyperventilation simulating the hyperventilation that occurred during the 7 sprints. No alterations were made to the composition of the inspired air. Twenty min after the last period of hyperventilation, the subjects took a 6-min asthmagenic run.

(5) The subjects performed 7 30-sec sprints at 2.5-min intervals and 20 min after the completion of the last sprint were subjected to a standard histamine challenge [7]. The concentration of histamine was gradually increased at 3-min intervals from 0.03mg/ml until a fall of 20 per cent or greater from the base-line FEV_1 occurred. The PD_{20} (the concentration of histamine necessary to produce a 20 per cent fall in FEV_1) was calculated.

Protection was calculated as mean fall after the control 6-min run minus mean fall in the 6-min run after sprints expressed as a percentage of the mean fall in the control test. Comparison of the results was made by Student's t test for paired data.

TABLE I. Protective effect on exercise-induced bronchoconstriction of 30-sec sprints 2.5 min apart and performed 20 min before a 6-min run (Results expressed as mean ± 1SD)

	PEFR			FEV_1			FEF_{25-75}		
	Base line % predicted	% fall	% protection	Base line % predicted	% fall	% protection	Base line % predicted	% fall	% protection
6-min run	90.8±13.9	25.8±11.1		88.4±14.7	22.0±12.8		66.0±24.0	35.2±18.6	
6-min run preceded by 2 sprints	87.8±10.9	17.5±13.9	32*	89.8± 9.4	17.5±12.8	21	64.0±11.6	27.1±21.1	23
6-min run	88.0±16.2	30.8±17.6		88.4±15.0	27.3±16.2		66.0±25.0	37.9± 8.5	
6-min run preceded by 4 sprints	99.2±12.7	17.5±13.2	43*	89.8±10.9	18.7±11.9	32*	6.50±13.7	23.5±16.9	38
6-min run	91.7±30.2	22.8± 6.6		84.1±26.3	23.0±10.4		58.5±32.6	37.3±14.0	
6-min run preceded by 7 sprints	94.9±30.3	10.4± 6.2	55*	87.5±31.2	6.9± 6.6	70*	66.6±36.3	18.9± 6.2	49*

* p<0.05

TABLE II. Protective effect on exercise-induced bronchoconstriction of 7 30-sec sprints 2.5 min apart performed before a 6-min run (Results expressed as mean ± 1SD)

	PEFR			FEV_1			FEF_{25-75}		
	Base line % predicted	% fall	% protection	Base line % predicted	% fall	% protection	Base line % predicted	% fall	% protection
6-min run	87.6±16.5	27.5±6.1		89.6±13.7	23.3± 2.9		61.4±18.2	39.5±18.2	
7 sprints 10 min before 6-min run	85.4±17.0	17.5±9.8	36*	87.4±17.0	15.3± 7.3	34*	58.0±16.7	24.7±14.2	38*
6-min run	91.7±30.2	22.8±6.6		84.1±26.3	23.0±10.4		58.5±22.6	37.3±14.0	
7 sprints 20 min before 6-min run	94.9±30.3	10.4±6.2	55*	87.5±31.2	6.9± 6.6	70*	66.6±36.3	18.9± 6.2	49*
6-min run	87.6±16.5	27.5±6.1		89.6±13.7	23.3±10.4		58.0±16.7	39.5± 6.6	
7 sprints 30 min before 6-min run	87.1±16.4	11.2±5.4	59**	89.2±13.0	8.8± 8.1	62**	63.4±22.4	11.1±17.1	72**

* p<0.05

** p<0.01

RESULTS

From Table I it can be seen that the protective effect of seven short sprints was greater than that of four sprints and that two sprints gave relatively little protection. The sprints themselves did not produce significant bronchoconstriction in any of the subjects.

Although there was significant protection from seven sprints 10min before the 6-min run (Table II), the protection with a 20-min interval was substantially better. However, waiting until 30min had elapsed added little further benefit. Similar bronchodilatory effects were seen with seven 30-sec sprints undertaken 2min and 10min after an asthmagenic run (Figure 1). The bronchodilatory effect was relatively small.

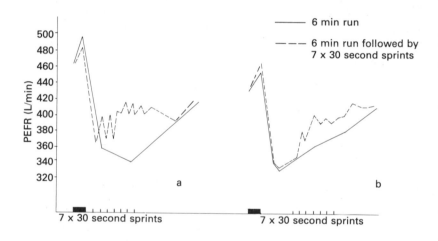

Figure 1. Time course of bronchoconstriction after a 6-min run (unbroken lines) and the bronchodilatory effect of 7 30-sec sprints begun 2min (a) and 10min (b) after the completion of the run (dashed lines)

Seven 30-sec periods of hyperventilation of room air provided no protective effect against exercise-induced bronchoconstriction (Table III). Similarly, 7 30-sec sprints 20min before a histamine challenge had no significant protective effect. The per cent predicted FEV_1 before the initial histamine challenge was 88.8 ± 8.7 and base-line PD_{20} was 1.5 ± 1.4mg histamine/ml. The per cent predicted FEV_1 before the seven sprints was 84.8 ± 10.1. If that value was taken as baseline for the second histamine test, the PD_{20} was 1.0 ± 1.3mg histamine/ml. If the base-line FEV_1 for the second hist-

TABLE III. Effect of 7 30-sec periods of hyperventilation of room air 2.5-min apart 20min before a 6-min run (Results expressed as mean ± 1SD)

	PEFR		FEV$_1$		FEF$_{25-75}$	
	Base line % predicted	% fall	Base line % predicted	% fall	Base line % predicted	% fall
6-min run	96.8±12.7	30.5±11.5	86.3±12.7	23.5±11.5	74.3±22.0	38.7± 9.1
6-min run preceded by 7 hyperventilations	96.8±11.9	29.5±26.5	85.3±10.9	18.6±16.2	69.3±12.7	29.4±27.7

amine test was taken as the value after the sprints but before the histamine challenge, the PD_{20} was 1.2±1.6mg histamine/ml.

DISCUSSION

These observations, together with those reported elsewhere [3], demonstrate that non-bronchoconstricting short sprints afford protection against exercise-induced bronchospasm. The results suggest that the effect is greater at 20 to 30min than at 10min but that the difference is not great. At least four sprints seemed necessary to give a degree of protection that would be beneficial for sporting activities. It was possible to reverse bronchoconstriction with short sprints but not to any great extent — this probably is an expression of the phenomenon of 'running through' the bronchoconstriction that has been noted by some asthmatics.

Hyperventilation of room air gave no protection. While it has been shown that hyperventilation of cold dry air is more likely to induce bronchoconstriction than is hyperventilation of room air [8], in this series of experiments we chose to use room air as the plan was to simulate normal sporting conditions. It is possible that hyperventilation of cold dry air would have a significant protective effect.

It seems unlikely that depletion of bronchoactive mediators could be the sole mechanism underlying the refractory period that follows exercise. If such was the mechanism, protection 10min after short sprints should be greater than that at 20 or 30min. It also seems unlikely that refractoriness of smooth muscle is a major factor as the short sprints afforded no protection against histamine-induced bronchoconstriction.

The results reported here suggest that exercise itself may have an important role in protecting against exercise-induced bronchoconstriction. Hyperventilation gave no protection as has been shown previously [9]. Further, the short sprints were shown to have a bronchodilator effect. This latter finding in particular would suggest that exercise results in the release of some bronchodilator agent, perhaps catecholamines. However, if the release of catecholamines is the sole explanation, it is unlikely that the refractoriness would be greater at 30min than at 10.

Tohmer and Cryer [10] have suggested that there is a biphasic response by beta-adrenergic receptors to an increase in beta agonists. During the first hour after infusion of a beta agonist the number of available binding sites progressively increased. After four hours, the number of binding sites fell below the base-line level. It is possible that a similar phenomenon occurs with exercise. The initial exercise could result in an increase in catecholamines [11] which, in turn, could result in an increase in the number of available receptors on bronchial smooth muscle and mast-cell membranes. This could inhibit spasm of the smooth muscle and the release of histamine. The greater the number of sprints and the longer the period between the sprints and the asthmagenic run, the greater might be the increase in the number of available beta-adrenergic receptor sites. Refractoriness may thus be related to an increment in available beta-adrenergic receptor sites induced by the release of catecholamines during the sprints.

Acknowledgments

This work was supported by grants from the National Health and Medical Research Council and Asthma Foundation of Victoria, Australia.

References

1   Jones RS, Butson MH, Wharton MJ.
    The effect of exercise on ventilatory function in the child with asthma.
    Br J Dis Chest 1962; 56: 78–86

2   McNeill RS, Wairn JR, Millar JS, Ingram CG.
    Exercise induced asthma.
    Q J Med 1966; 35: 55–67

3   Schnall RP, Landau LI.
    Protective effect of repeated short sprints in exercise-induced asthma.
    Thorax 1980; 35: 828–832

4   Godfrey S.
    Exercise induced asthma – clinical, physiological and therapeutic implications.
    J Allergy Clin Immunol 1975; 56: 1–17

5   Orehek J, Gayrard P, Grimand C, Charpin J.
    Effect of maximal respiratory manoeuvres on bronchial sensitivity of asthmatic
    patients as compared to normal people.
    Br Med J 1975; 1: 123–125

6   Weng TR, Levison H.
    Standards of pulmonary function testing in children.
    Am Rev Respir Dis 1969; 99: 879–894

7   Chai H, Farr RS, Froehlich LA et al.
    Standardisation of bronchial inhalation challenge procedures.
    J Allergy Clin Immunol 1975; 56: 323–327

8   Deal ECJ, McFadden ER Jr, Ingram RH Jr et al.
    Role of respiratory heat exchange in production of exercise induced asthma.
    J Appl Physiol 1979; 46: 467–475

9   Stearns DR, McFadden ER Jr, Breslin FJ, Ingram RH Jr.
    Reanalysis of the refractory period in exertional asthma.
    J Appl Physiol 1981; 50: 503–508

10 Tohmer JF, Cryer PE.
    Biphasic adrenergic modulation of beta adrenergic receptors in man.
    J Clin Invest 1980; 65: 836–840

11 Barnes PJ, Brown MJ, Silverman M, Dollery CT.
    Circulating catecholamines in exercise and hyperventilation induced asthma.
    Thorax 1981; 36: 433–440

DISCUSSION

AAS
(Oslo, Norway)

The first of Dr Gillam's tests involved quite a number of forced expiratory manoeuvres. Did he have any controls to show that this did not affect the exercise responses after 60 minutes?

GILLAM

I am sure many of you are aware that repeated spirometry manoeuvres can induce bronchoconstriction. In this study we actually ruled out two of the subjects because they showed bronchoconstriction after repeated forced expiratory manoeuvres. So this factor was controlled.

RICHARDSON
(Bromley, UK)

Instead of the heart rate in the tests being up to a maximum of 170 beats/min, would it not be preferable for the rate to be up to x times (say, 2½ times) the resting rate, in view of the wide range of normal resting heart rates?

GILLAM

In the standardisation of exercise tests for asthmatics, most people believe that for children the heart rate should exceed 170 beats/min or approximately two thirds of the $\dot{V}O_2$ $_{max}$. Resting heart rate is subject to a variety of factors including the state of training of the individual, viral infection, sympathomimetic drugs and environmental and nervous stimuli. I believe that the resting heart rate may, therefore, be an unreliable measurement on which to base the exercise provocation. If one wished to standardise the cardiac load, a fixed percentage of maximum heart rate may be useful since this would allow adjustments to be made in relation to age.

BURGE
(Birmingham, UK)

The group who obtained no protection from the first exercise test had developed helium-unresponsiveness before the second test. Were the patients in this group developing a late asthmatic reaction to the first test at the time of the second test?

GILLAM   No. I do not think so.

STRÖMBERG (Norrköping, Sweden)   If vagal mechanisms are important in exercise-induced asthma can the diving reflex explain some of the differences between running and swimming in exercise-induced asthma? Would spraying the face with cold water during running modify the exercise-induced asthma response?

GILLAM   As far as I am aware nobody has actually investigated the diving reflex in relation to exercise-induced asthma. Maybe Dr Bar-Or might like to answer that question since he has carried out studies on the relationship between body cooling and the resulting broncho-constriction.

BAR-OR (Hamilton, Canada)   We have no data on immersion of the face and exercise-induced asthma. However, the children in our swimming studies did not immerse their faces so I doubt very much whether the diving reflex *per se* would explain the protective nature of swimming. Their heads were out of the water virtually all the time.

HOLGATE (Southampton, UK)   Does Dr Phelan know if short sprints of 30 seconds also protect against isocapnic hyperventilation-induced asthma?

PHELAN   We have completed a study in the laboratory but regrettably I do not have the data with me.

DAHL   I would like to comment on that, with reference to late reactions after exercise testing. About two years ago we studied 10 patients with highly reproducible dual reactions after allergen challenges; when we produced in them a comparable fall in the immediate reaction after an exercise test we never found them to have a late reaction.

BAR-OR   Some data in the literature indicate that sprints *can* induce an increase in bronchial resistance. Dr Phelan, which function did you measure to assess the effect of sprint *per se?*

PHELAN   We measured at peak flow, FEV_1 and FEF_{25-75}. We did not measure airways resistance.

Chapter 11

^{81m}Kr GAS INHALATION TESTS FOR EXERCISE-INDUCED BRONCHOSPASM

Y Iikura, H Inui, T Masaki, K Nishikawa,
T Shimada*, K Kawakami**

National Children's Hospital, and
*Jikei Medical College, Tokyo, Japan

SUMMARY

To determine the role of airway obstruction after exercise, we have studied the changes in lung function and in lung images by means of ^{81m}Kr gas inhalation. We further observed the differences between air and HeO_2 inhalation, and the different lung image distributions after exercise-induced bronchoconstriction and allergen provocation inhalation tests.

Inhalation of ^{81m}Kr gas allowed us to detect uneven distribution images very clearly. Broncho-obstruction which occurs after exercise is likely to occur in the large airways. The ^{81m}Kr gas image differs depending on the workload being performed and the degree of the patient's asthma. Comparisons between the exercise load test and the allergen provocation test showed that the exercise load test produced a greater difference in ^{81m}Kr gas distribution with respect to air and HeO_2. In comparison with children, adults showed more severe image defects 15 minutes after exercise and slower recovery from the state.

INTRODUCTION

An important feature of bronchial asthma is hyperreactivity of the bronchus and many studies have been performed which make use of this characteristic. They include the acetylcholine provocation test, the methacholine test and tests to measure the degree of bronchospasm induced by various exercise loads and allergen inhalation provocation. Clinically, the stimuli produce reactions such as dyspnoea or impairment of lung function. However, this does not mean that the mechanisms responsible for the reactions are similar.

In this study we shall focus our attention on the obstruction of the airways in the early response to exercise loads and allergen inhalation provocation tests. We have found differences between responders and non-responders using flow rates at 50 per cent of vital capacity ($\dot{V}_{50}$) [1] and also in the main site of obstruction [2–4]. However, it is very difficult to quantify the degree of obstruction. Furthermore, it is difficult to detect changes in the bronchus by means of a measurement of lung function which is usually performed through the mouth. We therefore performed an ^{81m}Kr gas (which has a half-life of only 13 seconds) inhalation test in order to detect the image defects and obstructions in the airways caused by exercise-induced bronchospasm.

SUBJECTS

The subjects of our study were 38 inpatients and outpatients aged between eight and 16 years who were currently undergoing treatment at the National Children's Hospital, Tokyo, and 34 outpatients aged between 18 and 45 years from the Allergy Department of Jikei Medical University, Tokyo.

We compared the performance of these subjects with that of six healthy adults who underwent a similar exercise load. None of the subjects had experienced any form of asthmatic attack in the previous 10 days.

All subjects were examined to ensure that their forced expiratory volume in one second (FEV_1) was at least 80 per cent of their vital capacity, and any medicines were prohibited for 12 hours before the test.

METHODS

Exercise load We used the Master one-step method at a speed of 24 steps/minute. We exercised the children for six minutes or until the pulse rate rose to above 170 beats/minute. The exercise for the adults lasted for three to five minutes until the pulse rate rose above 150 beats/minute.

Allergen inhalation test The inhalations lasted for three minutes.

Lung function tests These were performed using an electronic flow volume meter. To detect the changes in flow volume, we used the following equations (1) and (2):

$$\text{Per cent rise in FEV}_1 = \frac{\text{FEV}_1 \text{ (after)} - \text{FEV}_1 \text{ (before)}}{\text{FEV}_1 \text{ (before)}} \qquad (1)$$

$$\text{Per cent fall in FEV}_1 = \frac{\text{FEV}_1 \text{ (before)} - \text{FEV}_1 \text{ (after)}}{\text{FEV}_1 \text{ (before)}} \qquad (2)$$

Airway scintigraphy for ^{81m}Kr gas inhalation

Inhalation technique The patients inhaled 10ml of ^{81m}Kr gas as a bolus from residual volume level and functional residual capacity level (Figure 1). After the inhalation we measured the gas distribution image by means of a scinticamera and fed the results into a computer.

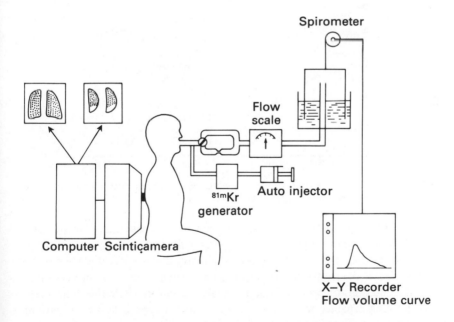

Figure 1. Diagrammatic representation of the ^{81m}Kr gas inhalation test

We made the patients inhale by maximum first inhalation and by slow inhalation (0.25/second or slower); when a count of 30,000 was reached, they stopped breathing so that we could obtain the lung image. We connected the system to a spirometer. When the lung capacity reaches a certain point the ^{81m}Kr gas is automatically exhaled through the mouth.

Computer processes

We fed the scintigraphic data into a Cyntipack 1200 Computer and obtained the data shown in Figure 2. We then compared the intensity of flow dependency (I) using the equation:

$$I = (C/D)/(A/B) \qquad (3)$$

The outer lines of Figure 2 show the areas obtained before the provocation test was computed by the Cyntipack with six or seven inhalations of ^{81m}Kr gas. Furthermore, we divided the ^{81m}Kr gas image patterns into two groups – maximum first inhalation and slow inhalation – and labelled them A to D.

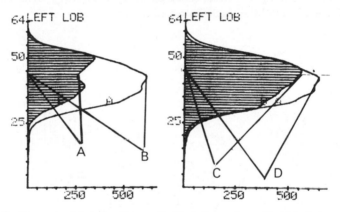

Figure 2. Computer inhalation images. On the left, maximum first inhalation; on the right, slow inhalation. I = (C/D)/(A/B) (see text)

We termed the pattern type A dominant if the image defect was greater in the maximum first inhalation compared with that of the slow inhalation indicating that it is mainly the central airways that are affected (Figure 3). However, if the slow inhalation showed a greater defect than the maximum first inhalation and provided that the image disappeared with high lung levels (total lung capacity minus 400ml) we termed it type B dominant pattern indicating involvement mainly of the peripheral airways (Figure 4).

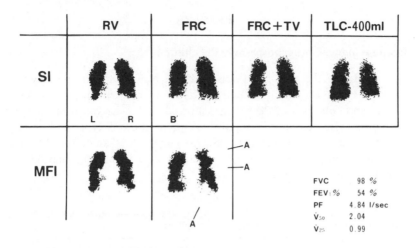

Figure 3.   Type A dominant pattern: exercise-induced bronchospasm in an 18-year-old girl (SI = slow inhalation; MFI = maximum first inspiration; RV = residual volume; FRC = functional residual capacity; TV = tidal volume; TLC = total lung capacity; FVC = forced vital capacity; PF = pulmonary flow)

	FRC	FRC+TV	TLC-400ml
SI			
MFI			

FVC   85 %
FEV₁%   60.4 %
PF   3.91 l/sec
V̇₅₀   1.54
V̇₂₅   0.77

Figure 4.   Type B dominant pattern: exercise-induced bronchospasm in a 16-year-old girl (SI = slow inhalation; MFI = maximum first inspiration; RV = residual volume; FRC = functional residual capacity; TV = tidal volume; TLC = total lung capacity; FVC = forced vital capacity; PF = pulmonary flow)

RESULTS

Exercise-induced bronchospasm in the children

The results of the test on exercise-induced bronchospasm are shown in Table I. Fourteen out of 20 patients had a 15 per cent or greater fall in FEV_1, and four out of 20 patients showed no ^{81m}Kr gas image changes before or after exercise load, five of them showed type A dominant pattern, four showed an image relatively close to that of type A, four showed an image relatively close to that of type B and only one showed type B dominant pattern.

TABLE I.   Comparison of the results of the exercise-induced bronchospasm and allergen inhalation provocation tests in the children

Test	Change in FEV_1	Number	^{81m}Kr gas image pattern	I (intensity of flow dependency)
Exercise	$\geqslant 15\%$	14	Type A (5) Type A > type B (4) Type A < type B (4) Type B (1)	1.10 ± 0.13
	$< 15\%$	6	No change (4) Type B*→type B (2)	
Allergen (mite)	$> 15\%$	18	Type A (1) Type A > type B (4) Type A < type B (4) Type B (5)	1.48 ± 0.81

* Type B* = type B + defects observed before exercise

This proved that after an exercise load, the airway changes take place over a wide area. The intensity of flow dependency value (1.10 ± 0.13) due to the differences in maximum first inhalation and slow inhalation was obtained using equation (3).

Allergen inhalation test in the children

The results of the allergen inhalation test in the children are also shown in Table I. The ^{81m}Kr gas image pattern differed from that in exercise-induced bronchospasm. Five patients showed type B dominant pattern, eight showed a pattern close to that of type B, four showed a pattern close to that of type A and only one showed type A dominant pattern. The difference in the intensity of flow dependency value was more evident in this test (1.48 ± 0.81).

Exercise-induced bronchospasm in the adults

The test results (clinical signs and ^{81m}Kr gas image defects) for the adult group are given in Table II. This shows that 21 of those with mild exercise-induced bronchospasm (84%) and all of those with moderate and severe exercise-induced bronchospasm had defects in the gas image. A comparison of the dominant patterns five minutes after exercise showed that 16 patients had type A dominant patterns and eight type B dominant; six had mixed types A and B patterns. A comparison between clinical severity of the asthma and ^{81m}Kr gas image pattern showed that 13 out of 16 of those with mild exercise-induced bronchospasm had type A dominant pattern and three out of eight with moderate and severe exercise-induced bronchospasm had type B dominant pattern.

TABLE II. Results of the exercise tests in the adult patients

Severity of asthma	Audible wheezing	> 15% decrease in FEV_1	Defects in ^{81m}Kr gas image
Mild	9/25 (31%)	13/23 (56%)	21/25 (84%)
Moderate	3/7 (43%)	4/7 (57%)	7/7 (100%)
Severe	2/2 (100%)	2/2 (100%)	2/2 (100%)
TOTAL	14/34 (41%)	19/32 (59%)	30/34 (88%)

DISCUSSION

We have compared the obstruction to the airways produced by exercise-induced bronchospasm and allergen inhalation provocation tests by means of ^{81m}Kr gas inhalation, which allowed us to identify where the passages were obstructed.

The cross section of the airways increases from central to peripheral. For example, the $2cm^2$ area of the lobal bronchi becomes $300cm^2$ at the respiratory bronchioles. At the same time, the flow slows down and Reynold's number changes from over 10,000 to under 10. Furthermore, if the flow is laminar, the loss of pressure will be proportional to that of flow ($\dot{V}$). However, if the flow is turbulent, the loss will be proportional to the square root of $\dot{V}$.

Using the slow inhalation method, the type A dominant pattern of obstruction had a laminar flow. But with the maximum first inhalation method, the flow became turbulent. Such a change causes an increase in the area of image defect that takes place mainly in the central airways. On the other hand, the type B dominant pattern of obstruction affected the small airways and was due more to the decrease in compliance than to increase in resistance. This is why the image defects can be seen more clearly with the slow inhalation method. With the maximum first inhalation method, the swing in pleural pressure increases in an attempt at equalisation. Thus, the image defects disappear with the use of the maximum first inhalation method. With an obstruction at the extreme periphery, the pattern shows little change in flow. From these data we can show that the sites of obstruction in exercise-induced bronchospasm and allergen provocation are as indicated in Figure 5.

In other research, we have shown, by the use of HeO_2, that the obstruction caused by allergen provocation tests was much more peripheral than that obtained by exercise load [5]. The difference in the ^{81m}Kr gas image defect with respect to air and HeO_2 after exercise load was seen in eight out of nine patients. In contrast, only one patient showed a defect as a result of the allergen provocation test [5].

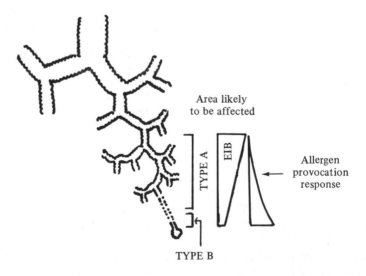

Figure 5. Bronchi affected by exercise-induced bronchospasm and allergen provocation

CONCLUSION

From our research we conclude that bronchospasm may occur in both the small and the large airways in exercise-induced asthma, but that it is the central airways that are most likely to be affected. In contrast, the peripheral airways are more usually obstructed in allergen inhalation provocation tests. However, the site of exercise-induced bronchoconstriction depends on the nature of the last attack of asthma and the clinical severity of the disease.

References

1   Despas PJ, LeRoux M, Macklem PT.
    Site of airway obstruction in asthma as determined by measuring maximal expiratory flow breathing air and helium-oxygen mixture.
    J Clin Invest 1972; 51: 3235–3243

2   Benatar SR, Konig P.
    Maximal expiratory flow and lung volume changes associated with exercise-induced asthma in children and the effect of breathing a low density gas mixture.
    Clin Sci 1974; 46: 317–319

3   Mildon A, LeRoux M, Hutcheon M, Zamel N.
    The site of airway obstruction in exercise induced asthma.
    Am Rev Respir Dis 1976; 113: 409–414

4   Chan Young M, Abboud R, Tsao MS, Maclean L.
    Effect of helium on maximal expiratory flow in patients with asthma before and during induced bronchoconstriction. *Am Rev Respir Dis 1976; 113:* 433–443

5   Iikura Y, Nishikawa K, Kawakami K et al.
    [81m]Kr gas tests of exercise and allergen challenge for asthmatic children.
    Respiration 1981; 42, Suppl 1: 57

Chapter 12

EXERCISE-ASSOCIATED VENTILATORY INSUFFICIENCY IN ADOLESCENT ATHLETES

H E Refsum, E Fønstelien

Laboratory of Clinical Physiology,
Ullevål Hospital, Oslo, Norway

SUMMARY

During the past year we have encountered several well-trained adolescent athletes who regularly develop severe respiratory stridor when they exert themselves towards maximal achievement in sports which make high demands on cardiopulmonary function. The stridor sets a definite limit to their performance, but disappears in the course of a few minutes' rest. It is not accompanied by clinical signs of bronchospasm.

A healthy 15-year-old girl track-and-field runner and cross-country skier who developed marked exertional stridor was tested at rest and while running on a treadmill at increasing speeds, until stopped by marked stridor. At rest her vital capacity, maximal voluntary ventilation, forced expiratory volume in one second (FEV_1), maximal inspiratory and expiratory flow rates and oesophageal pressures were all slightly below the expected average, but her flow-volume curve had a completely normal shape. On exercise there was a greater than expected rise in respiratory rate and a lower than expected rise in tidal volume. At the lower levels of exercise there were essentially normal relationships between the intensity of the exercise and inspiratory and expiratory flow rates and oesophageal pressures, and normal-shaped spontaneous flow-volume curves. At the highest levels of exercise, leading to increasing stridor, demanding that she stop the exercise, there was no further rise in inspiratory and expiratory flow rates, a definite fall in tidal volume and a sharp further rise in the oesophageal pressure excursions. At this time the inspiratory flow rate was the same as, and the inspiratory oesophageal pressure only slightly lower than, the maximal values observed during forced inspiration at rest. The expiratory flow rate increased slowly during the early phase of expiration and reached a maximum towards the end of expiration. This led to a spontaneous expiratory flow-volume curve resembling the mirror image of the curves observed at lower intensities of exercise. The observations correspond to those found in obstruction of the upper airways. The several possible causative or contributing mechanisms include a relative under-development of the dimensions of the upper airways as compared with the circulatory system.

INTRODUCTION

In healthy subjects engaged in exercise of the heavy endurance type, with high demands on oxygen intake, the limit of performance is usually set by the cardiovascular capacity not by the ventilatory capacity. However, recently we have encountered several healthy, well-trained adolescent athletes who regularly develop severe inspiratory and expiratory stridor when they exert themselves towards maximal achievement; the limit of their performance is definitely dependent on their ventilatory capacity. Their ventilatory distress is due to a restriction of air flow in the upper respiratory tract, and although it disappears in the course of a few minutes' rest, it is easily reproduced by repeated exertion.

This 'exercise-associated ventilatory insufficiency' is probably not a rare condition but seems to have been ignored in the medical literature. Probably it is confused with exercise-induced asthma, but it is clearly distinguishable by the fact that it is not associated with any evidence of bronchoconstriction, neither during nor after exercise.

CASE HISTORY

A girl, aged 15 years, has participated in track and field and cross-country skiing competitions since the age of 11 years. During the past four years she has been training under the supervision of an experienced coach for one to two hours, five days per week throughout the year. She is highly motivated, and is one of the higher ranking skiers in her age-group. She has always been in good health. Until the onset of the present condition, she never experienced any form of ventilatory distress. There is no history of allergy in the family.

Her ventilatory distress started at the age of 14 years during a period of rapid growth, and has followed an essentially similar pattern for one and a half years: she is capable of running at a high steady-state level for several minutes, but as soon as she tries to increase the speed to the maximum, as for instance in a spurt, she gets the feeling of a flap developing in her neck, in particular obstructing inspiration. She develops increasing stridor and is forced to slow down. The stridor disappears relatively suddenly, in the course of one to three minutes of rest, and is not accompanied by hoarseness or coughing. However, once induced, it reappears regularly on repeated exercise.

During track and field running the ventilatory distress usually develops before any feeling of fatigue and stiffness in the legs, whereas during other types of exercise for which she is less trained – as, for instance, bicycling – she may be forced to stop exercising on account of muscular fatigue, without developing ventilatory problems. The ventilatory distress is more easily provoked when the humidity of the air is low and in the summer half of the year; it is less easily provoked in very humid weather and during the winter half of the year. There is no obvious relation to pollen pollution. She has never experienced ventilatory problems at rest.

Physical examination

The girl is slender, well built, slightly less mature than the average girl of her age, and without obvious evidence of disease. Her height is 170cm and her weight 50kg. Laryngoscopy and bronchoscopy revealed nothing abnormal. There was no abnormal bulging during coughing and forced breathing. Fluoroscopy and x-ray of larynx and trachea, antero-posterior and lateral, at rest, during coughing, hyperventilation, Müller-Valsalva manoeuvre, and at the end of exercise-provoked stridor uncovered no obvious abnormalities of size, shape or movement. The chest x-ray and immunological allergy tests were all normal.

Ventilatory function studies

The values for the girl's vital capacity (3.2L), forced expiratory volume in one second (3.1 L) and maximal voluntary ventilation (125 L/min) were all slightly lower than the average for her age and height.

During the past nine months she has repeatedly been tested on a treadmill with an upward inclination of $10°$, at stepwise increases of running speeds up to 200m/min. Usually she is able to run for four minutes at each speed before developing stridor. She then has made repeated runs of shorter duration until incapable of continuing. Physiological measurements have been performed during short pauses between the running periods – usually within five to ten seconds of stopping exercise – and during the recovery period afterwards.

Results

The runs regularly provoked stridor, most severe after repeated runs approaching maximal performance. The stridor, which can be heard at a long distance, is both inspiratory and expiratory, and originates in the neck region. It always disappears within a few minutes after stopping exercise. Frequent auscultation during the period of stridor and throughout the recovery period has never revealed signs of bronchoconstriction, and repeated measurements of vital capacity (VC) and forced expiratory volume in one second (FEV_1) from two to 20 minutes after the end of the exercise have never shown values below the pre-exercise level.

Figure 1 shows flow recordings from five consecutive runs at increasing speed and during recovery, 90 seconds after the last run. At the three slowest speeds there was no stridor, while at 175 and 185 m/min there was a marked stridor, which, however, had disappeared after 90 seconds of rest. The recordings show marked changes in the expiratory flow curve: at 100 m/min there is a normal, early peak; at 125 m/min the well-defined peak has disappeared, and the flow rate remains high throughout the major part of the expiration; at 150 m/min there is a second peak at the end of expiration. At 175 and 185 m/min the early rise has been reduced and the peak toward the end of expiration is now marked. The inspiratory flow pattern shows no particular changes, but it should be noted that the peak flow rate is essentially the same at 150, 175 and 185 m/min. Ninety seconds after the end of exercise a normal-shaped flow pattern has been re-established.

Figure 2 shows spontaneous tidal flow-volume curves recorded under corresponding conditions. There was no stridor at 125 and 150 m/min, but it was marked and severe at 160 and 170 m/min. At 125 m/min the curve is of normal shape, with maximal expiratory flow rate early in expiration. At 150 m/min the flow rate remains high throughout the expiration; at 160 m/min the flow rate is higher at the end of expiration, and at 170 m/min the flow rate is low during the early part of expiration but increases toward a definite maximum at the end of expiration. Thus, simultaneously with the development of stridor, the expiratory curve has changed to a mirror image of the normal curve. Further, it may be noted that both the expiratory and inspiratory flow rates are about the same at 150, 160 and 170 m/min, and that the tidal volume is lower at the highest speeds than at 150 m/min, in particular at 170 m/min, coinciding with the most severe stridor.

Figure 3 shows spontaneous tidal flow-volume curves and forced maximal flow-volume curves at increasing exercise. There was no stridor at speeds up to 150 m/min but there was stridor of varying degree at 175 m/min. With increasing speed the spontaneous tidal flow volume curve fills up an

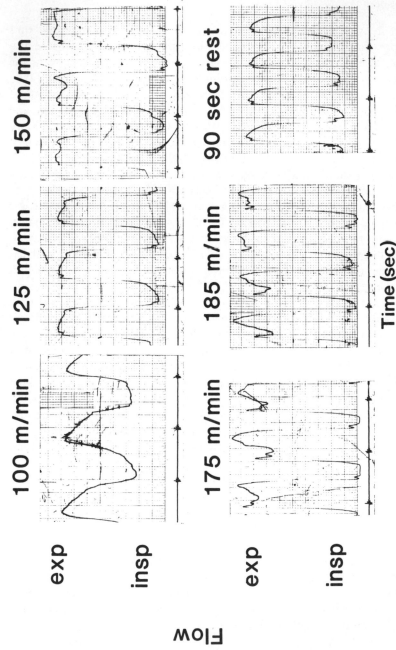

Figure 1. Flow recordings at increasing running speeds in the 15-year-old girl with exercise-associated ventilatory insufficiency

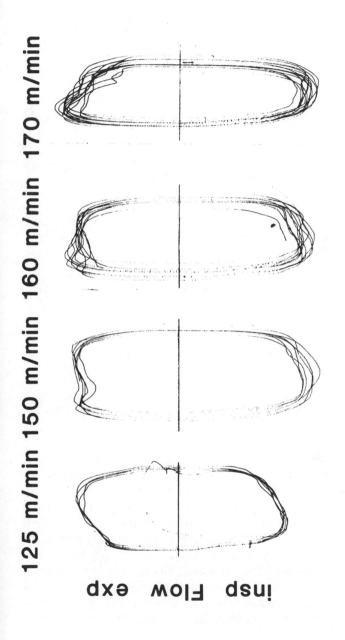

Figure 2. Tidal flow-volume curves at increasing running speeds in the 15-year-old girl with exercise-associated ventilatory insufficiency. Expiration starts at the right

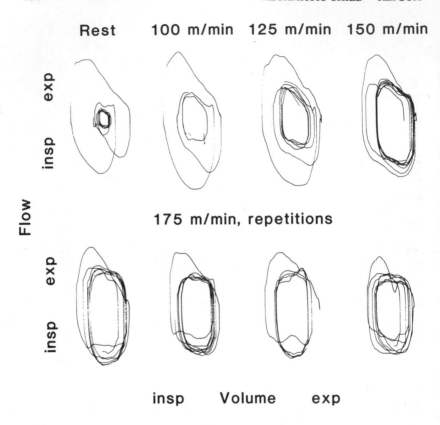

Figure 3. Tidal and forced maximal flow-volume curves at rest and at increasing running speeds in the 15-year-old girl with exercise-associated ventilatory insufficiency.
Expiration starts at the left

increasing part of the forced curve, the area of which is slightly reduced.
The spontaneous tidal curve is of normal shape, with an early expiratory
peak, until it reaches the boundaries of the forced curve. Then the expiratory curve forms a plateau, partly with the maximum in the late part of
expiration. It may be noted that the pattern of the forced, maximal
expiratory curve remains essentially unchanged, with an early peak of the
same magnitude as before the onset of stridor and definitely higher than
that of the spontaneous expiratory flow rate. The spontaneous inspiratory
flow rate, however, is the same as, or exceeds, the forced inspiratory flow
rate during the period of stridor. In fact, the spontaneous inspiratory flow
rate is the same as the forced maximal flow rate recorded before exercise.

Thus, during the stridor the inspiratory reserves seem to be exhausted, although there are still expiratory reserves. It may be added that there is no tendency for the spontaneous curve to move toward the maximal inspiration position of the forced curve.

For comparison, Figure 4 shows corresponding observations from a normally-reacting, well-trained 20-year-old girl, running until exhaustion without stridor. The spontaneous tidal flow-volume curve shows the same pattern throughout the test, with an early expiratory peak. This reaches the boundary of the mid-expiratory phase of the forced maximal flow-volume curve, whereas the spontaneous inspiratory flow rate at maximal exercise has not, by far, reached the forced inspiratory flow rate. Thus, in contrast to the girl with stridor there are still ample inspiratory reserves at maximal exertion.

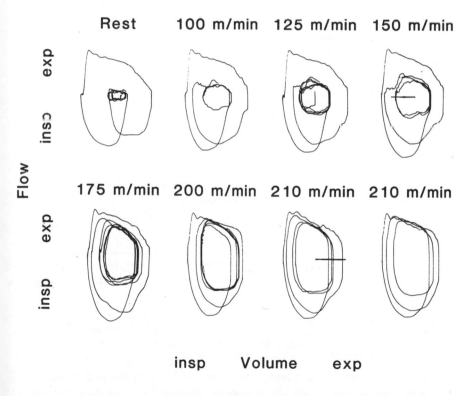

Figure 4. Tidal and forced maximal flow-volume curves at rest and at increasing running speeds in a 20-year-old girl without ventilatory problems. Expiration starts at the left

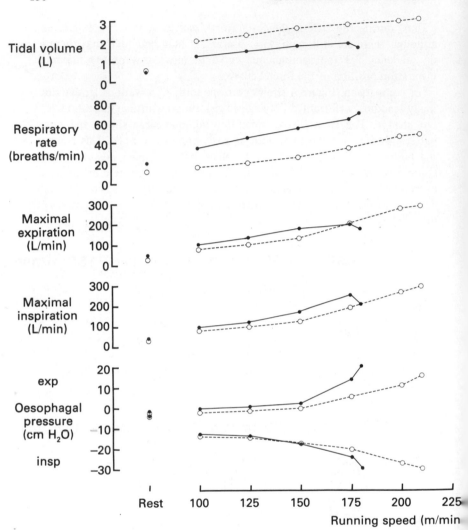

Figure 5. Respiratory frequency, tidal volume and maximal inspiratory and expiratory flow rates and oesophageal pressures at rest and increasing running speeds in the 15-year-old girl with exercise-associated ventilatory insufficiency (●) and the 20-year-old girl without ventilatory problems (○)

Figure 5 shows further comparisons between the two girls. In the control subject all measurements show smooth, gradual increases of a normal magnitude. The girl with stridor, however, shows an extraordinarily high respiratory rate of about 70 breaths/min at the end of the test, compared with 45 breaths/min in the control, and a relatively low tidal volume throughout the study. Otherwise, she shows essentially the same changes with increasing speed as the control, until she develops stridor at 175 m/ min. At this point both the inspiratory and expiratory flow rates and the tidal volume have reached a maximum, and further running at 185 m/min leads to a decline in these measurements, whereas the oesophageal, inspiratory and expiratory pressures rise sharply. In the girl with stridor the maximal spontaneous inspiratory and expiratory flow excursions during exercise were 100 and 75 per cent of the forced maximal values at rest, while the maximal spontaneous inspiratory and expiratory oesophageal pressures during exercise amounted to 85 and 60 per cent of the forced maxima at rest. In the control girl, the corresponding sets of figures for inspiratory and expiratory flow rates and inspiratory and expiratory oesophageal pressures were 70 and 70 per cent and 60 and 10 per cent, respectively. The ratio between maximal spontaneous ventilation and maximal voluntary ventilation was 90 per cent in the girl with stridor and 70 per cent in the control girl. Altogether, the girl with stridor had probably reached the limits of her ventilatory capacity, while the control girl had still ample reserves.

The end-tidal carbon dioxide tension, reflecting the arterial carbon dioxide tension, remained within the lower range of normal throughout the exercise. Thus there was no evidence for hyperventilation and excessive elimination of carbon dioxide.

So far, the inhalation before exercise of various spasmolytics and mucous membrane decongestant agents have not increased her stridor threshold or changed the flow-volume pattern during exercise.

DISCUSSION

The spontaneous tidal flow-volume curve at the onset of stridor shows two very characteristic, unusual features (Figures 1–3): the shape of the expiratory part changes from the usual picture with an early peak flow, through a curve with a prolonged maximum to one with an early, low maximum and a late peak flow (Figure 2). The inspiratory flow rate reaches the maximum obtainable during forced inspiration (Figure 3). These findings correspond with the usual observations in obstruction of the upper respiratory tract. The appearance of the pattern of obstruction may be due to exercise-provoked changes of the airways, such as bulging of weak parts of the laryngeal and tracheal walls and membrane flaps, mucous-membrane changes or laryngeal spasm, but may equally well be due to a permanent obstruction due to disease or to narrow undersized airways leading to evidence of obstruction only at increased air flow rates.

The failure of the laryngoscopic, bronchoscopic, fluoroscopic and roentgenographic examinations to show any abnormalities most probably rule out the anatomical possibilities. The fact that, even during severe stridor, the forced maximal flow-volume curve shows an early peak expiratory flow rate which is exactly the same as during rest (Figure 3) most probably excludes the possibility of an exercise-provoked laryngeal spasm.

The lack of evidence for pathological or pathophysiological causes for the stridor, together with the observation that the stridor starts when the spontaneous inspiratory flow rate reaches the maximal forced inspiratory flow rate strongly suggest that some part or parts of the upper respiratory tract, larynx or trachea, though seemingly of normal dimensions, are undersized for the high ventilatory demands of this well-trained, highly motivated athlete. This is supported by the fact that her bellows function is rather below expectations.

The fact that her problems started during a period of rapid growth may suggest that this relative ventilatory insufficiency is due to a temporary, growth-dependent mis-matching of the ventilatory and the circulatory systems. Such a mis-matching may well have been accentuated by the intensive training for sports with its heavy demands on cardiovascular function, since the growth of the heart and the peripheral muscles probably reacts more rapidly and effectively to heavy training than the cartilaginous structures of the upper respiratory tract. However, once the ventilatory resources have been maximally utilised during exercise and severe aerodynamic disturbances have been provoked, acute *secondary* changes in the mucous membrane may possibly have been induced which may, in turn, have contributed to further accentuation of the ventilatory insufficiency.

The subjective feeling of an inspiratory flap in the neck on the appearance of the stridor needs no structural, anatomical explanation. The lack of any way of further increasing the inspiratory flow rate, together with onset of turbulent air flow and eddy-formation probably lead to a sudden, marked increase in the resistance to, and effort of, breathing as reflected by the sharp rise in the oseophageal pressure (Figure 5) and a consequent feeling of acute obstruction.

The observation that the expiratory part of the forced maximal flow-volume curve remains unaffected during the period of stridor, while the spontaneous expiratory curve shows a picture of upper respiratory tract obstruction (Figure 3), probably demonstrates a frequency dependency of the resistance to flow. This may also explain the rapid changes and the variability of the distortions of the spontaneous flow-volume curve and the forced inspiratory curve during the stridor (Figures 1 and 3). Otherwise, the implications of the high respiratory rate are unclear — whether this is a primary, contributing factor or a consequence. The possibility exists that the high rate is accompanied by disturbances of the central and/or peripheral co-ordination of the switching from inspiration to expiration, with consequent disturbances of the air-flow dynamics.

Acknowledgments

We are grateful to NOS Stangeland MD, Department of Ear, Nose and Throat Diseases; NP Boye MD, Section of Allergy and Lung Diseases, Department of Internal Medicine; A Skjennald MD and A Høiseth MD, Department of Roentgenology, Ulleval Hospital, for help with the endoscopic and roentogenological examinations.

DISCUSSION

BAR-OR (Hamilton, Canada)	Dr Refsum, have you considered the possibility of a conversion-hysteria in your patient?
REFSUM	Yes, but at the moment I find it unacceptable. She is a very nice and natural girl, with no neurotic symptoms at all.
BRENNAN (Sheffield, UK)	Did the girl have an adolescent diffuse thyroid swelling? A mild goitre of this nature could, to some extent, be drawn into the thorax with strong respiratory efforts.
REFSUM	We saw no swelling on inspection, but we have done no special studies to elucidate this possibility.
HUGHES (London, UK)	Have you tried the effect of any pharmacological agents such as inhaled beta stimulants, ipratropium bromide or even spraying a local anaesthetic on the larynx of this patient?
REFSUM	We have been trying various inhalants, but they do not seem to have influenced the stridor threshold or the flow-volume curves. Nor did the girl herself feel any difference.
OSEID (Chairman)	We have had eight patients in our Institute during the past winter with similar clinical findings to those in Dr Refsum's patient. We shall be studying them further. Of interest is that four of them are competitive girl swimmers at fairly high level and they developed this stridor while swimming. There were two adolescent skiers, a boy and a girl, who developed these symptoms while skiing outdoors in the cold climate. And there was a girl who had no symptoms when running outdoors in the summer but only when running outdoors in the cold part of the winter. She also

developed a very severe stridor. We have given ipratropium bromide by inhaler to all these patients for a
long time to prevent this stridor, and in six out of the
seven adolescents we have had quite good therapeutic
success. Whether the success is due to suggestion or
whether the inhaler actually had some pharmacological
effect I would not like to say, but in four of the
patients the symptoms were completely abolished.

JENSSEN
(Trondheim,
Norway)

What advice did you give to the girl with regard to her
future sporting activities?

REFSUM

We told her to try to breathe in another way. But
that, as you will know, is easier said than done. She
has an unusually high respiratory rate during exercise,
and we have tried to persuade her to breathe more
slowly, but without success. However, she is a very
competent skier and I told her "You are perhaps first
of all a skier, and I think you should concentrate on
that. Then we will see how matters develop when you
grow further". I gave this advice because in skiing
you usually do not achieve such very high ventilation.
You have the chance to rest a little more during cross
country skiing than during track and field events. As
you know, 800 and 1500 metres with spurts are very
tough on ventilation. So we have advised her just to
concentrate on the sports which she can perform
without major ventilatory problems. We have advised
both the girl herself and her parents that she is completely healthy and that this will do her no harm.

FITCH
(Nedlands,
Australia)

Could Dr Refsum be describing 'breathing from the
top' or a failure to expire before attempting another
full inspiration? This is something I find not uncom-
monly in athletes, particularly when they are under
pressure. Instead of fully exhaling, and then inhaling,
they breathe out only partially before attempting
another full inspiration. That is why it is termed
'breathing from the top'. Nevertheless I appreciate

that laryngeal factors must be associated. The phenomenon is not uncommon in certain adolescents, more
especially in girls. But although I have submitted
some to submaximal exercise challenge, I have not
been able to reproduce the phenomenon. It happens
principally late in a contest or event – not infrequently
when a goal is missed, a race is lost or some other
stressful situation happens during near-maximal
exertion. There may, as Professor Bar-Or said, be
some psychosomatic provocation, but it is very real
and very disturbing to the athlete, her team mates
and team officials.

REFSUM   If I understand you correctly, you think she may be
over-filling her lungs? If you look at her flow-volume
curves, you will see that her spontaneous tidal flow-
volume curve was situated more on the expiratory
side than on the inspiratory side. In fact, she was
breathing just in the same way as the normal control.
There was no tendency to move up towards maximum
inspiration, which we usually see in patients with
obstructive disease, such as in asthma or emphysema.

PART III

STANDARDISATION OF EXERCISE TESTS

Chairman: Professor O Bar-Or, Hamilton, Canada

Chapter 13

THE IMPORTANCE OF STANDARDISING EXERCISE TESTS IN THE EVALUATION OF ASTHMATIC CHILDREN

Sandra D Anderson, Robin E Schoeffel

Royal Prince Alfred Hospital, Camperdown, NSW, Australia

SUMMARY

The importance of standardising challenge tests for the assessment of exercise-induced asthma has been recognised since the early 1970s. Godfrey and his colleagues, Connolly, Anderson and Silverman all clearly demonstrated the effect of varying the duration, intensity and type of exercise in children with asthma. At that time the standard exercise test recommended for obtaining an optimal response was one in which the subject performed running exercise for six to eight minutes, at an intensity sufficient to raise the heart rate above 170 beats/min during the last four minutes of exercise. Frequent measurements of flow rates and volumes were made within 15 minutes of the cessation of exercise. The recent observations by workers in Denver and Boston describing the relationship between heat loss from the airways and the asthmatic response has introduced a further dimension into standardisation.

The primary cause of loss of heat from the airways under ambient laboratory conditions is the level of ventilation achieved during exercise. This in turn is determined by the type, duration and intensity of the exercise. Thus these factors still remain of prime importance in evaluating the asthmatic response to exercise. Further consideration must also be given to a correction factor for differences in body size, particularly with regard to total loss of heat and water from the airways during exercise. This correction will permit longitudinal studies of changing sensitivity to exercise-induced asthma in asthmatic children.

Differences between challenge tests with regard to duration, intensity, type of exercise and the nature of the inspired air have all contributed to the wide variation in the reported incidence, severity, and reproducibility of exercise-induced asthma. Further, the failure to standardise challenges has led to differences in the interpretation of the effects of drugs. When exercise challenge tests become standardised, it will be possible for valid comparisons to be made of the incidence, severity and variability of responses with and without medications.

INTRODUCTION

The measurement of bronchial hyperreactivity in response to exercise is frequently used as a non-immunological test to identify patients with asthma. The importance of standardising the duration, intensity and type of exercise was reported in the early 1970s by a number of workers [1–3]. The more recent recognition that there is a relationship between heat loss from the airways and the asthmatic response [4, 5] has introduced a further dimension into the standardisation of exercise testing.

To define an abnormal airway response, to determine its severity within the asthmatic population and to assess its reproducibility, standardisation of exercise challenge is essential. Under ambient laboratory conditions loss of heat from the airways is determined by the level of ventilation [6] which, in turn is dependent on the type, duration and intensity of the exercise.

Within the asthmatic population exercise of the same intensity in relation to maximum working capacity results in different levels of ventilation and consequent heat loss. For this reason a correction factor for body size should be considered, permitting longitudinal studies of changing sensitivity to exercise challenge throughout childhood [6, 7].

Differences in duration, intensity and type of exercise and the nature of the inspired air between exercise tests have all contributed to the wide variation in the reported incidence, severity and reproducibility of exercise-induced asthma. Furthermore, failure to standardise challenges has been responsible for differences in the interpretation of the effects of drugs. We propose here to identify some important aspects of exercise challenge testing under normal laboratory conditions of temperature and humidity.

DEFINITION OF EXERCISE-INDUCED ASTHMA

The identification of abnormal bronchial reactivity and its severity is determined by the method used to measure changes in airways resistance in response to exercise.

Measurements of changes in specific conductance (sGaw), maximum mid-expiratory flow rate (MMEFR) and the flow rate at 50 per cent of the vital capacity ($\dot{V}_{50}$) have all been cited as more sensitive tests of exercise-induced asthma than changes in peak expiratory flow rate (PEFR) or forced expiratory volume in one second (FEV_1) [8, 9]. In most cases, however, the sensitivity of these measurements has been judged upon the percentage reduction from the pre-exercise level observed in asthmatic subjects. The greater the percentage fall of a measurement, it has been said, the greater its sensitivity for the identification of exercise-induced asthma. This concept, however, ignores the fact that normal non-asthmatic subjects also have greater changes in sGaw, MMEFR and $\dot{V}_{50}$ than PEFR or FEV_1 [10, 11] (Table I).

TABLE I. Mean per cent fall (+ 2SD) in six tests of pulmonary function in normal subjects after six minutes of treadmill running exercise (Data from Wilson and Evans [11] for adults*; other values are for children and are from Anderson [10]) (FVC = forced vital capacity)

Test	Mean per cent fall
PEFR	9.4
MMEFR	18.8
FEV_1	11.5
FVC	13.2
sGaw	50.2
$\dot{V}_{50}$	16.9*

In our laboratory, we define an abnormal response to exercise as a reduction in flow rates, volumes or conductance (expressed as a percentage of the pre-exercise level) greater than the mean plus two standard deviations of the reduction observed in normal non-asthmatics performing an exercise challenge under the same conditions. Thus for the percentage reduction is sGaw to be regarded as abnormal (that is, within the asthmatic range) a value of 50 per cent or more is required; for PEFR the reduction need be only 10 per cent.

The airway responses in normal subjects probably represent one extremity of a continuous spectrum of reactivity within the population. The changes in airways resistance are small compared with those in asthmatics and are not associated with either hyperinflation or hypoxaemia which normally accompany exercise-induced asthma.

For the laboratory diagnosis of exercise-induced asthma we prefer the measurement of PEFR for several reasons. Peak expiratory flow rate is dependent on a maximal inspiration; however, in contrast to FEV_1 or

MMEFR its measurement requires only a short maximal expiration since the value is registered within the first 500ml. Thus PEFR may be measured easily during exercise to assess bronchodilatation. Further, the transitory nature of exercise-induced asthma requires that frequent measurements of pulmonary function are made after exercise, especially in children. Peak expiratory flow rate may be measured at brief intervals: we recommend 1, 3, 5, 7, 10 and 15 minutes after exercise. Asthmatics rarely cough after a peak flow manoeuvre but frequently do so after the prolonged expiration required to record FEV_1 or MMEFR.

The changes in PEFR after exercise correlate well with changes in FEV_1 [12] and with $\dot{V}_{50}$ (Figure 1). Once exercise-induced asthma has been

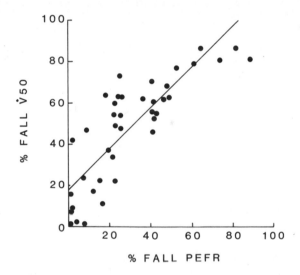

Figure 1. Individual data for the per cent fall in flow rates at 50 per cent of the vital capacity ($\dot{V}_{50}$) in relation to the per cent fall observed in peak expiratory flow rate (PEFR) in asthmatic subjects who exercised after placebo and salbutamol aerosol (r = 0.84; p < 0.001)

diagnosed in a patient other measurements such as $\dot{V}_{50}$ or sGaw may be useful for determining the site of action of a drug or the response to repeated exercise challenge. These measurements may also be useful in cases where a fall in PEFR is not detected; however, changes should be compared with the response observed in normal non-asthmatic subjects.

The choice of a measurement must take into account its reproducibility. The coefficient of variation for repeated measurements of some commonly

TABLE II. Coefficient of variation for repeated measurements of lung function in seven asthmatic and 18 normal children

Test	Normal children	Asthmatic children
PEFR	4.1%	11.0%
FEV_1	4.3%	11.2%
FVC	8.3%	7.7%
MMEFR	12.0%	36.3%
sGaw	8.3%	18.4%

used pulmonary function tests are given for asthmatic and normal subjects in Table II. The greater variation observed between measurements in the asthmatics must be considered when selecting the one to be used to diagnose exercise-induced asthma or to assess the efficacy of a drug.

The changes in PEFR and FEV_1 in non-asthmatic children have been well defined in separate studies of large numbers of subjects. A 10 per cent reduction in PEFR and FEV_1 has now generally been accepted as the upper limit of the normal fall after exercise [13, 14].

INCIDENCE OF EXERCISE-INDUCED ASTHMA

Using the criterion of a reduction in PEFR of 10 per cent or more of the pre-exercise level after exercise, that is

$$\text{Per cent fall in PEFR} = \frac{\text{Pre-exercise value for PEFR} - \text{lowest value for PEFR after exercise}}{\text{Pre-exercise value for PEFR}} \times 100$$

we have demonstrated exercise-induced asthma in 77 per cent of 313 children who had clinically recognised asthma (Figure 2). Each child performed six to eight minutes of treadmill running exercise, under ambient laboratory conditions ($18-25°C$, $7-11$ mg H_2O/L).

To determine the level of exercise required to induce an adequate heart rate we adjusted the slope and speed of the treadmill to induce a predicted oxygen consumption of $32-36$ ml/kg [15], which represented $60-80$ per cent of the maximum working capacity. The intensity of exercise was adjusted to increase the heart rate above 170 beats/min.

We do not know whether another measurement of lung function or cooling the inspired air would have elicited a positive response in the 23

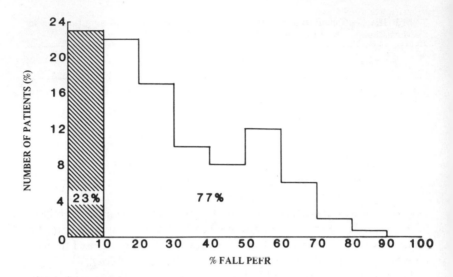

Figure 2. Incidence and severity of the fall in peak expiratory flow rate (PEFR) in 313 clinically recognised asthmatic children who ran on a treadmill for six to eight minutes. The temperature of the laboratory varied from 18–25°C and the water content from 7–11mg H_2O/L

per cent of the asthmatic children with negative tests [9, 16]. For patients who give a history of exercise-induced asthma, which is not demonstrable under ambient conditions, it may be necessary to dry or cool the inspired air and ensure a high level of ventilation to confirm the diagnosis. Since nasal breathing is less likely to induce exercise-induced asthma than mouth breathing [17] we now use a nose clip for routine diagnostic challenges.

INFLUENCE OF RESTING LEVELS OF AIRWAYS RESISTANCE

When exercise-induced asthma is observed it is not necessarily associated with abnormal lung function before exercise. In the 241 patients in whom we recorded exercise-induced asthma, 131 (54%) had resting levels of PEFR greater than 80 per cent of predicted normal. Of these 131 patients, 88 (67%) had a fall in PEFR after exercise of more than 20 per cent of the pre-exercise level and required treatment to control their symptoms. In the 110 patients who had flow rates below the normal range before exercise (that is, less than 80% predicted) 75 per cent had exercise-induced asthma of sufficient severity to require prophylactic treatment. Thus the severity of exercise-induced asthma cannot be predicted from the resting level of PEFR when the per cent fall index is used (Figure 3). By contrast, a negative exercise test in an asthmatic child is likely to be associated with normal function. In the 72 children who did not have exercise-induced asthma, 56 (78%) had a PEFR within the normal predicted range before exercise.

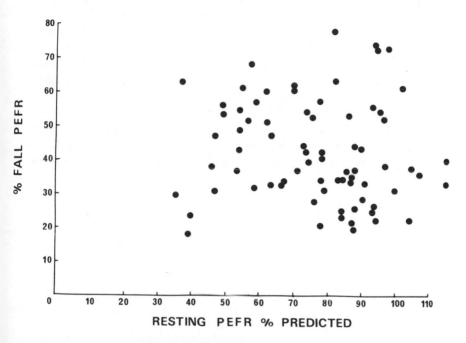

Figure 3. Individual data for the per cent fall in peak expiratory flow rate (PEFR) after running exercise in relation to the pre-exercise values for PEFR expressed as a percentage of predicted normal in asthmatic subjects (● = placebo)

With regard to pharmacotherapy for exercise-induced asthma, only a single medication is usually required (a beta-sympathomimetic aerosol or sodium cromoglycate) when falls in flow rates are less than 25 per cent. In severe cases (falls > 50%) it is difficult to predict how much therapy is needed. For some patients the standard dose of aerosol is sufficient, while for others who have the same degree of obstruction after exercise, two to three times the clinically recommended dose of an aerosol or combination therapy may be necessary to prevent the exercise-induced asthma.

FACTORS DETERMINING THE SEVERITY OF
EXERCISE-INDUCED ASTHMA

Under ambient laboratory conditions, the most important determinant of the airway response is the level of ventilation achieved and sustained during exercise [7, 11]. For a given individual the higher the level of ventilation the greater the loss of heat from the airways and the greater the subsequent increase in airways resistance. It is for this reason, no doubt, that a dose-response relationship for exercise-induced asthma with changing duration and intensity of exercise was observed previously [2]. The maximum response was recorded after six to eight minutes of running exercise at 60–85 per cent of the maximum working capacity.

By measuring the ventilation, the temperature of the inspired and expired air and water vapour content we have made continuous measurements of respiratory heat and water loss during cycling exercise [6]. Under ambient conditions the maximum losses of both heat and water occur between the

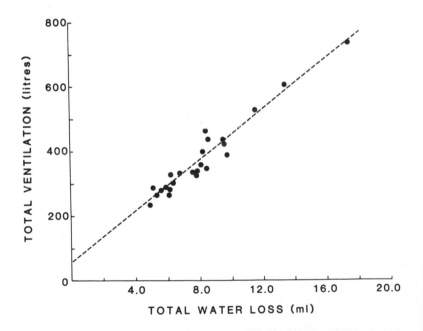

Figure 4. Total ventilation during exercise in relation to the amount of water lost during exercise in asthmatic children cycling under ambient laboratory conditions. The expired air was assumed to be fully saturated at the temperature measured (r = 0.96; p < 0.001)

fifth and seventh minutes of a steady-state exercise which may account for the maximal response previously observed after six to eight minutes [2]. Sophisticated technology is not required for the measurement of heat and water loss in the assessment of exercise-induced asthma. Under the ambient conditions of a laboratory 80—90 per cent of the heat lost is due to the loss of water from the respiratory tract. The amount of water lost is linearly related to ventilation, assuming the expired air to be fully saturated with water vapour [6] (Figure 4).

Although for a given individual there is a good correlation between water and heat loss and airway response (Figure 5), within the asthmatic popu-

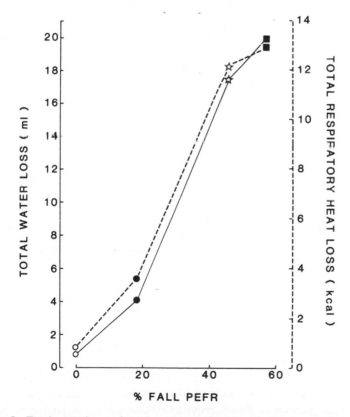

Figure 5. Total water loss and total respiratory heat loss during exercise in relation to the per cent fall in peak expiratory flow rate (PEFR) after exercise in a 17-year-old boy who performed cycling exercise at 73 per cent of his maximum working capacity for eight minutes at four different inspired air conditions (1 kcal = 4.2 kJ)

lation there is a wide variation in the sensitivity to loss of heat and water under ambient conditions [6] (Figure 6). When values for the loss of heat and water are corrected for body size the variation is reduced [6].

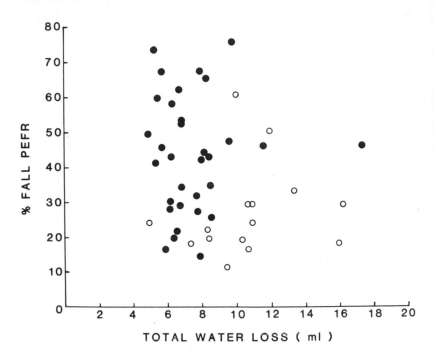

Figure 6. Individual data for the per cent fall in peak expiratory flow rate (PEFR) in relation to the amount of water lost in asthmatic children (•) and adults (o) during exercise by cycling for six to eight minutes under ambient conditions

For our investigations into the efficacy of drugs, we customarily exercise our patients by having them run for eight minutes under normal laboratory conditions. Under these conditions we usually observe a mean fall in PEFR greater than 35 per cent [12, 19]. This response is similar to that reported by other workers who exercised their patients for a shorter duration (3–4 min) while inspiring air at subfreezing temperatures [17]. It is, however, unnecessary to condition the inspired air, increasing the duration of exercise may be all that is required to increase the response. Further it may be possible to construct a dose-response curve merely by varying the duration (and thus ventilation and water loss) while maintaining the intensity of the exercise and constant inspired air conditions [7].

If the level of ventilation is high enough the type of exercise used may not matter [7, 20]. However, the recent studies of Bar-Yishay and his colleagues [21] demonstrated that even under matched conditions of heat loss, the exercise of swimming is less liable to induce asthma than that of running.

Several other factors determine airway response to exercise and must not be overlooked. They include the time since the last medication and the interval since the last attack of exercise-induced asthma. When measuring exercise-induced asthma [22] and a minimum of three or four hours after aerosol medication and of 24 hours after oral medications.

There are now several studies that document a refractory period after exercise-induced asthma [22] and a minimum of three or four hours should elapse before exercise is repeated. The variation in response to repeated running tests for patients exercising at the same intensity and duration in the same laboratory is given in Table III. Small variations do occur in temperature and relative humidity and keeping these factors con-

TABLE III. Mean values and SEM for per cent fall in PEFR in asthmatic children who performed two identical running tests on three occasions at different time intervals (NS = not significant)

	Test I		Test II
Time interval		40 minutes	
No. subjects		26	
Mean per cent fall in PEFR	37.6		23.7
SEM	2.8		3.2
p		< 0.001	
Coefficient of variation		65%	
Time interval		2 hours	
No. subjects		20	
Mean per cent fall in PEFR	39.3		36.0
SEM	3.4		3.5
p		NS	
Coefficient of variation		32%	
Time interval		7−28 days	
No. subjects		13	
Mean per cent fall in PEFR	43.0		50.5
SEM	5.2		4.3
p		NS	
Coefficient of variation		22%	

stant may reduce the variation noted within 28 days. Environmental variation, however, is unlikely to account for the variation observed within a
day.

In our studies on drug action we ask patients not to take drinks, such as
tea, coffee and Coca-Cola, that contain caffeine. When studying the
effects of drugs that do not induce bronchodilatation – for example,
sodium cromoglycate – we also find it useful to instruct the patient to
take their bronchodilator aerosol at a specified time (say 6–8 hours beforehand) and to keep this a standard interval for all tests in that patient. When
determining the efficacy of a drug we use the index of Godfrey and König
according to which a drug is regarded as efficacious if it provides greater
than 50 per cent protection and/or completely blocks exercise-induced
asthma (fall less than 10 per cent for PEFR). Other factors relating to the
efficacy of drugs in protecting against exercise-induced asthma have been
given in detail elsewhere [19].

CONCLUSION

We are all aware that normal values for biochemical and haematological
tests in blood or plasma fall within a range. There is also a need similarly
to define the limits of the normal airway response to exercise. Only thus
will it be possible to define an abnormal response. Sophisticated technology
is available to measure the loss of heat and water from the airways, the
initiating stimulus in exercise-induced asthma. We consider, however,
that for the diagnosis of exercise-induced asthma and the assessment of its
treatment it is sufficient to control the level of ventilation by the duration
and intensity of exercise and by maintaining constant inspired air conditions. When exercise challenge tests become standardised, it will be
possible to make valid comparisons of incidence, severity and variability of
response with and without medication.

References

1   Anderson SD, Connolly N, Godfrey S.
    Comparison of bronchoconstriction induced by cycling and running.
    Thorax 1971; 26: 396–401

2   Silverman M, Anderson SD.
    Standardization of exercise tests in asthmatic children.
    Arch Dis Child 1972; 47: 882–889

3   Godfrey S, Silverman M, Anderson SD.
    Problems of interpreting exercise induced asthma.
    J Allergy Clin Immunol 1973; 52: 199–209

4 Chen WY, Horton DJ.
   Heat and water loss from the airways and exercise induced asthma.
   Respiration 1977; 34: 305–313

5 Strauss RH, McFadden ER, Ingram RH et al.
   Influence of heat and humidity on the airway obstruction induced by exercise
   in asthma. *J Clin Invest 1978; 61:* 433–440

6 Anderson SD, Schoeffel RE, Follet R et al.
   Sensitivity to heat and water loss at rest and during exercise in asthmatic patients.
   Eur J Respir Dis 1982. In press

7 Kivity S, Souhrada JF.
   Hyperpnea: the common stimulus for bronchospasm in asthma during exercise
   and voluntary isocapnic hyperpnea. *Respiration 1980; 40:* 169–177

8 Buckley JM, Souhrada JF, Kopetzky MT.
   Detection of airway obstruction in exercise-induced asthma.
   Chest 1974; 66: 244–251

9 Schachter EN, Kreisman H, Littner M et al.
   Airway responses to exercise in mild asthmatics.
   J Allergy Clin Immunol 1978; 61: 390–398

10 Anderson SD.
   Physiological aspects of exercise-induced bronchoconstriction. PhD Thesis 1979.
   University of London

11 Wilson BA, Evans JN.
   Standardization of work intensity for evaluation of exercise-induced bronchoconstriction. *Eur J Appl Physiol.* In press

12 Anderson SD, Seale JP, Rozea P et al.
   Inhaled and oral salbutamol in exercise-induced asthma.
   Am Rev Respir Dis 1976; 114: 493–500

13 Anderson SD, Silverman M, Konig P, Godfrey S.
   Exercise-induced asthma. A review.
   Br J Dis Chest 1975; 69: 1–39

14 Kattan M, Keens TG, Mellis CM, Levis H.
   The response to exercise in normal and asthmatic children.
   J Pediatr 1978; 92: 718–721

15 Silverman M, Anderson SD.
   Metabolic cost of treadmill exercise in children.
   J Appl Physiol 1972; 33: 696–698

16 Strauss RH, McFadden ER, Ingram RH, Jaeger JJ.
   Enhancement of exercise-induced asthma by cold air.
   N Engl J Med 1977; 297: 743–747

17 Shturman-Ellstein R, Zeballos RJ, Buckley JM, Souhrada JF.
   The beneficial effect of nasal breathing in exercise-induced bronchoconstriction.
   Am Rev Respir Dis 1978; 118: 65–73

18 Deal EC, McFadden ER, Ingram RH, Jaeger JJ.
   Hyperpnea and heat flux: initial reaction sequence in exercise-induced asthma.
   J Appl Physiol 1979; 46: 476–483

19   Anderson SD, Seale JP, Ferris L, Schoeffel RE.
      An evaluation of pharmacotherapy for exercise-induced asthma.
      J Allergy Clin Immunol 1979; 64, part 2: 612–624

20   Miller GJ, Davies BH, Cole TJ, Seaton A.
      Comparison of the bronchial response to running and cycling in asthma using
      an improved definition of the response to work. *Thorax 1975; 30:* 306–311

21   Bar-Yishay E, Gur I, Inbar I et al.
      Differences between swimming and running as stimuli for exercise-induced
      asthma. *Eur J Appl Physiol.* In press

22   Edmunds AT, Tooley M, Godfrey S.
      The refractory period after exercise-induced asthma: its duration and relation
      to the severity of exercise. *Am Rev Respir Dis 1978; 117:* 247–254

Chapter 14

STANDARDISATION OF THE EXERCISE TEST IN ASTHMATIC CHILDREN

A Bundgaard

Rigshospitalet, Copenhagen, Denmark

SUMMARY

It is important to standardise the exercise test when two or more tests are made on the same patient — for example, when comparing different pre-treatments of exercise-induced asthma.

The inhaled air should be at identical temperature and relative humidity from one test to another and the total ventilation during the challenge should also be identical from day to day. (Identical ventilation is obtained by identical work load from day to day.) The work load must be sufficient to induce a fall in the ventilatory capacity greater than 20 per cent without at the same time inducing a severe attack of asthma. It makes no difference whether the exercise is performed on a bicycle ergometer, a treadmill or as a step test, as long as the workload is reproducible. The duration must be longer than four minutes. Assessments of the ventilatory capacity should be done immediately before and immediately after the exercise and at regular intervals up to 10—15 minutes after the exercise challenge. The assessment of the changes in ventilatory capacity must include the highest and the lowest readings in the study period.

The exercise should be performed at the same time of day (also it has to be shown that the challenges are comparable as soon as the base-line value is the same as when the exercise was first performed). Standardisation must also take account of the time interval since the latest intake of medicine.

INTRODUCTION

If the purpose of the exercise test is to confirm the diagnosis of bronchial asthma, the child should take no anti-asthmatic medicine by mouth during the 24 hours before the challenge. Inhaled medications should be avoided for six hours beforehand. The exercise should be performed in a room with a temperature $<25°C$ and a relative humidity <50 per cent. Free running, treadmill running or work on the bicycle ergometer may be used for six minutes' exercise. The velocity of running or the work load should be kept constant during the exercise, but high enough to result in a work load $>80-90$ per cent of the maximal oxygen consumption. This will be reached if the heart rate is >160 beats/min after two minutes of exercise. The lung function can be assessed by measuring the peak expiratory flow rate (PEFR), the forced expiratory volume in one second (FEV_1), although airways resistance (Raw) may be the best. The readings should be done immediately before and immediately after the exercise and then at $1, 3, 5,$ 10 and 15 minutes after the exercise. If the difference between the lowest reading after exercise and the higher of the readings immediately before and immediately after exercise is >20 per cent, the exercise test confirms the diagnosis of asthma.

If the purpose of the exercise test is to compare the effects of different variables, such as temperature or medication, attention should be paid to the following: the last dose of oral medicine should be taken at the same time before exercise every day. No medication must be inhaled during the four hours before the exercise. The temperature and relative humidity in the room where the exercise is performed must be standardised and the work load of the six minutes' exercise challenge must be identical from day to day. Lung function may be assessed by measurement of PEFR, FEV_1 or Raw. The base-line value must be at a level at which the patient is known to have exercise-induced asthma, and must show a day to day variation of $<15-20$ per cent. All patients with known asthma should be admitted, no matter what the results of their placebo test or their test on the day of inclusion in the study. Readings of lung function should be made at base line, immediately before and after the exercise and at $1, 3, 5,$ 10 and 15 minutes after exercise. The fall in lung function after exercise can be calculated as the percentage difference between the lowest of the readings after exercise and the higher of the readings immediately before and immediately after exercise. The staff should have great experience of patients with exercise-induced asthma and remain the same from day to day.

STANDARDISATION

To confirm the diagnosis of exercise-induced asthma

Pre-exercise medication The last dose of regular oral anti-asthmatic medication (for example, steroids, $beta_2$-agonists, theophylline) should be taken at the same time before each exercise test. No anti-asthmatic medication should be inhaled for four hours before the challenge (for example, $beta_2$-agonists, sodium cromoglycate, atropine).

Ambient conditions The temperature of the test room should vary by not more than 2–3°C and by not more than 10 per cent in relative humidity from day to day.

Equipment and work load Identical equipment should be used from day to day. The treadmill should be at an inclination of 10° and the rate of pedalling on the bicycle ergometer should be 60rpm. The speed of the treadmill and the load of the bicycle ergometer must be high enough to induce a post-exercise decrease in each patient and therefore they should be individually adjusted.

Duration of the exercise test The test should last for six minutes.

Lung function This is assessed by measurement of PEFR or FEV_1.

Readings The base-line value must be at a level at which the exercise will induce variations >20 per cent (for example, if the PEFR is high in a particular patient, exercise may only occasionally induce variations in PEFR, and also if the PEFR is very low only small changes will be recorded after exercise). The next readings are taken immediately before the exercise and immediately after cessation of the exercise. Post-exercise readings are then taken at 1, 3, 5, 10 and 15 minutes.

Calculation The per cent fall should be calculated as the lowest reading after exercise compared to the higher of the readings immediately before and immediately after exercise as shown in equation (1):

$$\frac{\text{Higher PEFR immediately before/after exercise} - \text{lowest PEFR after exercise}}{\text{Higher PEFR immediately before/after exercise}} \quad (1)$$

Inclusion in the study All patients with asthma are included in the study, no matter what the results of the exercise test on the placebo day or on the day of inclusion, so long as the base-line criteria are fulfilled. The patient must be in a stable phase of the disease.

Staff   Those in charge of the exercise tests should be experienced and remain unchanged throughout the study.

To compare the effects of variables

Medicine before exercise   No anti-asthmatic medicine should be taken within 24 hours of starting the exercise test (for example, steroids, theophylline and $beta_2$-agonists – including sustained-release tablets). No anti-asthmatic medication should be inhaled during the four hours before the exercise test (for example, steroids, $beta_2$-agonists, sodium cromoglycate, atropine etc).

Ambient conditions   A climatic chamber is required in which the temperature and relative humidity remain identical from day to day.

Equipment and work load   Identical equipment should be used from day to day. The treadmill should be at an inclination of $10°$ and the rate of pedalling on the bicycle ergometer should be 60rpm. The speed of the treadmill and the load of the bicycle ergometer must be high enough to induce a post-exercise decrease in each patient and therefore they should be individually adjusted.

Ventilation   The total ventilation must be the same from challenge to challenge.

Duration of the exercise test   The test should last for six minutes.

Lung function   This should be assessed by measurement of PEFR, FEV_1, Raw, sGaw or residual volume. (The last three may be difficult to measure at the recommended reading intervals.)

Readings   The base-line value must be at a level at which the exercise will induce variations >20 per cent. The next readings are taken immediately before the exercise and immediately after cessation of the exercise. Post-exercise readings are then taken at 1, 3, 5, 10 and 15 minutes.

Calculation   The per cent fall should be calculated as the lowest reading after exercise compared to the higher of the readings immediately before or immediately after exercise as shown in equation (1) above.

Inclusion in the study All patients with asthma are included in the study, no matter what the results of the exercise test on the placebo day or on the day of inclusion, so long as the base-line criteria are fulfilled. The patient must be in a stable phase of the disease.

Staff Those in charge of the exercise tests should be experienced and remain unchanged throughout the study.

DISCUSSION

Standardisation of the exercise test in asthmatic children has been considered by several authors during the past 10 years [1–6].

Standardisation of work load or ventilation

Although it has been known for many decades that hyperventilation alone can induce asthma, only during the past 10 years or so has evidence appeared that hyperventilation induces the same impairment in lung function as does exercise [7–11]. It has not been shown that exercise-induced asthma is identical to the asthma induced by hyperpnoea but they are

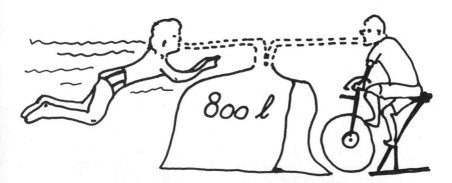

Figure 1. The importance of ventilation during swimming was compared to that during work on a bicycle ergometer by dosing the inhaled air from a large bag. In this way the inhaled air was identical from day to day. The results indicated that the exercise-induced asthma was on average similar. No bronchodilatation was found after swimming

clinically very much alike – except that hyperventilation does not produce the phase of improvement in lung function which is often found after exercise. This improvement seems to be constant after exercise on the bicycle but is also found after swimming [12–14] (Figure 1).

The good correlation between hyperventilation- and exercise-induced asthma should stress the importance of identical provocation and work load from challenge to challenge when comparing different exercises. It may be more important to reproduce the ventilation, as the correlation is poor between the total ventilations recorded during two different exercises – treadmill-running and work on the bicycle ergometer (unpublished observations).

Room temperature and relative humidity

It is well documented that warm air of high water content decreases the asthmatic's responses to exercise and that cold air worsens the impairment in lung function induced by exercise. The temperature and the humidity in

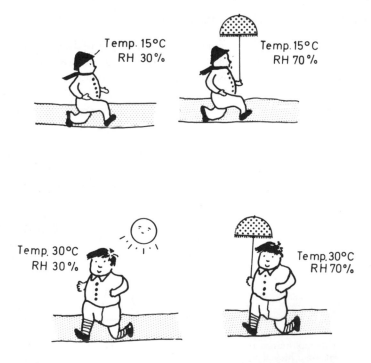

Figure 2. The study of the effects of four different weather conditions

these studies has reached extremes (for example, from +80°C to −50°C). The temperature in a great part of Europe lies between 10 and 25°C with relative humidities near to 50 per cent during most seasons, apart from a few winter months. The importance of temperatures between 15 and 30°C and relative humidities between 30 and 70 per cent was therefore studied. It was found that only when both the temperature and the relative humidity were high (30°C, 70%), was there a significant decrease in the response to exercise. The effect of a high temperature (30°C) and a low relative humidity (30%) was no different from that of a low temperature (15°C) and a high relative humidity (70%) or from that of a low temperature (15°C) and a low relative humidity (30%) (Figure 2). It seems therefore that a variation in the temperature of a few degrees and a variation in the relative humidity of 10−20 per cent has little influence on the changes in lung function after exercise [14].

Study design and calculation

Every day, when the patient arrives at the laboratory, the base-line value should be recorded during a period of up to 30 minutes. Then the pre-exercise medication can be given and the exercise performed. In our exercise studies, we most often find an increase in the ventilatory capacity after exercise. It is therefore recommended that the ventilatory capacity is measured immediately after the exercise. Some of the methods − for instance Raw in a body plethysmograph − demand some minutes of calibration before the assessment can be done and may therefore be unsuitable. Forced ventilations on the other hand may change the ventilatory capacity in asthmatics. Readings taken more than 15 minutes after the cessation of exercise add no further information to the results of the test (Figure 3).

How should the response be calculated? The possibilities include the Jones lability index, fall from base line, exercise lability index and top-bottom index. As it has been found that the top-bottom index is the most specific and sensitive [15], it is the one I prefer to use (see equation (1) above).

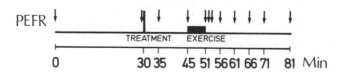

Figure 3. The effects of different drugs may be compared in a study of this design

Should readings be taken during the exercise? It has been found that the PEFR after 1, 2, 3, 4, 5 and 6 minutes of exercise is 461, 492, 497, 497, 496 and 478 L/min, respectively (average in eight asthmatics), which is a difference of about five per cent (unpublished observations). Readings can be taken during exercise but are rather difficult. If the ventilation is controlled during the exercise, readings cannot be taken.

Methods and inclusion of patients

All studies must, if possible, be done double-blind. It is very easy to blow in different ways, and – in our experience – makes for unreliability when assessing lung function by forced expirations in open studies.

The response to exercise in the same patient varies by about 20 per cent from day to day.

Therefore, if you are convinced that a patient has exercise-induced asthma, he should be included. Every time a group of patients does an exercise test, some will – by virtue of natural variability – have a negative test. If you exclude patients who, for this reason, have a negative exercise test on the day of the placebo test or on the day of inclusion, bias will enter the study.

References

1   Silverman M, Anderson SD.
    Standardization of exercise tests in asthmatic children.
    Arch Dis Child 1972; 47: 882–889

2   Godfrey S, Silverman M, Anderson SD.
    Problems of interpreting exercise-induced asthma.
    J Allergy Clin Immunol 1973; 52: 199–209

3   Eggleston PA, Guerrant JL.
    A standardized method of evaluating exercise-induced asthma.
    J Allergy Clin Immunol 1976; 58: 414–425

4   Eggleston PA.
    Exercise challenge.
    J Allergy Clin Immunol 1979; 64: 604–608

5   Cropp GJA.
    The exercise bronchoprovocation test.
    J Allergy Clin Immunol 1979; 64: 627–633

6   Johnson JD.
    Statistical considerations in studies of exercise-induced bronchospasm.
    J Allergy Clin Immunol 1979; 64: 634–641

7   Chan-Yeung MMW, Vyas MN, Grzybowski S.
    Exercise-induced asthma.
    Am Rev Respir Dis 1971; 104: 915–923

8   Simonsson BG, Skoogh BE, Ekstrom-Jodal B.
    Exercise-induced airways constriction.
    Thorax 1972; 27: 169–180

9   Zeballos RJ.
    The role of hyperventilation in EIA.
    Am Rev Respir Dis 1978; 118: 877–884

10 Kilham H, Tooley M, Silverman M.
    Running, walking and hyperventilation in EIA.
    Thorax 1979; 34: 582–586

11 Bundgaard A, Ingemann-Hansen T, Schmidt A, Halkjaer-Kristensen J.
    The importance of ventilation in EIA.
    Allergy 1981; 36: 385–389

12 Bundgaard A, Ingemann-Hansen T, Schmidt A, Halkjaer-Kristensen J.
    EIA after walking, running and cycling.
    Scand J Clin Lab Invest 1982; 42: 15–18

13 Bundgaard A, Schmidt A, Ingemann-Hansen T et al.
    Exercise-induced asthma after swimming and bicycle exercise.
    Eur J Respir Dis 1982; 63: 245–248

14 Bundgaard A, Ingemann-Hansen T, Schmidt A et al.
    Influence of temperature and relative humidity of inhaled gas
    in exercise-induced asthma. *Eur J Respir Dis 1982; 63:* 239–244

15 Bundgaard A.
    Incidence of EIA in adult asthmatics.
    Allergy 1981; 36: 23–26

Chapter 15

STANDARDISATION OF EXERCISE TEST PROTOCOLS FOR THE EVALUATION OF EXERCISE-INDUCED ASTHMA

O Inbar

Wingate Institute, Netanya, Israel

SUMMARY

Two types of treadmill exercise were performed by 10 asthmatic subjects (mean age 32.4 ± 8.9 years). One type of exercise was a steady-state, submaximal effort lasting approximately seven minutes. The other was a short, supramaximal effort designed to exhaust the subjects within 50 seconds. Ventilatory studies as well as measurements of gas exchange, arterial blood lactate and pH were undertaken before and after exercise. The submaximal exercise caused the expected increase in airways resistance (Raw) (19%) and a decrease in the forced expiratory volume at one second (FEV_1) (21%) and maximum mid-expiratory flow (MMEF) (20%) measured 10 minutes after the exercise. In contrast, only the MMEF was reduced (26%) at 10 minutes after the short exhaustive exercise. It was concluded that short ($<$ one minute) and highly intensive exercise challenge may cause a drastic fall in MMEF with no changes in FEV_1 or Raw. It is postulated that the unequal ventilatory response to the two modes of exercise is responsible for a greater respiratory heat loss during the long submaximal exercise and consequently for the greater obstruction of the large airways. In addition the short exhaustive exercise performed in this study may serve as a simple and accurate tool for detecting small airway obstruction as measured by the MMEF.

INTRODUCTION

The study of exercise-induced asthma is complicated by the multiplicity of variants inherent in subjecting an individual to an exercise stress test. The exposure of a subject's airways to direct exogenous, pharmacological or immunological stimuli can effectively provoke alterations in pulmonary functions. Techniques based on this fact and commonly used by allergists, not only cannot be used in the investigation of exercise-induced asthma but emphasise the importance of carefully controlling several confounding factors. Since exercise-induced asthma occurs in approximately 85–90 per cent of all asthmatic children and since physical activity is an integral and important aspect of life, attempts should be made to better the understanding of the underlying mechanisms of this pathological reaction.

Such a goal, however, cannot be reached until the standardisation of exercise testing is uniformally accepted and applied by those studying the disease. At present, the use of exercise challenge for both clinical diagnosis and investigational purposes is severely compromised by numerous unresolved issues that cloud the phenomenon of exercise-induced asthma.

PREVIOUSLY ACCEPTED CONCEPTS

Many investigators appear to view the asthmatic response to exercise as an all-or-none event with a clear-cut endpoint that can be readily assessed by measuring a single aspect of pulmonary mechanics. However, as has recently been shown, this need not be so, as the type of changes that occur may depend upon such factors as the size of the airways involved, the site of any obstruction that may be present before exercise testing, the time interval between two or more consecutive exercise challenges, and several more effort-specific factors such as the type, intensity and duration of the exercise [1–4 and I Ben-Dov, E Bar-Yishay, S Godfrey, unpublished observations].

Several studies have demonstrated that, compared with various other types of exercise such as treadmill running, climbing stairs, walking, cycling or swimming, free-range running is the most provocative stimulus of exercise-induced asthma [5–8]. Experiments have also shown that running provokes the greatest asthmagenic response when it lasts for six to eight minutes and when the intensity approximates 60–85 per cent of the patient's maximal aerobic power. Exercise of shorter or longer duration or of lower or higher intensity was claimed to provoke a lesser degree of exercise-induced asthma [5–8]. It is interesting to note that despite the scarcity of experiments addressed to the above problems, their relatively small subject samples, and their use (in most cases) of a single (most often peak flow rate) criterion of pulmonary function change, their findings, conclusions and interpretations have been widely accepted and applied in the construction of exercise test protocols throughout the world. In fact, in attempting to answer some of the questions regarding the triggering of asthmatic attacks, some of the above-mentioned studies introduced more confusion than clarification. For example, factors such as hypocapnia, lactic acidosis, pH and hyperventilation which were thought, at the time, to play a role in the induction of exercise-induced asthma [9–11], could not be fitted into the 'exercise mode, duration and intensity' theory. Indeed, several more recent studies seem to negate some of the previously accepted dogmas concerning the importance of type [12, 13], duration [2, 14] and intensity [2, 12, 14] of the exercise in the provocation of exercise-induced asthma.

FURTHER DEVELOPMENTS

Additional insight into this problem has been gained recently when investigating the effects of a short (less than one minute) but highly intense physical effort on various lung functions [2]. In this study two types of treadmill running exercise were performed by 10 asthmatics. One was the commonly used submaximal, steady-state effort, lasting approximately seven minutes. The other was a short, supramaximal effort designed to exhaust the subjects within 50 seconds. Ventilatory studies as well as gas exchange, arterial blood lactate and pH were measured before and after exercise. It was found that the so-called classical exercise challenge (submaximal-long) caused the expected increase in airway resistance (Raw – 19%) and decrease in forced expiratory volume in one second (FEV_1 – 21%) and maximum mid-expiratory flow rate (MMEF – 20%) measured 10 minutes after exercise (Figures 1 and 2).

In constrast, and as can be seen in Figure 1, only the MMEF was reduced (26%) after the short, exhaustive effort. It was therefore suggested that even a highly intensive physical challenge, when lasting less than one minute does not affect conductance in the large airways, as indicated by the small changes in Raw and FEV_1. However, in contrast to previous findings [7, 8, 15], such exercise may cause a marked and selective obstruction of the small airways as illustrated by the sharp and exclusive fall in MMEF.

In addition to affording some clarification of the mechanisms underlying exercise-induced asthma, the above study [2] also drew attention to the possibility of utilising the chosen exercise protocol as a simple and reliable tool for selectively detecting pulmonary changes in the small airways. Such

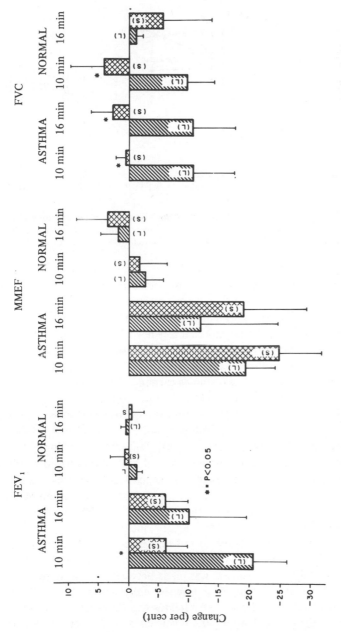

Figure 1.   Changes in dynamic ventilatory functions 10 and 16 minutes after the long (L) and short (S) exercise challenges in asthmatic and healthy populations ($\overline{X} \pm 1$ SEM) (Adapted from Inbar et al [2])

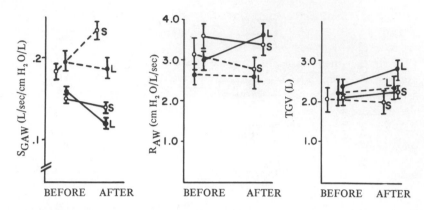

Figure 2. Changes in body plethsmographic measurements after the long (L) and short (S) exercise challenges in asthmatic (unbroken lines) and healthy subjects (broken lines) ($\overline{X} \pm 1$ SEM). TGV = total gas volume (Adpated from Inbar et al [2])

measures are strongly recommended if we are to achieve early detection of the disease [1].

Thus, it appears that the problem of standardisation of exercise testing is far from being solved and that more factors have yet to be delineated. One such was recently proposed and has been shown to play an important role in triggering exercise-induced asthma. This factor, termed respiratory heat exchange, was suggested by two studies carried out simultaneously by two different laboratories [16, 17]. Both studies pointed to the protective nature of breathing humid and/or warm air and to the asthmagenic effect of inhaling dry and/or cold air. Following suit, a comprehensive series of studies by Deal and his colleagues [18–20] demonstrated a close relationship between heat loss from the airway and real or simulated exercise-induced asthma, under a wide range of inspired-gas mixtures. Since the major determinants of respiratory heat exchange are the humidity and temperature of the inspired air on the one hand, and the flow rate or volume of the inhaled air on the other [19, 21], many of the once conflicting and inexplicable findings seemed to fall into place. For instance, differing and uncontrolled conditions of respiratory heat exchange could prevail in any study in which a comparison was made between two or more types or intensities of exercise, but in which minute ventilation or the condition of the inspired air was not strictly controlled (as was the case in most previous studies). This then would affect the occurrence and severity of exercise-induced asthma, thus permitting erroneous conclusions to be reached.

It seemed tempting to hypothesise, at this point, that all the factors already known to play a part in the onset of exercise-induced asthma might be encompassed by the new concept of respiratory heat exchange [22]. In fact there was some evidence to show that if respiratory heat loss attained a certain critical, but as yet undetermined, level exercise-induced asthma would be induced regardless of the type, duration or intensity of the exercise performed [19, 20]. Furthermore, it was demonstrated [18, 23] that asthmatic attacks could be provoked without using pharmaco-logical, immunological, or physical exercise stimuli, provided that a high enough minute ventilation prevailed and that the air temperature and humidity were sufficiently low. Although constituting a major advance, the introduction of the concept of respiratory heat exchange could not solve all the problems surrounding the mechanisms and pathophysiology of exercise-induced asthma nor that of the standardisation of exercise test protocols.

In a study carried out in our laboratory [24], nine asthmatic children between nine and 15 years old were given an exercise challenge consisting of an eight-minute tethered swim while inspiring relatively dry (25–30 per cent relative humidity), or humid (85–90 per cent relative humidity) air.

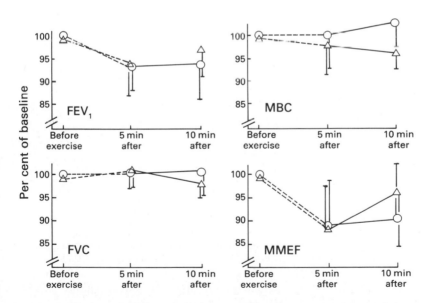

Figure 3. Changes in ventilatory functions after exercise in asthmatics exposed to humid (Δ) and dry (o) swimming ($\overline{X}$ ± 1 SEM). MBC = maximum breathing capacity; FVC = forced vital capacity (Adapted from Inbar et al [24])

They swam at a metabolic rate ($\dot{V}O_2$) of some 30ml/kg/min, minute ventilation ($\dot{V}E$) of approximately 34L/min and a heart rate of 160 beats/min, during both sessions. Ambient air and water temperatures were $28\pm2°C$ and $27 \pm 2°C$, respectively. As can be seen in Figure 3, no reduction in any of the pulmonary functions was found at five or 10 minutes after the swimming exercise in either condition of humidity. In contrast, a treadmill run of similar metabolic and ventilatory intensity, in the same patients, induced significant bronchoconstriction when room air was dried to a similar extent.

In yet another study, performed by my own group and that of S Godfrey, at Hadassa University Hospital in Jerusalem [25], it was found that the fall in FEV_1 was significantly greater after running than after swimming, when breathing either humid or dry air (drier than in the previous study – relative humidity $\approx$ 8%). Furthermore, it was demonstrated that at a standardised respiratory heat exchange, the difference between running and swimming was highly significant (p < 0.01; Figure 4).

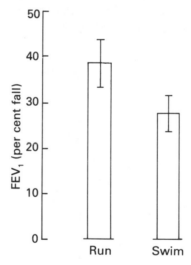

Figure 4. Mean ± SEM of the post-exercise fall in FEV_1 when performing running and swimming under hot, dry and humid conditions when the overall respiratory heat exchange levels were equalised (Adapted from Bar-Yishay et al [25])

The results of the above two studies, although not conclusive, suggest that some factors operating during swimming (efficiency of heat dissipation by water, body position, hydrostatic pressure on the chest cage, and so forth) are beneficial to the swimming asthmatic and may override the aggravating effects of inhaling dry air. These studies complicated the issue of exercise-induced asthma triggering mechanisms yet again by showing that the type of exercise (perhaps specific to swimming) and its intensity could play a role in determining the severity of exercise-induced asthma, even when the respiratory heat exchange was equalised, and that factors other than respiratory heat exchange may also be responsible for the onset of exercise-induced asthma. Further support for the yet uncovered complexity of the disease of asthma in general, and of exercise-induced asthma in particular, comes from several recent investigations. These studies have demonstrated that additional factors (to those already discussed), such as the refractoriness [2, 12, and unpublished observations of Ben-Dov et al and of Inbar et al] and the site of involvement in the airways [1, and Ben-Dov et al, unpublished observations] (pointing to the importance of the ventilatory functions used for evaluation), the interrelationships between some or all of the above-mentioned factors, and the level of activity of the autonomic nervous system [2, and Ben-Dov et al, unpublished observations] and the density of ionised air molecules (positive or negative) [Inbar et al, unpublished observations] may also play a part in the provocation of exercise-induced asthma.

CONCLUSIONS

There still exists some disagreement regarding the influence on exercise-induced asthma of various metabolic or neurogenic effort-dependent factors. The observed variable response to an exercise challenge can be used effectively in the clinical evaluation of the asthmatic patient and for the planning and following up of his treatment regimen.

Additional knowledge concerning the factors operating during an asthmatic attack should be taken into account when constructing an exercise test protocol. Some of these factors are summarised in Table I.

It is my belief that, since the asthmatic response to exercise challenge is highly specific (from both the patient's and the exercise standpoint), different kinds of exercise studies should be performed on each patient. Such a routine would enable the asthmagenic response to a variety of physical challenges, particularly to those encountered in the patient's daily life, to be measured.

Acknowledgments

I am grateful to Ronald Dlin MD for his assistance in putting this manuscript together. I also express my thanks to D Alvarez MD, HA Lyons MD, R Dotan, O Bar-Or MD and I Neuman MD, for their help in performing some of the original studies referred to in this paper.

TABLE I. Factors to be considered when performing an exercise test

Factor	General comments
Clinical status	Free of acute bronchospasm
Treatment status	No medications for at least 12 hours before testing
Respiratory heat exchange	Must be strictly controlled especially when large airway calibre is being studied. Could be manipulated by controlling air temperature and humidity as well as the flow volume of the inhaled air
Environmental conditions (other than air temperature and humidity)	Normal levels of pollens, moulds, dust, spores and air ions (both positive and negative) in the testing environment
Type of exercise	Any conventional and unskilled type of exercise, except swimming
Intensity of exercise	For the determination of the calibre of large airways the exercise should be of submaximal intensity with control of total air flow rather than of precise intensity of exercise. If the small airways are being evaluated, intensity of exercise should be close to the patient's maximum for the duration of the test
Duration of exercise	For challenging the large airways, the exercise test should last from three to eight minutes depending upon its severity (the more severe, the shorter the test). For evaluation of small airways, the exercise should last no longer than one minute and no less than 30 seconds and should lead to exhaustion
Pulmonary function measurements	Should always include tests capable of detecting changes in the diameter of large as well as small airways
Timing of pulmonary function measurements	Prior to, and five to ten minutes after cessation of the exercise challenge
Interval between two consecutive exercise tests	A minimum of three to four hours and a maximum of five to seven days are recommended

References

1   McFadden ER Jr, Kiker R, Holmes B, deGroot WS.
    Small airway disease. An assessment of the tests of peripheral airway function.
    Am J Med 1972; 57: 171–182

2   Inbar O, Alvarez DX, Lyons HA.
    Exercise-induced asthma – a comparison between two modes of exercise stress.
    Eur J Respir Dis 1981; 62: 160–166

3   Bergman NA.
    New tests of pulmonary functions: physiologic basis and interpretation.
    Med Intell Anesthesiol 1976; 44: 220–229

4   Haynes RL, Ingram RH Jr, McFadden ER Jr.
    An assessment of the pulmonary response to exercise in asthma and an analysis
    of the factors influencing it. *Am Rev Respir Dis 1976; 114:* 739–752

5   Anderson SD, Connolly NM, Godfrey S.
    Comparison of bronchoconstriction induced by cycling and running.
    Thorax 1971; 26: 396–401

6   Fitch KD, Morton AR.
    Specificity of exercise-induced asthma.
    Br Med J 1971; 4: 577–581

7   Godfrey S.
    Exercise-induced asthma – clinical, physiological and therapeutic implications.
    J Allergy Clin Immunol 1975; 56: 1–17

8   Silverman M, Anderson SD.
    The standardization of exercise tests in asthmatic children.
    Arch Dis Child 1972; 47: 882–889

9   Crompton GK.
    An unusual example of exercise-induced asthma.
    Thorax 1967; 23: 165–167

10 Rebuch AS, Read J.
    Exercise-induced asthma.
    Lancet 1968; i: 429–431

11 Vassalo CL, Gee JB, Domm BM.
    Exercise-induced asthma. Observations regarding hypocapnia and acidosis.
    Am Rev Respir Dis 1972; 105: 42–49

12 Edmunds AT, Tooley M, Godfrey S.
    The refractory period after exercise-induced asthma: its duration and relation
    to the severity of exercise. *Am Rev Respir Dis 1978; 117:* 247–254

13 Strauss RH, Haynes RL, Ingram RH Jr et al.
    Comparison of arm versus leg work in induction of acute episodes of asthma.
    J Appl Physiol 1977; 42: 565–570

14 Godfrey S.
    Exercise Testing in Children – application in health and disease 1974.
    London: Saunders

15 Jones RS, Buston MH, Wharton MJ.
    The effect of exercise on ventilatory function in the child with asthma.
    Br J Dis Chest 1962; 56: 78–86

16   Bar-Or, O, Neuman I, Dotan R.
     Effects of dry and humid climates on exercise-induced asthma in children and
     preadolescents. *J Allergy Clin Immunol 1977; 60:* 163–168

17   Chen WY, Horton DJ.
     Heat and water loss from the airways, and exercise-induced asthma.
     Respiration 1977; 34: 305–313

18   Deal EC Jr, McFadden ER Jr, Jaeger JJ.
     Hyperpnea and heat flux: initial reaction sequence in exercise-induced asthma.
     J Appl Physiol 1979; 46: 476–483

19   Deal EC Jr, McFadden ER Jr, Ingram RH Jr, Jaeger JJ.
     Esophageal temperature during exercise in asthmatic and non-asthmatic subjects.
     J Appl Physiol 1979; 46: 484–490

20   Deal EC Jr, McFadden ER Jr, Ingram RH Jr et al.
     Role of respiratory heat exchange in production of exercise-induced asthma
     J Appl Physiol 1979; 46: 467–475

21   Strauss RH, Ingram RH Jr, McFadden ER Jr.
     The role of circulating hydrogen ion and lactate in the production of exercise-
     induced asthma. *Fed Proc 1977; 36:* 606

22   McFadden ER Jr, Ingram RH Jr.
     Exercise-induced asthma. Observations on the initiating stimulus.
     N Engl J Med 1979; 301: 763–769

23   Kivity S, Souhrada JF.
     Hyperpnea: the common stimulus for bronchospasm in asthma during exercise
     and voluntary isocapnic hyperpnea. *Respiration 1980; 40:* 169–177

24   Inbar O, Dotan R, Dlin RA et al.
     Breathing dry or humid air and exercise-induced asthma during swimming.
     Eur J Appl Physiol 1980; 44: 43–50

25   Bar-Yishay E, Gur I, Inbar O et al.
     Differences between swimming and running as stimuli for exercise-induced
     asthma. *Eur J Appl Physiol 1982.* In press

DISCUSSION

JENSSEN (Trondheim, Norway)	The incidence of exercise-induced asthma in children (and adults) when provoked by appropriate methods is undoubtedly very high. Dr Anderson, do you know what is the incidence of exercise-induced asthma in asthmatic children performing normal physical activities? The goal is not to make athletes out of all asthmatics — or is it?
ANDERSON	I work in a clinical laboratory where children are referred from the outpatient clinic. I would suggest that one of the reasons that exercise tests are asked of the laboratory is because the patient has given a history of exercise-induced asthma during a normal daily activity. Consequently, I would imagine that there is a good correlation between the recognition by the children of shortness of breath and the exercise-induced asthma that we record.
JONES (Liverpool, UK)	I agree that standardisation is important in order to make it possible to compare the results from one laboratory with those from another. Would you agree, though, that greater sensitivity is possible by using the corridor for the exercise and varying the level of the exercise: this improves its diagnostic value and reduces your figure of 23 per cent of non-responders. In other words, do you agree that you have to sacrifice some sensitivity in order to achieve standardisation?
ANDERSON	I was taught never to run in a hospital. But when I went to the Institute for Diseases of the Chest in London I was allowed to run in the corridors. On return to a hospital environment I was no longer permitted to do so, but I do absolutely agree and the children will support me. Much as they may say that they are worse on a treadmill I think you would increase the incidence and the severity of the response by making them run round the Oval — though this would be hard to prove.

DAHL   What is a false positive exercise test?
(Aarhus, Denmark)

BUNDGAARD   That was in the design of our study. We made a clinical
                         assessment of our patients as to whether they had
                         asthma or not and we compared that assessment with
                         the response to the exercise test. Out of some 100
                         patients we only had one who had a positive exercise
                         test and he was not diagnosed clinically as an asth-
                         matic but as a bronchitic. He was the false positive.

CORRIS   How important is it to perform exercise tests at the
(Newcastle, UK)   same time of day?

BUNDGAARD   We have studied that point and have done exercise
                         tests at 7am, 12 noon, 5pm and 10pm on the same day
                         with the same base-line values every time and the
                         response was exactly the same. I do not think there is
                         any diurnal variation in the response.

PIERSON   Dr Inbar, what were the kinetics of recovery in air
(Washington,   flow obstruction for the short versus the long exercise
USA)   test? Were they similar or different?

INBAR   All we did in this regard was to take the measurements
                         10 minutes and 16 minutes after the exercise. All
                         values, regardless of the mode of exercise, were
                         reduced — that is, the situation was improved — at
                         16 minutes as compared to 10 minutes after the
                         exercise challenge.

BAEVRE   How easily is the short test carried out on children? Is
(Bergen, Norway)   it not too strenuous, too mentally disturbing to carry
                         out a test that leads to exhaustion within about one
                         minute?

INBAR   I think it is much more difficult to perform such a
                         strenuous test with an adult population than with
                         children. We have had quite a lot of experience in
                         dealing with this type of exercise challenge and we

have found that young children can perform the strenuous exercise repeatedly 30 or 60 minutes apart. The recovery rate in children is probably faster than that of senior adults.

VÄLIMÄKI
(Turku, Finland)

What is the optimal work load in relation to body size? And is the increase in loading best done step-wise, single step, multi-step or triangular?

INBAR

Dr Anderson has had more experience than I in this area, but as a brief comment I would say that whether or not the specific load is relative to the body weight is not of prime importance in exercise-induced asthma challenge. What is important in this regard is respiratory heat loss. So what one should measure and control is $\dot{V}E$ (provided temperature and humidity are controlled and constant) rather than specific intensity or load of the exercise being used.

ANDERSON

What Michael Silverman and I did was to study a number of normal children and relate the gradient and the speed of the treadmill to their oxygen consumption [reference 2 in my paper]. If you aim for an oxygen consumption between 32 and 36ml per kilogram of body weight (and our graphs will tell you what speed and slope you need to obtain that consumption on the treadmill) then the ventilation induced by that will be sufficient to lose the necessary heat.

BUNDGAARD

We have recently studied the spontaneous ventilation when two bicycle ergometer tests or two treadmill runs were done. There were large variations in spontaneous ventilation although the work load was exactly the same and the temperature and humidity were the same. I would prefer, if anything, to standardise the total ventilation during exercise.

BAR-OR
(Chairman)

In this regard what about exercise of a very low intensity which may last 20 minutes and not induce any bronchoconstriction?

ANDERSON   I think one of the unresolved questions *is* that variation
                in ventilation. I agree that total ventilation is import-
                ant but the time that you do it in is also important.
                For our children we have about 400 litres of venti-
                lation in seven to eight minutes. But if you ventilate
                those 400 litres in half an hour you will not produce
                exercise-induced asthma.

INBAR   One thing suggested by the study I have presented is
                that there are still unanswered questions related to
                the effect of respiratory heat loss on exercise-induced
                asthma. For example, what is the threshold tempera-
                ture level which triggers the exercise-induced asthma?
                The short exercise induced very high rates of venti-
                lation but relatively small total air flows. It could be
                that the high rate of ventilation brought the tempera-
                ture of the respiratory system to the triggering level
                (unknown for the moment). But the length of time
                that this threshold temperature was maintained was
                insufficient to cause an exercise-induced asthma. So
                there seem to be several still unanswered questions
                concerning respiratory heat exchange.

STERN   Is the apparently lower prevalence of exercise-induced
(Leicester, UK) asthma in adults simply due to the fact that few
                adults exercise enough to know?

ANDERSON   When I was asked to talk about children I had to
                separate my 782 subjects into children and adults.
                Having done that, I can assure you that the incidence
                is markedly higher in adults – 85 per cent among the
                adults compared with 77 per cent among the children.

BUNDGAARD   The figures I presented were actually from incidence
                studies in adults and the incidence in adults is similar
                to the incidence in children.

BAR-OR   Two aspects of this discussion seem to me to be very
                important. One is that we should not regard our
                protocols as being above criticism. The other is the

cost effectiveness of standardisation. I think the point made by Dr Bundgaard that although theoretically we should standardise exactly for temperature, humidity and so on, it may be too costly. Therefore we have to keep a perspective and whilst striving to standardise we should still consider how much variance we will get by not standardising enough — but, again, more work needs to be done in this particular area.

PART IV

THE INFLUENCE OF DRUGS ON EXERCISE-INDUCED ASTHMA

Chairman: Professor K Aas, Oslo, Norway

Chapter 16

THE EFFECT OF DRUGS ON EXERCISE-INDUCED ASTHMA

W E Pierson

University of Washington, Seattle,
Washington, USA

SUMMARY

The treatment of exercise-induced asthma has been significantly improved with the development of new pharmacological agents and delivery systems. Major categories of drugs used for exercise-induced asthma include $beta_2$-adrenergic agonists, sodium cromoglycate, and methylxanthines and their derivatives. In addition, anticholinergic drugs, antihistamines, calcium antagonists, alpha-adrenergic blockers and carbon dioxide have all been shown to have a significant effect on exercise-induced bronchospasm.

Exercise-induced asthma has become a useful assay system for assessing the clinical effectiveness of many new pharmacological agents. The implications of drug treatment of exercise-induced asthma are highly significant for children, adolescents and competitive athletes.

INTRODUCTION

Exercise-induced asthma in children and adolescents is a handicap that can dramatically alter the course of a young life [1]. The serious limitations often imposed can be detrimental to the physical and psychological development of the young patient, but they need no longer be suffered [2].

The recognition of exercise-induced asthma, the incidence of which is significantly increased in patients with atopic disease, has led to improved treatment during the past decade [3], particularly as a result of the arrival of numerous new drugs [4]. The recognition that a child, adolescent or athlete suffers from exercise-induced asthma now permits an appropriate pharmacological agent to be selected which can modify or reduce the symptom and have a dramatic effect on the prognosis and expectations of that patient.

Various drugs have been evaluated for their efficacy in either reducing or eliminating exercise-induced bronchospasm [5]. Exercise test systems also have become useful for evaluating the clinical efficacy of drugs in the treatment of asthma [6]. The major classes of drugs used in the management of exercise-induced asthma include beta-adrenergic agonists, sodium cromoglycate and methylxanthines. Other compounds have been evaluated and show varying degrees of potential for therapeutic use in exercise-induced asthma [3].

BETA$_2$-ADRENERGIC AGONISTS

The beta$_2$-adrenergic agonists have been evaluated extensively; they include such drugs as salbutamol, fenoterol, terbutaline, metaproterenol, isoproterenol, isoetharine, tornalate and others. The mode of action of this group of sympathomimetic amines appears to be directed primarily at the beta$_2$-adrenergic receptor and, secondarily, to increasing intracellular cyclic adenosine monophosphate (cyclic AMP). These drugs also may influence the control of the calibre of the airway by secondary effects on the intrinsic bronchial nerves. The available formulations include aerosols, syrups and tablets. Generally, aerosols have the most rapid onset of action and achieve their maximum effectiveness with a markedly lower dose than the other formulations. Although the syrups and tablets have slower onsets of action, the duration of their action is comparable to or longer than that of the aerosols. However, a greater incidence of tremor, nausea and irritability has been reported with the syrups and tablets which is most probably due to the higher dose required for pharmacological effect [7]. The syrups and tablets are, however, particularly valuable in very young children, who are unable to master the administration of aerosol medications.

Newer agents such as hexoprenaline sulphate, reproterol, carbuterol, fenoterol and tornalate are also pharmacologically effective in controlling exercise-induced bronchospasm [8—10]. The new time release systems for transcutaneous administration will be even more advantageous in protecting patients from exercise-induced bronchospasm by prolonging the duration of action of the drug [11].

SODIUM CROMOGLYCATE

The effect of sodium cromoglycate has been well studied in the past decade [12,13]. The drug is effective primarily in patients with atopic asthma whose exercise-induced bronchospasm is mainly situated in the larger airways [14]. Sodium cromoglycate is usually administered by Spinhaler in powdered form with a lactose carrier. An aerosol formulation has been shown to be effective, especially in the treatment of young patients [15]. The pharmacological action of this drug is to stabilise the mast cells with consequent reduction in the release of mediators which are responsible for secondary bronchoconstriction [16]. However, it has recently been shown that sodium cromoglycate also has an effect on the response to exposure to sulphur dioxide and exercise [17]. Sodium cromoglycate usually is most effective when the larger airways are constricted [18].

XANTHONES

Several orally active xanthone compounds have been shown to be effective in modifying exercise-induced asthma [19,20].

METHYLXANTHINES

The methylxanthine group of drugs, which includes theophylline, aminophylline and dyphylline, has been thoroughly evaluated in the modification of exercise-induced bronchospasm [21—23]. Their mode of action appears to be blockade of phosphodiesterase breakdown of intracellular cyclic AMP thereby reducing the release of mediators by the pulmonary mast cells. The effect of the methylxanthines on myogenic control of airway musculature has not been clearly demonstrated.

The methylxanthines are available in several formulations: suspensions, elixirs, tablets, time-release preparations and intravenous preparations (aminophylline). The use of a rapid-acting suspension or tablet has been shown to be effective [24] as has the use of sustained-release preparations in allowing asthmatic patients with hypersensitive airways to participate in strenuous exercise [25]. The individualisation of the dosage of theophylline has been markedly improved with the introduction of a single-point kinetic system which establishes the patient's individual theophylline clearance rate [26].

The rapid-acting theophylline preparations should be taken 30−60 minutes before strenuous exercise. However, the sustained-release preparations have little effect when taken one to two hours beforehand.

Dyphylline has been shown to have some effect in the blockade of exercise-induced asthma, but less than that of theophylline or aminophylline [27]. One advantage of the drug, however, is that the side effects of nausea and irritability of the gastrointestinal tract and central nervous system appear to be less severe than with theophylline.

Aminophylline tablets are effective against exercise-induced bronchospasm when administered an adequate time before exercise.

Thus the major disadvantage of the methylxanthine preparations is the need to take them 30−60 minutes before exercise to ensure their effectiveness. Frequently this is impractical in the treatment of exercise-induced asthma in children and adolescents.

ANTICHOLINERGIC DRUGS

Several investigators in Europe and the United States have shown that atropine and ipratropium bromide are effective in the blockade of exercise-induced bronchospasm [28−30]. However, they have been less universally effective in clinical trials in children and adolescents than the beta-adrenergic agents, theophylline and sodium cromoglycate. There have been reports of dramatic effects on the blockade of exercise-induced bronchospasm, but these effects appear to be selective − that is to say, patients with atopic asthma and other atopic respiratory diseases and moderate to severe exercise-induced asthma do not always respond to anticholinergic drugs [31].

Patients with marked receptor reactivity to air pollutants and/or cold stimulus, experience relief with the use of the anticholinergic agents [32,33]. However, the role of these agents in altering either myogenic airway control or the release of chemical mediators does not lead to significant therapeutic benefit in many patients [34].

CALCIUM ANTAGONISTS

There has been a great interest recently in calcium antagonists blockading the release of chemical mediators [35]. The role of calcium antagonists in myocardial cellular stabilisation is well known but their impact on exercise-induced asthma has also been evaluated. Nifedipine, for example, has been shown to blockade exercise-induced bronchospasm [35]. But besides their therapeutic importance, calcium antagonists also offer the prospect of increasing our understanding of the aetiology of exercise-induced asthma. Studies must nevertheless be extended to children and adolescents with exercise-induced asthma to establish the safety and efficacy of these agents in this age group.

ALPHA-ADRENERGIC BLOCKING AGENTS

The alpha-adrenergic blocking agents had not been regarded as effective until recently, when prazosin was shown to modify exercise-induced bronchospasm in young adult patients [36]. Other alpha-adrenergic blocking agents have not proven to be particularly effective [37].

ANTIHISTAMINES

The role of antihistamines has not been important in the control of exercise-induced bronchospasm. Nevertheless, azatadine has been shown to have a significant inhibiting effect on exercise-induced bronchospasm when administered by oral inhalation. The mode of action of this drug may be by inhibiting the release of histamine which appears to play a role in exercise-induced bronchospasm [38]. Azatadine also has a certain anticholinergic activity, and its effectiveness in the suppression of exercise-induced bronchospasm may be due to this characteristic.

Ketotifen, another antihistamine, which has a protective effect in asthma in children, has less effect in blocking exercise-induced bronchospasm [39,40].

PROSTAGLANDINS

Prostaglandin E_2 has been shown to diminish exercise-induced bronchospasm [41]. Other arachidonic acid blocking agents are currently being developed, and may prove to have advantages in the treatment of exercise-induced bronchospasm. However, further evaluation, especially in children and adolescents, is awaited.

CORTICOSTEROIDS

Corticosteroid compounds, both in aerosolised and systemic forms, have uniformly failed in the management of exercise-induced bronchospasm. Clinical studies of corticosteroids in aerosolised formulations as well as in syrup and tablet form have shown that these drugs appear to have no beneficial effects in the pharmacological management of exercise-induced bronchospasm in children and adolescents [42,43].

GASES

Carbon dioxide has been shown to reduce postexercise bronchoconstriction when administered during or immediately after exercise [44]. The mode of action appears to be a direct bronchodilating effect, since hypocapnia has not been demonstrated to be an aetiological factor in exercise-induced bronchospasm [45]. The administration of oxygen during exercise also has decreased the magnitude of the asthmatic response after strenuous exercise [46]. The use of either carbon dioxide or oxygen in the treatment of children or adolescents with exercise-induced asthma is usually impractical owing to their lack of availability.

ANTIFILARIAL AGENTS

Diethylcarbamazine pamoate, which inhibits the release of slow-reacting substance of anaphylaxis (SRS-A – an arachidonic acid metabolite), effectively inhibits exercise-induced bronchospasm. Its clinical usefulness has been limited, particularly in children [47].

SPECIAL CONSIDERATIONS

The drugs for the control of exercise-induced asthma must be chosen carefully to accommodate to the patient's needs and with due consideration of the drug's pharmacology, speed of onset and site and duration of action. In addition, the patient's age and ability to manage the delivery system (aerosol, Spinhaler) may determine which formulation is the most suitable for the management of their exercise-induced asthma.

A significant consideration in the pharmacological management of exercise-induced asthma is the restrictions placed on the use by competitive athletes of certain classes of compounds. A knowledge of the drugs approved by the International Olympic Committee and any national athletic federation is essential before administering a drug to a competing athlete. This is particularly important if disqualification for 'doping' is possible, which could seriously jeopardise the career of an asthmatic athlete [48,49].

SUMMING UP

The use of drug therapy for exercise-induced asthma can greatly help asthmatic patients to pursue normal activities, including recreational and competitive sports. This is particularly important in adolescents and children, whose very development, socially, psychologically and physically, is enhanced if they are capable of performing normal levels of exercise.

It is, however, important to tell both patients and parents that there is no evidence that the use of pharmacological agents will lead to increased athletic performance. Pharmacological intervention merely allows the patient to compete somewhere near physiological parity with his or her non-asthmatic contemporaries.

The continued development and assessment of drugs for exercise-induced asthma is not only exciting but constantly evolving. It is imperative that any new agents are evaluated not only in the treatment of adult patients but also in that of adolescents and children before clinical use. This will ensure that the correct paediatric dosing is established and that safety and efficacy are beyond doubt.

References

1   Oseid S, Aas K.
    Exercise-induced asthma.
    Allergy 1978; 33: 227–228

2   Eggleston PA.
    Exercise-induced asthma. In Bierman CW, Pearlman DS, eds.
    Allergic Diseases of Infancy, Childhood and Adolescence 1980: 605.
    Philadelphia: Saunders

3   Kawabori I, Pierson WE, Conquest LL et al.
    Incidence of exercise induced asthma in children.
    J Allergy Clin Immunol 1976; 58: 447–455

4   Anderson S, Seale JP et al.
    An evaluation of pharmacotherapy for exercise-induced asthma.
    J Allergy Clin Immunol 1979; 64: 612–624

5   Bierman CW, Pierson WE, Shapiro GG.
    Effect of drugs on exercise-induced bronchospasm.
    In Dempsey JA, Reed CE, eds. *Muscular Exercise and the Lung 1977:* 279.
    Madison: University of Wisconsin Press

6   Poppius H.
    Exercise provocation in the evaluation of drug therapy in asthma.
    Scand J Respir Dis (Suppl) 1979; 103: 69–71

7   Francis PWJ, Krastins IRB et al
     Oral and inhaled salbutamol in the prevention of exercise-induced bronchospasm.
     Pediatrics 1980; 66: 103–108

8   Anderson SD, Spiroglou M, Lindsay D.
     An evaluation of oral hexoprenaline sulphate (Ipradol) in exercise-induced
     asthma. *Med J Aust 1977; 2:* 825–827

9   Van As A, McDonald I, Gebhardt T et al.
     A comparative assessment of carbuterol, fenoterol and hexoprenaline in allergic
     asthma. *S Afr Med J 1978; 53:* 1011–1015

10   Prime FJ, Bianco S, Kamburoff PL.
     Inhibition of artificially-induced asthma by reproterol ('Bronchospasmin').
     Curr Med Res Opin 1979; 6: 364–370

11   Drill VA, Lazar P.
     New procedures for evaluating cutaneous absorption.
     In Shaw JE, Chandrasekaran SK, Campbell PS, Schmidt LG, eds.
     Cutaneous Toxicity 1977: 83–94. London, Toronto, Sydney: Academic Press

12   Godfrey S.
     The relative merits of cromolyn sodium and high-dose theophylline therapy in
     childhood asthma. *Pediatrics 1980; 65:* 97–104

13   Bernstein IL.
     Cromolyn sodium in the treatment of asthma: changing concepts.
     J Allergy Clin Immunol 1981; 68: 247–253

14   Eggleston PA, Bierman CW, Pierson WE et al.
     A double blind trial of the effect of cromolyn sodium on exercise-induced
     bronchospasm. *J Allergy Clin Immunol 1972; 50:* 57–63

15   Dahl R, Henriksen JM.
     Inhibition of exercise-induced bronchoconstriction by nebulised sodium cromo-
     glycate in patients with bronchial asthma.
     Scand J Respir Dis 1979; 60: 51–55

16   Gaddie J, Legge JS, Palmer KNV.
     The effect of disodium cromoglycate on pulmonary function in asthma.
     Br J Dis Chest 1972; 66: 254–260

17   Koenig JQ et al.
     Acute effects of inhaled SO_2 plus NaCl droplet aerosol on pulmonary function
     in asthmatic adolescents. *Environ Res 1982; 22:* 145–153

18   Silverman M, Andrea T.
     Time course of effect of disodium cromoglycate on exercise-induced asthma.
     Arch Dis Child 1972; 47: 419 – 422

19   Stenius B, Salorrine Y, Parrott D.
     The effect of inhaled RS 7540, a xanthone, on exercise-induced asthma.
     Scand J Respir Dis 1978; 59: 79–81

20   Lenney W, Milner AD, Tyler RM.
     BRL10833 in inhibiting exercise-induced bronchoconstriction in asthmatic
     children. *Br J Dis Chest 1978; 72:* 225–230

21   Shapiro GG, McPhilips JJ, Smith K et al.
     Effectiveness of terbutaline and theophylline alone and in combination in exer-
     cise-induced bronchospasm. *Pediatrics 1981; 67:* 508–513

22 Pollock J, Kiechel F, Cooper D et al.
Relationship of serum theophylline concentration to inhibition of exercise-induced bronchospasm and comparison with cromolyn.
Pediatrics 1977; 60: 840

23 Katz RM, Rachelefsky GS, Siegel S.
The effectiveness of the short and long-term use of crystallized theophylline in asthmatic children. *J Pediatr 1978; 92:* 663–665

24 Bierman CW, Shapiro GG, Pierson WE et al.
Acute and chronic theophylline therapy in exercise-induced bronchospasm.
Pediatrics 1977; 60: 845–849

25 Weinberger M.
Theophylline for treatment of asthma.
J Pediatr 1978; 92: 1–7

26 Shapiro GG, Koup JR, Furukawa CT et al.
Individualization of theophylline dosage using a single serum sample following a test dose. *Pediatrics 1982; 69:* 70–73

27 Simons FER, Bierman CW, Sprenkle AC et al.
Efficacy of dyphylline (dihydroxypropyltheophylline) in exercise-induced bronchospasm. *Pediatrics 1975; 56(Suppl):* 916–918

28 Rachelefsky GS, Tashkin DP, Katz RM.
Comparison of aerosolized atropine, isoproterenol, atropine plus isoproterenol, disodium cromoglycate and placebo in the prevention of exercise-induced asthma. *Chest 1978; 73(6) Suppl:* 1017–1019

29 Thomson NC, Patel KR, Kerr JW.
Sodium cromoglycate and ipratropium bromide in exercise-induced asthma.
Thorax 1978; 33: 694–699

30 Kamburoff PL.
Effects of different drugs on exercise-induced asthma (EIA).
Eur J Respir Dis 1980; Suppl 106: 65–69

31 Godfrey S, Konig P.
Inhibition of exercise-induced asthma by different pharmacological pathways.
Thorax 1976; 31: 137–143

32 Harries MG, Parkes PEG, Lessof MH et al.
Role of bronchial irritant receptors in asthma.
Lancet 1981; i: 5–7

33 Rasmussen FV, Madsen L, Bundgaard A.
Combined effect of an anticholinergic drug ipratropium bromide and disodium cromoglycate in exercise-induced asthma.
Scand J Respir Dis 1979 (Suppl); 103: 159–162

34 Deal EC, McFadden ER, Ingram RH et al.
Effects of atropine on potentiation of exercise-induced bronchospasm by cold air. *J Appl Physiol 1978; 45:* 238–243

35 Patel KR.
The effect of calcium antagonist, nifedipine in exercise induced asthma.
Clin Allergy 1981; 11: 429–432

36 Barnes PJ, Wilson NM et al.
Prazosin, an alpha$_1$ adrenoceptor antagonist, partially inhibits exercise-induced asthma. *J Allergy Clin Immunol 1981; 68:* 411–415

37   Seale JP, Anderson SD, Lindsay DA.
     A trial of an alpha adrenoreceptor blocker lindoramin in exercise-induced
     bronchoconstriction. *Scand J Respir Dis 1976; 57:* 261–266

38   Harries MG, Burge PS, O'Brien I et al.
     Blood histamine levels after exercise testing.
     Clin Allergy 1979; 9: 437–441

39   Østerballe O, Nielsen EAL.
     The protective effect of a new agent, ketotifen syrup, in the treatment of child-
     hood asthma. *Allergy 1979; 34:* 125–129

40   Petheram IS, Moxham J, Bierman CW et al.
     Ketotifen in atopic asthma and exercise-induced asthma.
     Thorax 1981; 36: 308–312

41   Souza LM, Silverman M.
     Prostaglandins in exercise-induced asthma.
     Clin Allergy 1981; 11: 506–507

42   Yazigi R, Sly RM, Frazer M.
     Effect of triamcinolone acetonide aerosol upon exercise-induced asthma.
     Ann Allergy 1978; 49: 322–325

43   Konig P, Jaffe P, Godfrey S.
     Effect of corticosteroids on exercise-induced asthma.
     J Allergy Clin Immunol 1974; 54: 14–19

44   McFadden ER, Stearns RH, Ingram RH et al.
     Relative contribution of hypocarbia and hypercapnea as mechanisms of post-
     exercise asthma. *J Appl Physiol 1977; 42:* 22–27

45   Katz RM, Whipp BJ, Heimlich EM et al.
     Exercise-induced bronchospasm, ventilation and blood gases in asthmatic
     children. *J Allergy 1971; 47:* 148–158

46   Schiffman PL, Ryan A, Whipp BJ et al.
     Hyperoxic attenuation of exercise-induced bronchospasm in asthmatics.
     J Clin Invest 1979; 63: 30–37

47   Sly RM, Matzen K.
     Effect of diethylcarbamazine pamoate upon exercise-induced obstruction in
     asthmatic children. *Ann Allergy 1974; 33:* 138–144

48   Committee on Drugs, American Academy of Pediatrics.
     The athlete and medication.
     Pediatrics 1973; 52: 886–887

49   Katz RM.
     Asthmatics don't have to sit out sports.
     Physician Sportsmed 1976; April: 45–53

Chapter 17

PHARMACOTHERAPY OF EXERCISE-INDUCED ASTHMA

E A Stemmann

Staedtische Kinderkliniken, Gelsenkirchen-Buer, FRG

ABSTRACT

Exercise of appropriate type and severity will induce an acute attack of asthma in asthmatic children. Most of these children will, however, show greatly improved exercise tolerance if an anti-asthmatic drug is administered beforehand but the response is variable and not predictable. Exercise-induced asthma seems to be provoked by different pathways either alone or in combination with each other.

Supposing that only five exist — mast-cell degranulation, release of histamine or acetylcholine, stimulation of adrenergic alpha-receptors or diminished response of adrenergic beta-receptors — there would be 31 different possibilities. Blocking the different pathways with anti-asthmatic drugs (sodium cromoglycate, antihistamines, anticholinergic drugs, alpha-blockers, or beta-stimulants) means that 31 different therapeutic regimens are possible. Therefore the only safe way to manage exercise-induced asthma is by the repeated use of provocation tests after medication — this will help to identify suitable treatment.

DISCUSSION

STRUNK
(Denver, USA)

We have a large number of patients with exercise-induced bronchoconstriction that is not blocked by either beta$_2$-agonists or sodium cromoglycate alone (or with theophylline), but is effectively blocked by the combination of a beta$_2$-agonist with sodium cromoglycate. Does anyone else have this experience?

PIERSON

I think others have described that phenomenon although I am not aware that it has been effectively studied. It would appear that there are patients who have a fairly severe combined small/large airway involvement that usually responds to that combination or treatment.

LEWIS
(Portsmouth, UK)

Some asthmatic toddlers (1—2 years) are excitable prior to asthma attacks, and the inhalation of salbutamol when they are in this overactive state may forestall an asthma attack. Does exercise-induced asthma occur in toddlers?

PIERSON

We have certainly seen instances if you assume that toddlers can walk. They were children under three years old who became excited and, especially if they had a respiratory infection, developed exercise-induced bronchospasm.

AAS
(Chairman)

If the problem is severe we use inhalation of a beta$_2$-adrenergic agent in the young age group, too, but we give it by nebuliser and face mask or by mouth tube.

HAIDER
(Bury, UK)

Dr Stemmann, how frequently did you estimate the serum levels of theophylline when you used this drug in suppository form? The pharmacokinetics of theophylline are such that one or two estimations only do not give a true idea of the serum level.

STEMMANN

The suppository was given on one occasion only four hours before doing the exercise test. When we did the exercise test we measured serum levels and they were low — 4–11ng/ml.

HAIDER We have used theophylline by inhalation and in some patients it proved to be an irritant, but in those who could tolerate it it had no effect on the exercise-induced asthma.

JOHNSON
(Dundee, UK)
Can any of the speakers comment on the possible use of the methylxanthines as aerosols?

STEMMANN I have no experience.

PIERSON I have no experience either, but I do not think that aerosolised methylxanthines would be effective in exercise-induced bronchoconstriction. We do, however, use nebulised beta$_2$-agonists delivered in humidified oxygen with a face mask. We find them very effective in the treatment of acute asthmatic attacks, especially in pre-school age children as it often avoids the need for injections and the delivery system is a comfortable one. In the home, however, it is quite a different problem.

AAS The difficulty is to decide whether a subclinical obstruction is being increased by the exercise or if it is true exercise-induced asthma.

FRANKLAND
(London, UK)
Exercise-induced angina is helped by the calcium antagonist nifedipine. Is there any reason to suppose that this drug has any beneficial effect on exercise-induced asthma?

HAIDER We have used both verapamil and nifedipine. Although the effect is just significant I would not recommend them for clinical use in the management of exercise-induced asthma.

GILL
(Dublin, UK)
Would the speakers comment on the duration of action of sodium cromoglycate versus that of beta$_2$ stimulation in prevention of exercise-induced asthma.

PIERSON   The *effective* duration of action is the important
                                 consideration and the newer beta$_2$-agonists have a
                                 much longer duration of action. The duration of action
                                 of salbutamol as regards repetitive exercise testing is
                                 probably in the range of four hours.

STEMMANN   The results with sodium cromoglycate at 30 minutes
                                 and four and six hours after giving the drug were good.
                                 We also tested salbutamol in tablet form, measuring
                                 the plasma levels. After four hours the drug was no
                                 longer active, but some drugs act for as long as six
                                 hours.

AAS   Professor Pierson mentioned that in some areas air
                                 pollution — whether industrial or natural — may be
                                 as important as exercise. This stresses the need to
                                 differentiate between the drug or drugs of choice
                                 under laboratory conditions and in real life. In the
                                 laboratory it is very much a question of a saturation
                                 effect, usually lasting 60 minutes. For training an
                                 effect of medium duration is required. But for daily
                                 living the effect may need to last for four to six
                                 hours. Furthermore Dr Stemmann emphasised the
                                 need for clinical flexibility after assessing the need
                                 of the patient.
                                    Dr Thompson's paper gave substance to this need
                                 for differentiation, showing that under laboratory
                                 conditions he could divide his nine patients into at
                                 least two groups with different types of responses. So,
                                 above all we need a detailed characterisation of the
                                 patient in question — and this is often lacking.

Chapter 18

RELATIONSHIP OF DRUG EFFECT AND SITE OF CONSTRICTION IN EXERCISE-INDUCED ASTHMA

N C Thomson

Western Infirmary, Glasgow, United Kingdom

SUMMARY

The mechanisms involved in exercise-induced asthma are unknown. Both reflex bronchoconstriction secondary to stimulation of vagal receptors and direct narrowing of the airway consequent upon degranulation of the mast cells have been postulated. In previous studies these hypotheses have been examined using different pharmacological agents, although the interpretation of the results may be influenced by a number of factors including the dose and type of drug administered and differences in lung function between subjects.

Circumstantial evidence for the occurrence of reflex bronchoconstriction in exercise-induced asthma is based on blocking efferent motor actions with anticholinergic drugs. The protective effect of these agents is variable although in some studies this may be a result of insufficient cholinergic blockade. In nine adult asthmatics the protective effect of ipratropium bromide (0.4mg) and placebo were tested. All drugs were administered by aerosol from a Wright nebuliser. Exercise testing consisted in steady-state running on an inclined treadmill for up to eight minutes. In five of nine subjects ipratropium bromide partially prevented exercise-induced asthma ($<15\%$ fall in forced expiratory volume in one second — FEV_1). In the remaining four subjects neither ipratropium bromide nor large doses of atropine sulphate (6mg) inhibited exercise-induced asthma. Thus, in some asthmatics the inability of anticholinergic drugs to prevent exercise-induced asthma is not due to insufficient vagal blockade.

In a separate study in 13 adult asthmatics, the protective effect of ipratropium bromide on exercise-induced asthma was related to intersubject differences in the main site of obstruction to airflow as assessed by maximal expiratory flow rate responses to the breathing of low density gas.

Subjects were pretreated with ipratropium bromide (1.3mg), sodium cromoglycate (13mg) and ipratropium bromide plus sodium cromoglycate. In eight of the 13 subjects the base line ratio of expiratory flow at 50 per cent vital capacity was over 1.2 and these were termed 'responders'; the remaining five subjects were termed 'non-responders'. Ipratropium bromide had a significantly protective effect in responders only, whereas sodium cromoglycate had an inhibitory effect on exercise-induced asthma in both groups. This result suggests that the effect of anticholinergic drugs in exercise-induced asthma may be influenced by intersubject differences in the main site of airflow resistance.

INTRODUCTION

It has been suggested that airway cooling is the primary stimulus in exercise-induced asthma, and that this depends on the level of minute ventilation, inspired air temperature and water content [1,2]. The severity of the response to exercise or isocapnic hyperventilation of cold air is also influenced by the level of bronchial responsiveness to histamine or methacholine [3,4]. In an individual asthmatic, however, the mechanism by which airway cooling produces bronchoconstriction after exercise is unknown. Both reflex bronchoconstriction secondary to stimulation of vagal receptors [5] and

TABLE I. Possible factors influencing the results of exercise tests

---

Exercise test

Type (minute ventilation, temperature of inspired air and water content)
Method of measuring response
Method of expressing results
Reproducibility

Pretreatment drug

Type
Dose
Method of administration
Mode of action
Site of action

Subjects studied

Characteristics
Lung function
Medications
Level of non-specific bronchial responsiveness (increased by, for example, recent respiratory tract infection or exposure to allergen)

---

direct airway narrowing following mast-cell degranulation have been postulated [6]. One method by which these hypotheses have been examined has
been to study the effect of different pharmacological agents in preventing
exercise-induced asthma. The results of these investigations may be influenced by a wide variety of factors (Table I). In this paper I shall consider
the effects on exercise of the dose of the pretreatment drug and intersubject differences in the main site of obstruction airflow.

DOSE OF CHOLINERGIC (MUSCARINIC) BLOCKING DRUG

Circumstantial evidence for the occurrence of reflex vagal bronchoconstriction in exercise-induced asthma is based on blocking efferent motor
actions with anticholinergic drugs. The protective effect of these agents
is variable [7,8] and Tinkelman and his colleagues [8] suggested that the
lack of effect in some studies may be due to inadequate cholinergic blockade.

We have examined this suggestion in nine adult atopic asthmatics with
reproducible exercise-induced asthma, in whom the protective effect of
ipratropium bromide (nebulised dose, 0.4mg) and placebo were tested.
All drugs were administered by aerosol from a Wright nebuliser 30 minutes
before exercise. Exercise testing consisted of steady-state running on an
inclined treadmill for between five and eight minutes. The treadmill was
situated in a draught-free room, the daily temperature of which was always
in the range 19–22°C. The humidity of the inspired air was not recorded.
The speed of the treadmill was adjusted so that the patient's pulse rate at
the end of the exercise was at least 170–180 beats/min. The response to
exercise was expressed as the maximum post-exercise fall in forced expiratory volume in one second (FEV_1) as a percentage of post-drug or post-
placebo base line.

Ipratropium bromide gave no significant protection compared to placebo
so far as the mean maximum percentage fall in FEV_1 after exercise was
concerned (Table II). However with ipratropium bromide, five out of the
nine subjects had less than a 15 per cent fall in FEV_1 after exercise, whereas with placebo all subjects had more than a 20 per cent fall in FEV_1 after
exercise. To determine if the lack of protective effect of ipratropium
bromide in the four subjects was due to insufficient cholinergic (muscarinic) blockade, they were exercised 30 minutes after inhaling atropine
sulphate (nebulised dose, 6mg). This, too, gave no significant protection
(Figure 1).

These results suggest that the lack of effect of anticholinergic drugs in
preventing exercise-induced asthma in some asthmatics is unlikely to be

TABLE II. Base line FEV$_1$ and maximum percentage fall after exercise in nine asthmatic subjects

| | PLACEBO | | | IPRATROPIUM BROMIDE | | |
| | Base line | | Per cent fall | Base line | | Per cent fall |
	B	A		B	A	
Mean	2.92(85%)	2.95(85%)	−36.9	2.95(85%)	3.32(98%)	−26.1
SEM	0.28	0.30	4.5	0.27	0.25	8.6
p value						NS

Base-line data are expressed as absolute values (L) and percentage of predicted (in parentheses)

B, before pretreatment; A, after placebo or ipratropium bromide. NS = not significant

p value refers to the difference between percentage fall after placebo and after ipratropium bromide

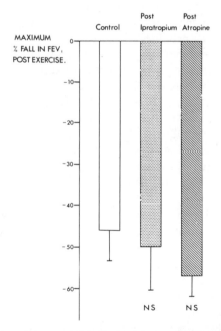

Figure 1. Maximum percentage fall in FEV$_1$ (mean ± SEM) after exercise following pretreatment with atropine sulphate (nebulised dose 6.0mg) in four asthmatics in whom ipratropium bromide (nebulised dose 4.0mg) gave no significant protection compared to placebo (control). (NS = not significant; refers to difference between percentage fall after placebo and after ipratropium or atropine)

due to insufficient vagal blockade. A nebulised dose of 3mg atropine sulphate — that is, half that administered in this study — has been shown to increase the mean provocation concentration of methacholine producing a 20 per cent decrease in FEV_1 (PO_{20}) from 0.66 ± 0.85 to 94.9 ± 0.73mg/ml [NC Thomson and his colleagues, unpublished observations] ($p<0.001$) (Figure 2). Thus, although the dose of an anticholinergic agent required to inhibit the effects of vagal impulses on smooth muscle of the airways is

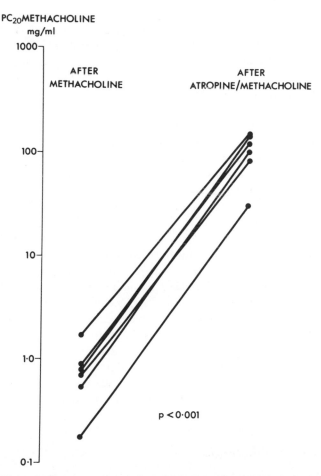

Figure 2. Effect of inhaled atropine sulphate (nebulised dose 3mg) on the provocation concentration of methacholine producing a 20 per cent decrease in FEV_1 (PC_{20}) in six asthmatics ($p<0.001$)

unknown, a dose sufficient to displace the response to methacholine by greater than two log-concentrations should have a similar effect on responses to acetylcholine released by vagal activity.

INTERSUBJECT DIFFERENCES IN THE MAIN SITE OF OBSTRUCTION TO AIRFLOW

In 1977, McFadden and his colleagues [9] suggested that the effect of pharmacological blockade on the response to exercise in asthmatics was influenced by intersubject differences in the predominant site of obstruction to the airflow as assessed by the response of the maximal expiratory flow rate to breathing gas of low density. These differences had previously been classified by Despas and his colleagues [10] : subjects who showed an increase in flow rate while breathing helium (a low-density gas), were thought to have the main site of limitation to flow in the large central airways – they were classified as responders. Those who showed no increase in flow rates were thought to have the main site of limitation in the smaller peripheral airways – they were classified as non-responders. Using this classification McFadden and his colleagues [9] found that ipratropium bromide prevented exercise-induced asthma only in those subjects with mainly central airways obstruction during exercise whereas the combination of sodium cromoglycate and ipratropium bromide had a protective effect in all the subjects studied. Sodium cromoglycate was not given alone.

These findings were re-examined in a group of 13 adult atopic asthmatics. The subjects were pretreated on four separate days with inhaled ipratropium bromide (nebulised dose, 1.3mg), sodium cromoglycate (nebulised dose, 13mg), ipratropium bromide plus sodium cromoglycate, and placebo. All drugs were administered by a Wright nebuliser in a random double-blind fashion. Further details of the methods have been published elsewhere [11]. In eight of the 13 subjects the mean base line maximal expiratory flow rate responses to breathing a low-density gas were in the responders; the remaining five subjects were non-responders. Ipratropium bromide had a significant protective effect in the responders only, whereas sodium cromoglycate had an inhibitory effect on exercise-induced asthma in both groups (Figure 3).

Interpretation of the findings

Thus the effectiveness of an anticholinergic agent in the protection from exercise-induced asthma appeared to be related to the main site of obstruction to airflow before exercise as assessed by maximal expiratory flow

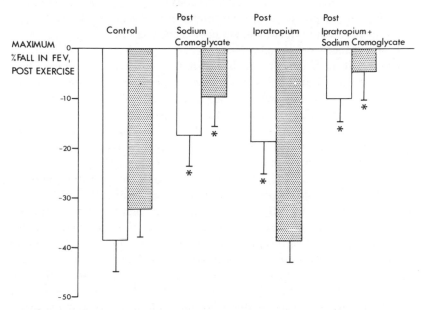

Figure 3. Maximum percentage fall in FEV_1 (mean $\pm$ SEM) after exericse following pretreatment with sodium cromoglycate, ipratropium bromide, ipratropium bromide plus sodium cromoglycate and placebo (control), in eight low-density gas responders (open columns) and five non-responders (hatched columns) (*$p<0.05$ – these values refer to difference between percentage fall after placebo and after pretreatment drugs in responders and non-responders)

rate responses to breathing a low-density gas – that is, cholinergic blockade had no protective effect in subjects in whom the main site of obstruction was in the smaller peripheral airways (non-responders). There are, however, several difficulties with the interpretation of these findings.

First, within the group of responders there was intersubject variability in the effect of ipratropium bromide; only four of the eight subjects had less than a 15 per cent fall in FEV_1 after ipratropium bromide. These differences may have been due to a change in the main site of airflow obstruction – that is, a responder before exercise became a non-responder after exercise. In their results, which showed ipratropium bromide to be effective in protecting from exercise-induced asthma, McFadden and his colleages [9] referred to subjects who were responders after exercise.

Secondly, Spiro and his colleagues [12] have recently reported that the helium-oxygen response after exercise varies from time to time in the same individual, which may indicate poor reproducibility of the test during exercise. Alternatively, a subject's response may vary physiologically – that is, from responder to non-responder or vice versa. If this is the case then the protective effect of an anticholinergic agent on exercise may possibly also change from time to time.

Thirdly, the interpretation of changes in flow rates while breathing a low-density gas mixture is more complex than originally suggested [13,14]. This measurement may assess the site of limitation of flow rather than the site of obstruction in the airways [13]. The association between the effectiveness of the protective effect of cholinergic blockade in exercise-induced asthma and helium-oxygen response in some individuals may be an indicator of some other important but unrecognised factor.

The interpretation of these findings in relation to the pathogenesis of exercise-induced asthma also depends on the mode of action of ipratropium bromide, atropine sulphate and sodium cromoglycate in these studies. Anticholinergic drugs could be acting in a number of ways. First, by acting directly on muscarinic receptors in smooth muscle, reflex vagal pathways would be blocked. Secondly, bronchodilatation after ipratropium or atropine might reduce bronchial responsiveness owing to a change in the base line calibre of the airways [15]. Thirdly, *in-vitro* studies have shown that anticholinergic agents can prevent the release of mediators from mast cells [16]. Fourthly, Breslin and his colleagues [17] have suggested that atropine may alter the sites and distribution of respiratory heat loss within the airways. The mode of action of sodium cromoglycate is also complex and is poorly understood [18]. The drug is thought to have a temporarily stabilising effect on the mast cell and so prevent the release of mediators [19]. It may also have effects on the autonomic nervous system [20] although these have not been demonstrated conclusively in man [21]. Because of the uncertainties surrounding the modes of action of both anticholinergic agents and sodium cromoglycate, the mechanism that causes exercise-induced asthma remains unclear – possibly more than one mechanism may be involved.

References

1   Strauss RH, McFadden ER Jr, Ingram RH Jr et al.
    Influence of heat and humidity on the airway obstruction induced by exercise
    in asthma. *J Clin Invest 1978; 61:* 433–440

2   Deal EC Jr, McFadden ER Jr, Ingram RH Jr, Jaeger JJ.
    Hyperpnea and heat flux: initial reaction sequence in exercise-induced asthma.
    J Appl Physiol 1979; 46: 476–483

3   Anderton RC, Cuff MT, Frith PA et al.
    Bronchial responsiveness to inhaled histamine and exercise.
    J Allergy Clin Immunol 1979; 63: 315–320

4   O'Byrne PM, Ryan G, Morris M et al.
    Asthma induced by cold air and its relationship to nonspecific bronchial responsiveness to methacholine. *Am Rev Respir Dis 1982; 125:* 281–285

5   Gold WM.
    The role of the parasympathetic nervous system in airways disease.
    Postgrad Med J 1975; 51 Suppl: 53–62

6   Anderson SD, Silverman M, König P, Godfrey S.
    Exercise-induced asthma.
    Br J Dis Chest 1975; 69: 1–39

7   Godfrey S, König P.
    Inhibition of exercise-induced asthma by different pharmacological pathways.
    Thorax 1976; 31: 137–143

8   Tinkelman OG, Cavanaugh MJ, Cooper DM.
    Inhibition of exercise-induced bronchospasm by atropine.
    Am Rev Respir Dis 1976; 114: 87–94

9   McFadden ER Jr, Ingram RH Jr, Haynes RL, Wellman JJ.
    Predominant site of flow limitation and mechanisms of post-exertional asthma.
    J Appl Physiol 1977; 42: 746–752

10 Despas PJ, Leroux M, Macklem PT.
    Site of airway obstruction in asthma as determined by measuring maximal expiratory flow breathing air and a helium-oxygen mixture.
    J Clin Invest 1972; 51: 3235–3243

11 Thomson NC, Patel KR, Kerr JW.
    Sodium cromoglycate and ipratropium bromide in exercise-induced asthma.
    Thorax 1978; 33: 694–699

12 Spiro SG, Bierman CW, Petheram IS.
    Reproducibility of flow rates measured with low density gas mixtures in exercise-induced asthma. *Thorax 1981; 36:* 852–857

13 Macklem PT.
    A revisit to the site of airway obstruction in asthma. In Hargreave FE, ed.
    Airway reactivity 1980: 20
    Mississauga: Astra Pharmaceuticals Canada Ltd

14 Berend N, Thurlbeck WM.
    Correlations of maximum expiratory flow with small airway dimensions and pathology. *J Appl Physiol 1982; 52:* 346–351

15 Benson MK.
    Bronchial hyperreactivity.
    Br J Dis Chest 1975; 69: 227–239

16 Kaliner M, Orange RP, Austen KF.
    Immunological release of histamine and slow reacting substance of anaphylaxis from human lung. IV Enhancement by cholinergic and alpha-adrenergic stimulation. *J Exp Med 1972; 136:* 556–567

17 Breslin FJ, McFadden ER Jr, Ingram RH Jr, Deal EC Jr.
    Effects of atropine on respiratory heat loss in asthma.
    J Appl Physiol 1980; 48: 619–623

18   Altounyan REC.
     Review of the clinical activity and modes of action of sodium cromoglycate.
     In Pepys J, Edwards AM, eds. *The Mast Cell 1979:* 199.
     London: Pitman Medical

19   Orr TSC, Pollard MC, Gwilliam J, Cox JSG.
     Mode of action of disodium cromoglycate studies on immediate type of hyper-
     sensitivity reactions using 'double sensitization' with two antigenically distinct
     rat reagins. *Clin Exp Immunol 1970; 7:* 745–757

20   Jackson DM, Richards IM.
     The effects of sodium cromoglycate on histamine aerosol induced reflex bron-
     choconstriction in the anaesthetized dog.
     Br J Pharmacol 1977; 61: 257–262

21   Thomson NC.
     The effect of different pharmacological agents on respiratory reflexes in normal
     and asthmatic subjects. *Clin Sci 1979; 56:* 235–241

Chapter 19

THE PRESENT STATUS OF BRONCHODILATORS IN THE TREATMENT OF EXERCISE-INDUCED ASTHMA

T-Ø Endsjø

Oslo, Norway

SUMMARY

A review of the literature leads me to the following four conclusions.

(1) Inhaled beta$_2$-agonists such as salbutamol, terbutaline, fenoterol and rimiterol are the most effective drugs in treatment and prophylaxis of exercise-induced asthma, whether used alone or in combination with sodium cromoglycate — especially in children.

(2) When given by mouth, beta$_2$-agonists do not give the same protection.

(3) Theophylline at serum levels between 10–20μg/ml give some protection.

(4) Inhaled atropine-like compounds such as ipratropium bromide have no convincing effect on exercise-induced asthma.

INTRODUCTION

The beneficial effect of bronchodilator drugs on the increase of airways resistance after exercise in children with bronchial asthma was described by Jones and his colleagues in 1963 [1]. Since about 95 per cent of these children suffer from exercise-induced asthma, its treatment is of the greatest importance.

Despite the many problems connected with the standardisation of methods, I believe it could be worthwhile to try to draw some conclusions from the published reports of the use of bronchodilators in the treatment of exercise-induced asthma, interpreting the findings in the light of my own experience.

REVIEW OF THE LITERATURE

In 1976 Godfrey and König [2] used standardised treadmill running for six minutes as the provocative stimulus in 15 asthmatic children. Their study has been frequently cited in subsequent publications. The following drugs were given in normal therapeutic doses: salbutamol in aerosol form to 13 children and in tablet form to two, theophylline in tablet form, sodium cromoglycate as inhaled powder, and atropine as an aerosol administered by face mask.

The lowest peak expiratory flow rate (PEFR) after exercise was compared with the PEFR measured immediately before exercise, but after the child had taken the active drug or placebo. The average falls in PEFR were: for placebo 45 per cent, for sodium cromoglycate 20 per cent, for atropine 25 per cent and for salbutamol 4 per cent. The authors concluded that exercise-induced asthma was blocked in all children by salbutamol, in 80 per cent by theophylline or sodium cromoglycate, but only in some 60 per cent by atropine.

This study, however, revealed a general problem. Out of the 15 patients, some eight or nine were obstructed, but their PEFRs became normal after bronchodilator medication and before the exercise test – this, of course, did not happen with sodium cromoglycate predmedication. In part, at least, this difference can explain why there are those who respond and those who do not respond to treatment of exercise-induced asthma with sodium cromoglycate, in contrast to the bronchodilators.

As confirmed by later workers, Godfrey and König found no correlation between bronchodilator activity at rest and the ability of a drug to block exercise-induced asthma.

Also in 1976, Fitch and Godfrey [3] concluded that "Salbutamol is the most effective prophylactic against exercise-induced asthma and is an ideal drug for asthmatic sportsmen". However, since then terbutaline, fenoterol and salbutamol in spray form have been found equally effective.

If sports activities are sufficiently strenuous, and carried out under appropriate conditions, exercise-induced asthma will probably occur in all asthmatics. Two puffs of a beta$_2$-agonist shortly before exercise, will satisfactorily prevent the exercise-induced asthma and the effect seems to last for three to four hours.

The publications concerned with oral beta$_2$-agonists and exercise-induced asthma have, to say the least, been highly contradictory. This may be due to methodological inconsistencies, but a recent convincing publication by Sly and his co-workers [4] has shown a good effect of oral terbutaline on exercise-induced asthma. Eighteen asthmatic youngsters were provoked by treadmill running two hours after the oral administration of 2.5–5.0mg of terbutaline; satisfactory protection was achieved in 14. The authors concluded that an oral beta$_2$-agonist was an effective alternative for patients who needed protection two to five hours after administration of the dose, or who preferred not to attract attention by using a metered dose inhaler.

In 1978, Gibson and his colleagues [5] found that a slight tolerance or tachyphylaxis towards salbutamol tablets, but not to salbutamol by inhalation, developed after several weeks. In this context, it is interesting to keep in mind that the inhaled dose is equivalent to only one-twentieth of the oral dose. The few failures to prevent exercise-induced asthma can usually be overcome by increasing the inhaled dose of the bronchodilator, but not by increasing the oral dose.

Bundgaard and Schmidt [6] investigated 18 adults whose reduction of pulmonary function after exercise was only partially prevented by two puffs (0.4mg) of fenoterol metered aerosol. However, inhalation of 2mg from a nebuliser provided complete protection.

Some 50 per cent of adult patients, and an even higher percentage of children and the elderly, use the metered aerosol incorrectly. Beta$_2$-agonists can be inhaled as a powder from a capsule, by means of a powder inhalator. Bundgaard and Schmidt [7] found that fenoterol given either as a powder or as a metered aerosol was equally effective against exercise-induced asthma provided the aerosol technique was good. Nevertheless the powder form appears to offer some clear advantages:

(1) the potentially injurious effects of the freon gas are avoided
(2) there is no irritant effect from a carrier substance (especially glucose)
(3) the inhalation technique is easy to learn
(4) it is easy to avoid over-dosage.

The atropine-like substances have found no place in the prevention of exercise-induced asthma. However, when the inhaled dose of ipratropium bromide was increased from 100 to 1000mg, on one occasion, exercise-induced asthma was significantly blocked in most of the patients [8].

When adults were given theophylline in doses from 125 up to 375mg, they experienced no significant effect on their exercise-induced asthma. Above this dosage level, inhibition was noted [9]. However, in some of these cases side effects were a limiting factor.

CONCLUSIONS

Inhaled beta$_2$-agonists are the most effective drugs against exercise-induced asthma, used either as powder or as aerosol.

When given by mouth, beta$_2$-agonists are also effective but their action is delayed.

Theophyllines give some protection, but rather high doses are necessary.

Ipratropium bromide has no convincing effect.

Nevertheless sodium cromoglycate, with its lack of systemic side effects, is the preferred drug for the pretreatment of exercise-induced asthma in children and young adults with mild or moderate bronchial asthma.

References

1   Jones RS, Wharton MJ, Buston MH.
     The place of physical exercise and bronchodilator drugs in the assessment of the asthmatic child. *Arch Dis Child 1963; 38:* 539–545

2   Godfrey S, König P.
     Inhibition of exercise-induced asthma by different pharmacological pathways. *Thorax 1976; 31:* 137–143

3   Fitch KD, Godfrey S.
     Asthma and athletic performance. *JAMA 1976; 236:* 152–157

4   Sly RM, O'Brien SR.
     The effect of oral terbutaline on exercise-induced asthma. *Ann Allergy 1982; 48:* 151–155

5   Gibson GJ, Greenakre JK, König P et al.
     Use of exercise challenge to investigate possible tolerance to beta-adrenoceptor stimulation in asthma. *Br J Dis Chest 1978; 72:* 199–206

6   Bundgaard A, Schmidt A.
     Medikamentel behandling af anstrengelsesudløst asthma. *Ugeskr Laeger 1981; 143/44:* 2876–2877

7   Bundgaard A, Schmidt A.
     Pretreatment of exercise-induced asthma by fenoterol delivered as inhalation powder and pressurized aerosol. *Ann Allergy 1982; 48:* 36–39

8   Hartley J, Davies B.
     Ipratropium bromide in exercise-induced asthma.
     J Allergy Clin Immunol 1978; 64: 612–624

9   Bierman CW, Shapiro GG, Pierson WE et al.
     Acute and chronic theophylline therapy in exercise-induced bronchospasm.
     Pediatrics 1977; 60: 845–849

Chapter 20

SODIUM CROMOGLYCATE AND BRONCHIAL HYPERREACTIVITY MEASURED BY STANDARDISED HISTAMINE PROVOCATION

O Löwhagen, E Millqvist, S Raak

Sahlgrenska's Hospital, University of Göteborg, Göteborg, Sweden

SUMMARY

As there is some evidence to support the belief that long-term treatment with sodium cromoglycate reduces non-specific bronchial hyperreactivity in asthmatic patients, the object of this study was to investigate the effect of sodium cromoglycate on the histamine bronchial reactivity over a period of four weeks.

A randomised, double-blind, placebo controlled, cross-over study was performed outside the pollen season in 14 adult patients with atopic bronchial asthma. Between the two treatment periods (sodium cromoglycate 20mg $\times$ 4 and placebo) there was a wash-out period of two weeks.

Standardised histamine provocation tests were performed before, during and at the end of each treatment period. Shifts in the individual dose-response curves were calculated and comparisons between active drug and placebo were analysed. These analyses revealed no significant change in bronchial response during treatment with either sodium cromoglycate or placebo.

We conclude that bronchial responsiveness to histamine seems not to be reduced by treatment with sodium cromoglycate in atopic asthmatic patients during the non-pollen season.

INTRODUCTION

The mechanism of action of sodium cromoglycate is still not clear [1, 2]. The inhibition of allergen-induced symptoms is well documented [3–8]; however, other effects, such as inhibition of asthma induced by exercise, sulphur dioxide or aspirin [9–15] can hardly be explained by mast-cell stabilisation. In some studies on sodium cromoglycate a reduction of non-specific bronchial hyperreactivity has also been reported [16–19].

The object of this present study was to evaluate the change in bronchial responsiveness to histamine during treatment with sodium cromoglycate in patients with atopic bronchial asthma by using a standardised histamine provocation model.

PATIENTS AND METHODS

Experimental design

The trial was a double-blind, crossover, randomised study comparing inhaled sodium cromoglycate (20mg $\times$ 4) and placebo. During the first week base-line pulmonary function (forced expiratory volume in one second — FEV_1) was recorded and a standardised histamine provocation (control) performed. The two treatment periods lasted for four weeks each and were separated by a wash-out period of two weeks.

Patients

Fourteen patients with atopic bronchial asthma, six men and eight women with a mean age of 31 years (range, 20–48 years) were selected for the study. The diagnosis was based on a history of allergy and a positive prick test, radioallergosorbent test (RAST) and allergen bronchial provocation test. None of the patients was in need of regular anti-asthmatic medication.

At the time of the study, most of the patients were free from asthma symptoms, the FEV_1 values being more than 80 per cent of predicted, except in one patient. None of the patients was receiving immunotherapy and none had had a recent respiratory infection.

Histamine provocation

Standardised histamine provocations [20, 21] were performed at the start, during and at the end of each treatment period. Dilutions of histamine chloride (range, 0.0075 — 16mg/ml) were performed before each provocation and nebulised by a Pari inhalerboy nebuliser (particle size, 0.5–5.5μm; nebuliser output 0.75ml/min). Two-fold increasing concentrations of histamine were inhaled through the mouth by tidal volume breathing for two minutes with an interval of five minutes between the doses. At least four doses were given in each provocation. The last dose should decrease the FEV_1 by more than 25 per cent of the base-line value. Lung function measurements – FEV_1, forced vital capacity (FVC), peak expiratory flow rate (PEFR) and maximum expiratory flow at 50 per cent of vital capacity (MEF_{50}) – were made before and two minutes after each dose of histamine. Measurements were also made at 10 and 20 minutes after the final dose. The higher of the two values was used in the statistical evaluation.

RESULTS

The results are given as changes in FEV_1. Representative dose-response curves in one patient are shown in Figure 1. The calculation of the provocation concentration at 25 per cent fall in FEV_1 (PC_{25}) is indicated. Mean base-line values for FEV_1 were 3.21, 3.20 and 3.24L during the placebo treatment period and 3.22, 3.28 and 3.32L during treatment with the active drug. The differences were not statistically significant.

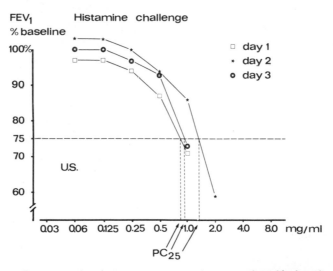

Figure 1. Representative dose-response curves in one patient (during the placebo period) provoked with histamine at the start (day 1), during (day 2) and at the end (day 3) of the treatment period. Five or six doses of histamine were given. Linear interpolation between the two last points gave the provocation concentration at 25 per cent decrease from the base line (PC_{25}) as indicated in the figure

The individual differences in PC_{25} before and after the two treatment periods are shown in Figure 2. After treatment with placebo, the PC_{25} was increased in eight and decreased in six patients. After treatment with

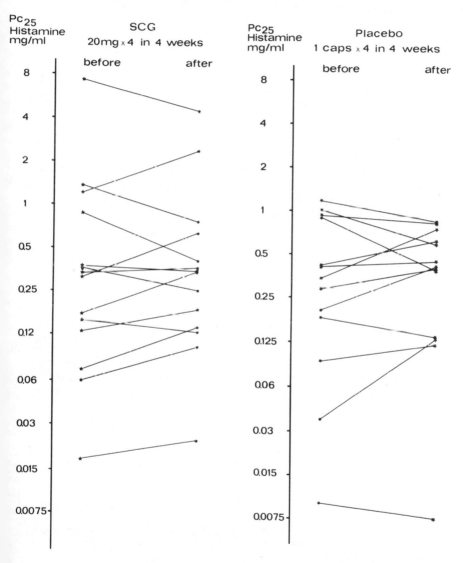

Figure 2. Provocation histamine concentration at 25 per cent decrease in FEV_1 (PC_{25}) before and after treatment with sodium cromoglycate (SCG) and placebo in 14 patients with atopic bronchial asthma

sodium cromoglycate, the PC_{25} was also increased in eight and decreased in six patients. Thus, there was no significant difference in effect between placebo and sodium cromoglycate. All individual changes in PC_{25} were within one dose step.

DISCUSSION

This study shows that treatment with sodium cromoglycate for four weeks does not change the bronchial responsiveness to histamine in atopic asthmatic patients during the non-pollen season.

Patients with mild bronchial asthma, who were allergic to one or several allergens, were selected. As exposure to the relevant allergens could mostly be avoided only a few patients had asthmatic symptoms during the study.

The base-line value for FEV_1 before each histamine provocation was more than 80 per cent of predicted in all patients except one. Control challenges before the study showed that all selected patients responded to low concentrations of histamine, the range for a greater than 20 per cent decrease in FEV_1 being 0.03–2mg/ml. In our provocation model these values are representative for asthmatic patients.

The reproducibility during the two treatment periods (placebo and active drug) was very good and in agreement with previous studies on patients with stable or mild asthma [20, 22].

We conclude, therefore, that sodium cromoglycate has no effect on non-specific hyperreactivity in asthmatic patients with mild symptoms during a period when they are not regularly exposed to the relevant allergens. At times of regular exposure, such as during the pollen season, secondarily increased bronchial hyperreactivity has been shown [16, 23] and studies are in progress to evaluate the inhibitory effect of sodium cromoglycate on this temporary increase in hyperreactivity.

References

1   Stokes FC, Morley J.
    Prospects for an oral Intal.
    Br J Dis Chest 1981; 75: 1–14

2   Brogden RN, Speight TM, Avery GS.
    Sodium cromoglycate (cromolyn sodium); a review of its mode of action, pharmacology, therapeutic efficacy and use. *Drugs 1974; 7:* 164–272

3   Altounyan REC.
    Inhibition of experimental asthma by a new compound, disodium cromoglycate, "Intal". *Acta Allergol 1967; 22:* 487

4 Muittari A.
Effect of disodium cromoglycate on exercise and allergen induced asthma.
Folia Allergol 1970; 17: 445

5 Kolatkin BM, Lee CK, Townley RG.
Duration and specificity of cromolyn sodium on allergen inhalation challenges in asthma. *J Allergy Clin Immunol 1974; 53:* 288–297

6 Booij-Noordh H, Orie NGM, De Vries K.
Immediate and late bronchial obstructive reactions to inhalation of housedust and protective effects of disodium cromoglycate and prednisolone.
J Allergy 1971; 48: 344–354

7 Pepys J.
Non-immediate asthmatic reactions. In Pauwels R, ed.
Fundamentals of Respiratory Disease, Bronchial Asthma Volume 1 1976.
Brussels: Belgian Society of Allergology and Clinical Immunology

8 Löwhagen O, Granerus G, Wetterqvist H.
Studies on histamine metabolism in allergen-induced asthma.
Allergy 1980; 35: 521–529

9 Godfrey S.
The physiological assessment of the effect of disodium cromoglycate in the asthmatic child.*Respiration 1970; 27, Suppl:* 353–356

10 Silverman M, Anderson SD.
Standardisation of exercise tests in asthmatic children.
Arch Dis Child 1972; 27: 882–889

11 Morton AR, Turner KJ, Fitch KD.
Protection from exercise induced asthma by pre-exercise cromolyn sodium and its relationship to serum IgE levels. *Ann Allergy 1973; 31:* 265–271

12 Silverman M, Turner-Warwick M.
Exercise induced asthma. Response to disodium cromoglycate in skin test positive and skin test negative subjects. *Clin Allergy 1972; 2:* 137–142

13 De Vries K, Gokemeijer JDM, Orie NGM et al.
The response of the bronchial tree to allergic and non-allergic stimuli in patients with generalized obstructive lung disease.
Bull Int Union Tuberc 1976; 51: 617–624

14 Sheppard D, Nadel JA, Boushey H.
Inhibition of sulfur dioxide-induced bronchoconstriction by disodium cromoglycate in asthmatic subjects. *Am Rev Respir Dis 1981; 124:* 257–259

15 Basomba A, Romar A, Pelaz A et al.
The effect of disodium cromoglycate in preventing aspirin induced bronchospasm. *Clin Allergy 1976; 6:* 269–275

16 Altounyan REC.
Changes in histamine and atropine responsiveness as a guide to diagnosis and evaluation of therapy in obstructive airways disease. In Pepys J, Frankland AW, eds.
Disodium Cromoglycate in Allergic Airways Disease 1970; 47–53.
London: Butterworth

17 Kerr JW, Govindaraj M, Patel KR.
Effect of alpha-receptor blocking drugs and disodium cromoglycate on histamine hypersensitivity in bronchial asthma. *Br Med J 1970; 2:* 139–141

18   Dickson W.
     One year's trial of Intal compounds in 24 children with severe asthma.
     In Pepys J, Frankland AW, eds.
     Disodium Cromoglycate in Allergic Airways Disease 1970; 105–109
     London: Butterworth

19   Jackson DM, Richards IM.
     Effect of sodium cromoglycate on histamine aerosol induced reflex broncho-
     constriction in the anaesthetized dog. *Br J Pharmacol 1977; 61:* 257–262

20   Löwhagen O, Lindholm NL.
     Standardized histamine provocation model – short and long term variation in
     bronchial response. *Eur J Respir Dis.* In press

21   Hegardt B, Löwhagen O, Svedmyr N, Granerus G.
     The protective property of equipotent bronchodilating doses of inhaled KWD
     2131 and terbutaline against allergen-induced bronchospasm. *Allergy.* In press

22   Juniper EF, Frith PA, Dunett C et al.
     Reproducibility and comparison of response to inhaled histamine and
     methacoline. *Thorax 1978; 33:* 705–710

23   Boulet LP, Thomson NC, Cartier A, Hargreave FE.
     Increased bronchial responsiveness to methacholine after natural exposure to
     pollen. *J Allergy Clin Immunol 1982; 69:* 25

Chapter 21

DOSE-RESPONSE STUDY OF SODIUM CROMOGLYCATE IN EXERCISE-INDUCED ASTHMA

K R Patel, K E Berkin, J W Kerr

Western Infirmary, Glasgow, United Kingdom

SUMMARY

Ten patients with exercise-induced asthma participated in a single-blind dose-response study comparing the protective effect of inhaled sodium cromoglycate in increasing concentrations from 2 to 40mg/ml. Saline was used as a control. Effects were assessed from the mean maximal percentage fall in forced expiratory volume in one second (FEV_1) after running on a treadmill for eight minutes. Slight bronchodilation was observed in base line FEV_1 after inhalation of sodium cromoglycate which reached statistical significance with the highest concentration (5.7%; $p<0.05$). After exercise, the mean maximal percentage falls in FEV_1 (SEM) after saline and sodium cromoglycate 2mg/ml, 10mg/ml, 20mg/ml and 40mg/ml were 37.3 (4.7), 17.3 (4.1), 10 (3.3), 7.6 (2.4) and 12 (2.9), respectively. Sodium cromoglycate inhibited the exercise-induced fall in FEV_1 at all the concentrations used in the study ($p<0.001$) and its inhibitory effect increased from 2 to 20mg/ml. The mean FEV_1 returned to base-line values within 15 minutes at higher concentrations of sodium cromoglycate (20 and 40mg/ml) and a small bronchodilator effect was noted at 30 minutes.

The findings suggest that the protective effect of sodium cromoglycate in exercise-induced asthma is dose-related. At higher concentration, the drug suppresses the release of chemical mediators from the mast cells in the lung and may also modify the bronchial reactivity to released mediators.

INTRODUCTION

Sodium cromoglycate suppresses the release of mast cell mediators [1] and is effective in inhibiting both the allergen- and exercise-induced bronchoconstriction in patients with allergic asthma [2–4]. Recently a low-dose pressurised aerosol delivering 1mg of sodium cromoglycate per inhalation has become available – this is a considerably smaller dose than the 20mg of dry powder obtained in a Spincap or the 20mg in 2ml of nebuliser solution. However, a properly conducted dose-response study of sodium cromoglycate in experimental asthma is lacking. Clinical and experimental studies have compared the effect of a pressurised metered-dose aerosol with that of the dry powder inhaled through a Spinhaler, and the effect of sodium cromoglycate powder with that of sodium cromoglycate nebuliser solution [5 and unpublished observations of B Blohm et al and N Knudsen]. There is considerable variation in the size of the particles and in the site at which the drug is deposited in the airways with different methods of administration. In addition, sodium cromoglycate in the powder form has a greater affinity for water [6] and this may lead to differences when aerosol and dry powder are compared to nebuliser solution if respiratory heat loss, airway cooling and humidity are considered to be important factors in exercise-induced asthma [7].

We have compared the effect of sodium cromoglycate nebuliser solution inhaled from a Wright nebuliser in increasing concentrations from 2 to 40mg/ml in 10 patients with allergic and reproducible exercise-induced asthma.

PATIENTS AND METHODS

Ten patients aged between 17 and 54 years (mean, 29 years SEM 3.2) with extrinsic asthma with reproducible exercise-induced attacks were studied. No patient was taking corticosteroids, antihistamines or anticholinergic drugs. Sodium cromoglycate and bronchodilators were discontinued for 24 hours before each test was carried out. The forced expiratory volume in one second (FEV_1) was measured on a water-sealed spirometer.

Exercise testing consisted of steady-state running on a treadmill for up to eight minutes at submaximal workload under controlled conditions of temperature and humidity. A series of five tests in each patient were completed within 10–14 days. The tests were performed in a single-blind fashion using physiological saline or sodium cromoglycate solution in various concentrations (2mg/ml, 10mg/ml, 20mg/ml or 40mg/ml) delivered through a Wright nebuliser driven by compressed air at a flow rate of 9L/min. All inhalations were carried out at tidal breathing for five minutes. The estimated dose of nebulised sodium cromoglycate was 2.4mg, 12mg, 24mg and 48mg, respectively, for each of the four concentrations. The FEV_1 was recorded at 30 minutes after inhalation and just before exercise and then at 2, 5, 10, 15 and 30 minutes after exercise. The results of exercising were expressed as the maximal falls in FEV_1 from post-drug base line. The treatments were analysed using analysis of variance for overall effect and Duncan's multiple range test and the Student's paired t test for the dose-response effect.

RESULTS

Tables I and II give the results. There was no significant difference in the mean base line FEV_1 values on the five days of exercise testing. Neither saline nor sodium cromoglycate at 2mg/ml, 10mg/ml and 20mg/ml had any significant effect on the mean FEV_1 at 30 minutes after inhalation of the drug before exercise. However, sodium cromoglycate at these concentrations did have a small bronchodilator effect. In contrast, sodium cromoglycate at 40mg/ml raised the mean base-line value by 0.21L (5.7%) and this bronchodilator effect was statistically significant ($p<0.05$).

After treadmill exercise the mean percentage falls in FEV_1 (SEM) after saline and sodium cromoglycate 2mg/ml, 10mg/ml, 20mg/ml and 40mg/ml were 37.3 (4.7), 17.3 (4.1), 10.3 (3.3), 7.3 (2.4) and 12.9 (2.9), respectively. Sodium cromoglycate inhibited the exercise-induced fall in FEV_1 at all the concentrations used in the study ($p<0.001$), an effect that was significantly greater at 10mg/ml, 20mg/ml and 40mg/ml than at 2mg/ml ($p<0.05$). The protective effect of sodium cromoglycate was greatest at 20mg/ml but this did not reach statistical significance when compared with the effects of 10mg/ml or 40mg/ml. The mean FEV_1 returned to base-line values within 15 minutes when sodium cromoglycate was used at 20mg/ml and 40mg/ml and a small bronchodilator effect was noted at 30 minutes. In contrast, the mean FEV_1 remained below the base-line values over 30 minutes of reading with lower concentrations of sodium cromoglycate (2mg/ml and 10mg/ml).

DISCUSSION

Sodium cromoglycate inhibited the exercise-induced asthma at all the concentrations used in the study and its protective effect increased with increasing concentrations from 2mg/ml to 20mg/ml. Furthermore, the mean FEV_1 returned to the base-line values within 15 minutes after

TABLE I. Effect of saline and sodium cromoglycate on the maximal fall in FEV_1 after exercise in 10 patients (base-line data before and after inhalation expressed as absolute values in litres)

No.	Sex	Age (years)	SALINE			SODIUM CROMOGLYCATE											
						2mg/ml			10mg/ml			20mg/ml			40mg/ml		
			B	A	Change	B	A	Change	B	A	Change	B	A	Change	B	A	Change
1	F	32	2.14	2.11	−0.75	1.76	1.91	−0.55	1.77	2.00	−0.23	1.74	1.80	−0.40	2.04	2.18	−0.07
2	M	28	2.61	2.61	−1.15	2.34	2.18	−0.87	2.64	2.40	−0.86	2.48	2.64	−0.53	2.41	3.21	−0.83
3	M	32	2.91	2.98	−0.67	2.95	3.11	−0.31	3.08	3.01	−0.13	2.91	2.98	−0.20	2.78	2.85	−0.31
4	M	17	3.85	3.45	−2.11	2.98	3.52	−0.34	3.62	3.92	−0.27	2.58	3.31	+0.10	3.58	4.05	−0.40
5	M	54	2.48	2.48	−0.47	2.14	2.38	−0.24	2.14	2.34	−0.16	2.28	2.21	−0.03	1.98	2.48	−0.17
6	M	24	4.10	4.08	−1.54	4.12	3.95	−0.55	4.02	4.12	−0.30	4.07	4.08	−0.20	3.88	4.05	−0.15
7	M	32	3.35	3.21	−0.77	3.18	3.68	−0.23	3.15	3.26	−0.38	3.38	3.65	−0.10	3.68	3.70	−0.50
8	M	22	5.39	5.39	−3.11	5.20	5.16	−1.98	5.12	5.16	−1.21	5.32	5.09	−0.54	5.19	5.02	−0.74
9	M	27	4.51	4.52	−1.14	3.98	3.82	−0.30	4.52	4.47	−0.17	3.50	3.60	+0.06	3.80	3.08	+0.08
10	F	22	3.08	3.01	−1.40	3.10	3.15	−0.27	3.10	3.08	−0.10	2.91	2.91	−0.07	2.81	2.81	−0.82
Mean		29	3.44	3.38	−1.31	3.18	3.29	−0.56	3.31	3.37	−0.38	3.12	3.23	−0.19	3.21	3.42	−0.39
SEM		3.2	0.32	0.32	0.25	0.33	0.31	0.17	0.33	0.32	0.11	0.32	0.30	0.07	0.32	0.28	0.10

B = base line before inhalation; A = base line after inhalation; Change = fall in FEV_1 from the base line after inhalation; SEM = standard error of mean

TABLE II. The mean percentage change in FEV_1 in 10 patients after inhalation of saline and sodium cromoglycate and at 2, 5, 10, 15 and 30 minutes after exercise

	Change in base line	After exercise					p	
		2 min	5 min	10 min	15 min	30 min	Saline versus SCG	SCG (2mg) versus SCG
Saline	−1.7	−21	−36	−35	−31	−24		
Sodium cromoglycate								
2mg/ml	+3.6	+ 2.5	−11.3	−11.0	− 6.2	− 3.0	0.001	
10mg/ml	+2.2	+ 1.2	− 8.2	− 8.5	− 6.9	− 4.2	0.001	0.05
20mg/ml	+2.1	+ 6.5	− 3.6	− 1.0	+ 2.2	+ 6.5	0.001	0.01
40mg/ml	+5.7	+ 1.5	− 5.9	− 4.0	+ 0.3	+ 3.3	0.001	0.05

SCG = sodium cromoglycate

exercise with higher concentrations of sodium cromoglycate (20mg/ml and 40mg/ml) with a slight bronchodilator effect noticeable at 30 minutes. Chung and Jones [8] reported that sodium cromoglycate had a broncho-dilator effect in children which was comparable to that of salbutamol. Our observations support the view that sodium cromoglycate has a broncho-dilator effect when used in higher concentrations, although this effect is rather small and of little therapeutic value.

Breslin and his colleagues [7] have reported that sodium cromoglycate attenuates the obstructive response observed in asthmatic patients after hyperventilation and cooling of the airways. However, these workers were unable to confirm the hypothesis that sodium cromoglycate, with its great affinity for water, acted as a series heat exchanger with the respiratory mucosa. The studies comparing inhaled dry powder with nebuliser solution are difficult to interpret because of the hygroscopic property of sodium cromoglycate and also because the dose of the drug and the site at which it is deposited in the airways may vary with different methods of administration. In the present study we used sodium cromoglycate dissolved in water and delivered with consistent technique to avoid these differences.

The mechanism of exercise-induced asthma remains unclear, both a vagal reflex and the release of mast-cell mediators have been suggested [4,9,10]. The vagal mechanism is apparently significant only in patients in whom the main site of airflow obstruction is in the large airways [4,10]. In contrast, sodium cromoglycate prevents exercise-induced asthma in most patients. Studies have shown that sodium cromoglycate also modifies and hastens recovery from histamine- and methacholine-induced bronchoconstriction in asthmatic patients and this effect may be mediated through cholinergic or irritant receptors [11,12]. The recovery of patients within 15 minutes of exercise when sodium cromoglycate is used at the higher concentrations is consistent with these observations. In addition, the protective effect of sodium cromoglycate in exercise-induced asthma is dose-related and may require adjustment for individual patients. Clearly, the dose-response curves of sodium cromoglycate to specific and non-specific bronchial challenge are required to clarify the additional properties of the drug and also to help in the understanding of its mechanism of action.

References

1   Orr TSC, Pollard MC, Gwilliam J, Cox JSG.
    Mode of action of disodium cromoglycate: studies on immediate type hypersensitivity reaction using 'double sensitisation' with antigenically distinct rat reagins. *Clin Exp Immunol 1970; 7:* 745−757

2   Davies SE.
    Effect of disodium cromoglycate on exercise-induced asthma.
    Br Med J 1968; 3: 593−594

3   Godfrey S, König P.
    Inhibition of exercise-induced asthma by different pharmacological pathways.
    Thorax 1976; 31: 137−143

4   Thomson NC, Patel KR, Kerr JW.
    Sodium cromoglycate and ipratropium bromide in exercise induced asthma.
    Thorax 1978; 33: 694−697

5   Jones RS, Chung JTN.
    Comparison of action of disodium cromoglycate powder and solution on bronchoconstrictor mechanisms in asthmatic children.
    In Pepys J, Edwards AM, eds. *The Mast Cell: its role in health and disease 1979:* 287. Tunbridge Wells: Pitman Medical

6   Cox JSG, Woodward GD, McCrone WC.
    Solid state chemistry of cromolyn sodium.
    J Pharm Sci 1971; 60: 1458−1465

7   Breslin FJ, McFadden ER, Ingram RH.
    The effect of cromolyn sodium on the airway response to hyperpnoea and cold air in asthma. *Am Rev Respir Dis 1980; 122:* 11−16

8   Chung JTN, Jones RS.
    Bronchodilator effect of sodium cromoglycate and its clinical implications.
    Br Med J 1979; 2: 1033−1034

9   McFadden ER, Ingram RH, Haynes RL, Wellman JJ.
    Predominant site of flow limitation and mechanism of post exertional asthma.
    J Appl Physiol 1977; 42: 746−752

10   Anonymous.
     Arms and bronchi.
     Lancet 1976; i: 287–289

11   Woenne R, Kattan M, Levison H.
     Sodium cromoglycate-induced change in the dose-response curve of inhaled
     methacholine and histamine in asthmatic children.
     Am Rev Respir Dis 1979; 119: 927–932

12   Woolcock AJ, Salome CM, Schoeffel RE.
     The effect of sodium cromoglycate on bronchial challenge with methacholine.
     In Pepys J, Edwards AM, eds. *The Mast Cell: its role in health and disease 1979:*
     271. Tunbridge Wells: Pitman Medical

DISCUSSION

HENRIKSEN (Aarhus, Denmark)	Dr Endsjø, have you any experiences of the problem of muscular incoordination after inhalation of beta$_2$-agonists before gymnastics and sports?
ENDSJØ	Yes, I have, but I think the incoordination is not peculiar to pre-exercise use. For this reason, I think that in many respects inhalation is an improvement over the powder form of beta$_2$-agonists. Some of these problems of incoordination can, I believe, be avoided with the use of the inhaler or perhaps with the terbutaline extension device which can be used as an inhaler.
BOLAND (Dublin, Ireland)	How safe is the use of beta$_2$-adrenergic agonists for preventing exercise-induced bronchoconstriction in relationship to the cardiovascular system?
ENDSJØ	A review of the literature indicates that the use of the usual doses over the short term would be quite safe. But I am more uncertain about long-term treatment.
ANDERSON (Camperdown, Australia)	Defining exercise-induced asthma as a 10 per cent fall in peak expiratory flow rate (PEFR), we have found that only 20 per cent of 126 asthmatics have derived protection from oral beta-sympathomimetic agents or oral theophylline. Their primary action is to bronchodilate at rest, not prevent a post-exercise fall.
ENDSJØ	Yes, I agree. I think this is yet another area where we encounter the heterogeneity of asthma. Any effect is probably just due to the relief of a subclinical obstruction and not a protective effect against exercise-induced asthma.
SPEIGHT (Newcastle upon Tyne, UK)	In view of its prolonged action, might not oral terbutaline have some advantage over inhaled salbutamol (or inhaled terbutaline) for athletes involved in prolonged exercise?

ENDSJØ

I think it is a good idea to put athletes with moderate and perhaps severe bronchial asthma, who like to compete and to undertake strenuous training, on a basic oral treatment of $beta_2$-agonists perhaps also giving a $beta_2$-agonist by inhaler a quarter to a half an hour before they start their exercise.

BIRRER
(Berne,
Switzerland)

Dr Löwhagen, which is of greater importance in provocation tests: absolute quantity of inhaled histamine or concentration of inhaled histamine?

LÖWHAGEN

In our test system we increase the quantity of histamine by increasing the concentration since the other factors defining the dose (nebuliser output, type of breathing and inhalation time) are kept constant. The absolute quantity of histamine reaching the bronchi is very difficult to assess so we have to determine the dose in this indirect (but standardised) way. Thus, the absolute quantity and concentration are related to each other and I do not know whether it is possible to differentiate their effects.

AAS
(Chairman)

The problem of dose-response in both testing and use of drugs is important. It is not only the total quantities and concentrations at each step that matter, but also the increments. How long do you allow between each concentration, for instance?

LÖWHAGEN

Yes, it is important. As we get a cumulative dose-response curve it is most important to have a constant interval between the doses and in our system it is exactly five minutes. This is the standardised procedure.

STRUNK
(Denver, USA)

Did you study methacholine sensitivity also? Does sensitivity to this drug correlate to the histamine sensitivity?

LÖWHAGEN

We often find a good correlation between the effects of histamine and methacholine, but more work has to

be done to see if there are differences between certain
types of asthma. The important points are to have a
standardised test and carefully defined patients —
what patients are we really studying? As I showed,
there is a possibility of adding to the definition
by determining the degree of bronchial hyperreactivity
to histamine or methacholine.

LEEGAARD   What are the chances that repeated histamine bronchial
(Oslo, Norway)   provocation tests themselves will induce enhanced
                  bronchial hyperreactivity and thus influence the dis-
                  ease itself?

LÖWHAGEN   We have repeated histamine provocation tests at short
                  intervals and have found no indication of enhanced
                  reactivity.

SPEIGHT   Does Dr Löwhagen have any information on the effects
                  of beclomethasone on bronchial hyperreactivity as
                  measured by histamine challenge?

LÖWHAGEN   No, but there is a study in progress. I think it is an
                  interesting drug in relation to bronchial hyperreac-
                  tivity.

WINSNES   Is there any information that poor control of asthma —
(Drammen,   that is, frequent asthmatic attacks — will increase
Norway)   bronchial hyperreactivity?

LÖWHAGEN   The general hypothesis today is that increased severity
                  of the asthma is also followed by an increased non-
                  specific hyperreactivity. We often notice that patients
                  tested, for example, during respiratory infections
                  have more severe symptoms and are also more hyper-
                  reactive.

EDWARDS   The patients in your study required no anti-asthmatic
(Loughborough,   therapy during the time of the study. Does this not
UK)   mean that their bronchial reactivity was not very
                  severe and that the degree of improvement possible
                  was also small?

LÖWHAGEN   One of the criteria for inclusion was that the patients
                   should be asymptomatic at the start of the study —
                   and that also meant that they had no need for regular
                   anti-asthmatic treatment. However, all patients had
                   an increased bronchial reactivity and there was a wide
                   range (PC_{25} between 0.0075 and 8mg/ml). So I think
                   we have a mixed group of asymptomatic asthmatics
                   with good possibilities for improvement.

RICHARDSON   Dr Patel, how much effect did the wide age range
(Bromley, UK)   from 17 years to 54 years have on the results?

PATEL   All our patients had reproducible asthma and positive
                   skin tests and in that respect there was nothing
                   different between patients. Most were under 30.

STERN   Could the bronchodilatation after exercise plus sodium
(Leicester, UK)   cromoglycate be due to the unmasking of an effect of
                   exercise, rather than true bronchodilatation by the
                   drug?

PATEL   It is possible. I would not like to postulate on the
                   mechanism of bronchodilatation with sodium cromo-
                   glycate.

BURGE   Was the sodium cromoglycate nebulised during expir-
(Birmingham,   ation as well as during inspiration? If so, the dose
UK)   during inspiration would be about one third of the
                   total dose that was given.

PATEL   Yes. What I mentioned was the dose that was nebulised,
                   but I am not sure how much of this got into the lung.
                   The range is between 8—16 per cent with the method
                   we use.

HARRIES   Have you shown a statistically significant difference
(London, UK)   in the protective effect of 10mg compared with 40mg
                   sodium cromoglycate?

PATEL   No.

HAIDER   Did you observe any difference in the duration of
(Bury, UK)   protective effect of sodium cromoglycate with differ-
                ent doses?

PATEL   Yes. We have conducted a trial which showed that the
                effect of 2mg wears off by four hours, whereas with
                20mg and 40mg there is still some protection at four
                hours. We have not taken the study beyond four hours.

McKENZIE   What *is* known about the site of deposition of the
(Romford, UK)   various presentations of sodium cromoglycate? What
                are the difficulties of labelling this compound and
                using lung scanning to try to answer this question?

PATEL   You can label sodium cromoglycate with ^{14}C. It is
                difficult to tag a gamma emitter on to sodium cromo-
                glycate without changing its characteristics. We
                thought of using radiolabelled Teflon discs of a similar
                particle size. There are differences in the physical
                properties of the sodium cromoglyate crystal com-
                pared with a Teflon disc and the results with Teflon
                discs may therefore not apply to sodium cromoglycate.

AAS   One of my tasks is to referee papers for publication in
                journals and I find it very frustrating to have to reject
                more than 80 per cent of the papers on this and similar
                subjects. Why? Because, for instance, the same statisti-
                cal rules for significance that were created for methods
                with less than one per cent range of reproducibility
                are adopted for biological tests in which there may be
                a 30 per cent range of reproducibility. Furthermore
                you have not calibrated your instrument − that is,
                the tests you use. We know how difficult it is to repeat
                tests in biology which means that we need more data
                on methods, precision, reliability and on reproduci-
                bility, both for the challenge as such and for the
                method of measuring lung function. So I would ask
                you to bear these points in mind when making your
                decisions about protocols.

PART V

**THE USE OF PHYSICAL ACTIVITY PROGRAMMES
IN THE HABILITATION AND REHABILITATION
OF ASTHMATIC CHILDREN**

Chairman: Dr A M Edwards, Loughborough, United Kingdom

Chapter 22

PHYSICAL ACTIVITY AS PART OF A COMPREHENSIVE REHABILITATION PROGRAMME IN ASTHMATIC CHILDREN

S Oseid

The Norwegian College of Physical Education and Sport; and Children's Asthma and Allergy Institute, Voksentoppen, Oslo, Norway

SUMMARY

Bronchial obstruction triggered by physical exercise represents a major clinical problem and a severe handicap to young asthmatic children, restricting their normal physical and psychological development.

Several studies indicate that the avoidance of exercise is unwarranted and detrimental for young children with asthma. Although exercise provokes bronchospasm in 80–90 per cent of the children studied, the severity of exercise-induced asthma can be reduced by physical activity programmes based on the following four principles: premedication with beta-adrenergic drugs and/or sodium cromoglycate, sufficient warm-up periods, interval training, and exercise with submaximal work loads.

Traditionally the treatment of asthmatic children has been orientated towards help during an attack. However, we feel it necessary to offer children with chronic diseases a form of treatment beyond the acute stage. We want to enable them to enjoy physical activity and to give them confidence and enthusiasm to take part in activities beyond that offered traditionally. We set out to show them that this is possible despite their asthma.

The use of programmes of physical activity, with the emphasis on group treatment, has played a major role in the total rehabilitation of our patients. The beneficial long-term effects observed in our studies were: increase in aerobic fitness, enhanced exercise tolerance with fewer asthmatic repercussions during and after exercise, improvement in bodily awareness, increased self-confidence and greater social and psychological independence.

INTRODUCTION

Bronchial obstruction triggered by physical exercise is of more than theoretical interest since it represents a major clinical problem and a severe handicap for young asthmatic children restricting their normal physical and psychological development [1].

Vigorous physical activity often leads to acute exacerbation of asthmatic symptoms, and the degree of bronchoconstriction is more pronounced if the child already suffers from clinical or subclinical chronic obstruction [2]. In some individuals exercise is apparently the only stimulus to provoke asthma, but that is rare. Consequently, the use of physical activity programmes in the habilitation and rehabilitation of asthmatic children has been controversial and regarded by many doctors as irrelevant or of minor value even when broadly based and attempting to deal with the complete life situation of the asthmatic child. The lack of scientific documentation has been an obstacle to its acceptance, and much of the criticism of the various approaches is therefore justified.

The physical benefits are mostly obvious and fairly easy to establish [3—5]. However, the psychological and social benefits which are probably of more importance with regard to prognosis, are more difficult to substantiate [4, 6]. But there is yet another very important aspect that is frequently forgotten — namely, the assessment of the intrinsic value of play and sport in themselves and perhaps even their cultural value.

THE NORWEGIAN APPROACH

The physical treatment of asthmatic children has for many decades traditionally been orientated towards help during an attack (as, for example, breathing control and the use of relaxation positions), postural drainage and isolated exercises to correct chest deformities. In Norway this was previously carried out in institutions situated either in the mountains or deep in the countryside. Programmes of management consisted of symptomatic medication and residence in a dry climate where air pollution was minimal. More active treatment or the initiation of rehabilitation programmes was not attempted. The children were kept in these institutions for prolonged periods, often with a deleterious effect on their psychological and intellectual development.

Today the care of asthmatic children in Norway to a great extent is organised through children's hospitals or children's units in regional hospitals. Besides, the University Hospital in Oslo, with the financial support from the Norwegian Red Cross Association, in 1971 built the specialised Children's Asthma and Allergy Institute, Voksentoppen – which in addition to basic research activities, diagnostic evaluation and introduction of broadly based programmes of treatment also functions as a habilitation and activity centre for asthmatic children referred from all parts of Norway.

In working with these asthmatic children, we feel it essential to offer them treatment beyond the acute stage. We want to enable them to enjoy physical activity and give them confidence and enthusiasm to take part in activities beyond those of the initial treatment programme. We expend considerable effort to show them that this is possible despite their asthma.

Treatment of the child with asthma by means of physical training programmes, with the emphasis on group treatment, has played a major role in the total rehabilitation of our patients. We initiate these programmes which can then be followed up locally, at school, in sport clubs, or with friends and members of the family supervised by health personnel or physical education instructors [4, 7].

Before they are included in these rehabilitation programmes most children undergo exercise tolerance tests and measurements of lung function. A bicycle ergometer or a treadmill is used to evaluate the degree of exercise-induced asthma and also, if required, the aerobic capacity. The results give guidance to the composition of the rehabiliation group and also, to a certain extent, to those activities that would be recommendable. The exercise tests also help us to evaluate which drugs should be given to the individual patient.

These studies have shown that nearly 80 per cent of the children referred to Voksentoppen develop exercise-induced asthma, which in our hospital is defined as a fall of at least 15 per cent in pulmonary function – measured by peak expiratory flow rate (PEFR) and forced expiratory volume in one second (FEV_1) – in the post-exercise period in individuals with an asthmatic predisposition.

In addition to our regular programmes in the Institute and at Voksentoppen School, which is closely connected with the Institute, different groups of children recruited from our outpatients department undergo regular physical training of one hour's duration two to three times per week for periods up to four to six months. The training is designed to improve endurance, muscle strength and joint flexibility. The training also includes a 14-day intensive programme at Beitostølen Health Sport Center, where every day the children participate in three training sessions, outdoors (skiing in the winter, hiking, ball games, canoeing and kayaking in the summer) and indoors (different activities in the gymnasium and in the swimming pool).

These programmes increase the aerobic capacity by 10–20 per cent [1], and the children also experience a considerable improvement of muscle strength, both statically and dynamically [1]. The dynamic muscle strength in the asthmatic children undergoing the training programmes was improved over that of a control group of similar age and degree of disability who did not take part in regular physical exercise.

The exercise tolerance tests, including lung function measurements, and in the absence of premedication, were performed before and after a training period of three and a half months' duration on 10 pre-pubertal asthmatic children. One would presume that a training effect would influence pulmonary function after exercise and indeed the fall in lung function produced by an ergometer test was considerably less after the training programme than before it. However, this does not necessarily mean that there has been any direct improvement of lung function – what it does mean is that as a result of improved aerobic capacity, the exercise tolerance limit has been increased so that, with identical work loads, there is a significantly smaller fall in lung function. The asthmatic child experiences this as a significant improvement of his physical fitness with fewer subjective symptoms and considerably less bronchial obstruction. An example of such an increase in exercise tolerance is shown in Figure 1. In this girl lung function studies were performed before and after 14 days of intense conditioning preceded by three and a half months of regular endurance training two to three times weekly.

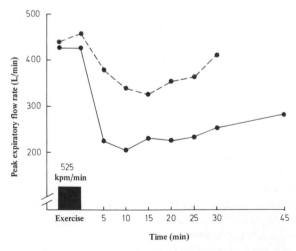

Figure 1. Peak expiratory flow rates in a 13½-year-old girl after exercise on a bicycle ergometer before (———) and after (– – – –) a 14-day conditioning programme

RELEVANCE OF PHYSICAL TRAINING PROGRAMMES FOR THE CHILD WITH ASTHMA

It must be remembered that in our Institute we are involved in the treatment of the more severe asthmatics. Not all asthmatic children have the problems mentioned here, since, as in other illnesses there are many degrees of disability. In spite of this, our experience supports our previous suggestions that even lesser degrees of asthma can lead to disability and social isolation with a harmful effect on the child's self-confidence and motor development.

We consider the following six points to be of great importance.

(1) Asthmatics need regular physical activity as do all children. They need, in fact, to be fitter than healthy children in order to have something to fall back on in bad periods.

(2) Asthmatics are often in poor physical condition and even small amounts of exercise can prove difficult without promoting wheeziness.

(3) Children with exercise-induced asthma benefit from a systematic programme of endurance and muscle strengthening exercises. Their exercise tolerance level thus is increased allowing them to take part more freely in physical activities with fewer asthmatic repercussions.

(4) It is also important that a child with asthma develops a positive attitude towards physical activity. The restrictions placed upon the child and the often over-protective parental attitude may result in social isolation. Physical activity is often associated with wheeziness, distress and defeat. The child eventually withdraws from any form of exercise that puts physical demands upon him and looks upon himself as physically inferior. The child is assigned to the category of a sick person.

(5) The need to feel that one belongs to a group is very important — especially for children. Asthmatics are often onlookers wanting to join in but unable to do so because of their disability.

(6) They are often exempted from gym at school. Therefore a physical training programme can be used as a 'springboard' to give them the necessary encouragement to take part in physical education at school or in games with their fellows at home or in sports clubs.

ORGANISATION OF THE ACTIVITY PROGRAMMES

Before taking part in group activities, asthmatic children must be given the opportunity to test their own limits under secure medical supervision. An exercise tolerance test is a valuable and objective method of assessing progress both for the child and the leader. Co-operation between the doctor and the group leader is therefore of great advantage whenever this can be arranged. Physical activity programmes also allow the child to discover how much he can tolerate before becoming wheezy.

How well a child functions physically is dependent upon confidence in his own capabilities. One of the objectives, therefore, is for the child to realise that: "I can take part despite my asthma". But how do we achieve our objectives? Group treatment is essential, as are the following basic conditions.

Premedication

Before all physical activity premedication with sodium cromoglycate or a beta-adrenergic drug is essential for most patients with exercise-induced asthma. Sodium cromoglycate should be administered (after the bronchodilator, if required) 5—10 minutes before starting activity, either by using the Spinhaler or the aerosol. Sustained-release theophylline preparations have also been reported to be of value in preventing exercise-induced asthma.

Long warm-up period of mild intensity

In order to prevent wheeziness, it is essential to have a longer and less strenuous warming-up period than is usual. This is especially important for those children with exercise-induced asthma, since beginning a session with activities that put strong demands upon the cardio-respiratory system invariably results in bronchial obstruction, despite premedication. The warm-up period of 10—15 minutes should include activities whose intensity the patient is able to control for himself, thereby discovering his own exercise tolerance level and its limits. The principles of interval training should also be applied in this warming-up period.

Interval training

It is generally accepted that interval training is especially useful for building up endurance. When working with asthmatics it is important that the more demanding work periods do not last longer than three minutes if bronchial obstruction is to be prevented. This does not mean that the child suddenly stops in the middle of an activity (this is both artificial and unnecessary) but that less strenuous work periods are interspersed with the more strenuous ones, though the child is not allowed to have complete rest periods which may induce exercise-induced asthma. Games, such as ball games and relay races, that contain natural interval periods are particularly useful. The training programmes should be as natural as possible, not continually reminding the child of his asthma. The group treatment should above all be enjoyable.

Training with a submaximal work load

To ensure that the work load is not too great, heart rates of 160–170 beats/min are aimed at in pre-pubertal children and up to 180 beats/min in younger children.

A training session should last 45–60 minutes. Circuit training, relay races, ball games, movement free dance, swimming, kayak paddling or canoeing and skiing are examples of activities that are beneficial for children with asthma.

ATTITUDES AND RESPONSES

A child's physical training is play.

Keeping this in mind, we should strive consciously to include play activities in the training programmes. The word 'training' is traditionally associated with the blood, sweat and tears of competition. But accepting play as a form of training, we can give the asthmatic child the opportunity of a more enjoyable form of training as a part of his natural development – something that is especially important for those who are reluctant to take part in physical activities. This does not mean that play reduces the demands put on the child. Learning correct swimming techniques, for example, makes pool activities more effective and more fun.

Reactions to group treatment vary. Some children react with tears, tantrums and may even resort to violent protest. Group treatment can be self-revealing and can result in the child provoking an asthmatic reaction, either consciously or unconsciously. Such reactions are often expressions of inadequacy, due to the lack of body awareness and self-confidence. The attitude we have towards our own body is one aspect of how we regard ourselves generally. Improving a person's bodily awareness gives him greater confidence in himself, as a person, and makes him more positive and secure in different situations.

The demonstration of the child's ability to participate in programmes of physical activity (play and sport) in institutions and at school will eventually reduce the overprotective attitude of parents, teachers – and doctors. If the programme is successful, the child gains self-confidence through physical activity, develops ability to socialise and thus integrates more easily with other children.

FOLLOW-UP

Our aim as therapists must be to make ourselves superfluous to the individual asthmatic – but only when he is ready for it. Our supporting function should be necessary for a limited period only, as we must work towards making the patient independent, both in relation to his asthma and to the community. He does belong, after all, at home and at school and it is there that he must fit in and function. We are often faced with the problem of 'follow-up' when the child returns home since it is important for these children to continue with physical activity in their home environment. We often try to persuade them to join some sort of club: athletics, football or swimming, for example. Modern or classical ballet classes are often good alternatives for girls. It is, therefore, necessary to inform the club leader or the physical education teacher at school how they best can help the child to function to the full extent of his ability.

In order to do this, we must involve the parents as early as possible. Both individual and group meetings with parents allow us to give them the information they need and have the right to expect. These meetings also give us the opportunity to learn of their experiences and of the problems involved in having a severe asthmatic in the family. It is important to put their expectations into words and, at the same time, to explain what the child is taking part in and why. Parental co-operation is an essential factor in the follow-up of these patients.

The demands imposed by a group training programme can be so great that both parent and child need all the support we can give them. Sometimes we succeed, sometimes not.

CONCLUSIONS

Treatment of the child with asthma through physical training programmes, with the emphasis on group treatment, has played a major role in the total rehabilitation of our patients.

We aim to provide programmes and recommendations for the child and the adolescent; the family; responsible professional people and the community.

The following beneficial long-term effects of these physical training programmes have been recorded: increase in aerobic fitness; enhanced exercise tolerance with fewer asthmatic repercussions during and after exercise; improvement of bodily awareness; increased self-confidence, and greater social and psychological independence.

References

1 Oseid S, Haaland K.
   Exercise studies on asthmatic children before and after regular physical training.
   In Eriksson BO, Furberg B, eds.
   International Series on Sports Sciences. Swimming Medicine IV 1978; 32–41.
   Baltimore: University Park Press

2 Oseid S, Aas K.
   Exercise-induced asthma.
   Allergy 1978; 33: 227–228

3 Fitch KD, Morton AR, Blanksby BA.
   Effects of swimming training on children with asthma.
   Arch Dis Child 1976; 51: 190–194

4 Oseid S, Kendall M, Larsen RB, Selbekk R.
   Physical activity programs for children with exercise induced asthma.
   In Eriksson BO, Furberg B, eds.
   International Series on Sports Sciences. Vol 6: Swimming Medicine IV 1978;
   42–51. Baltimore: University Park Press

5 Svenonius E, Kantto R, Arborelius M.
   Improvement after training of children with exercise-induced asthma.
   Acta Paediatr Scand 1982. In press

6 Graff-Lonnevig V, Bevegård S, Eriksson BO et al.
   Two years follow-up of asthmatic boys participating in a physical activity
   programme. *Acta Paediatr Scand 1980; 69:* 347–352

7 Oseid S.
   Exercise-induced asthma. A review.
   In Berg K, Eriksson BO, eds.
   International Series on Sports Sciences. Vol 10: Children and Exercise IX 1980;
   277–288. Baltimore: University Park Press

Chapter 23

SPORT, PHYSICAL ACTIVITY AND THE ASTHMATIC

K D Fitch

Department of Human Movement and Recreation Studies,
The University of Western Australia, Nedlands,
Western Australia

SUMMARY

Asthmatics have a unique relationship to physical activity. Exercise can be shown to provoke bronchoconstriction in most asthmatics and this has been utilised extensively to examine exercise-induced asthma during the past two decades. Paradoxically, regular physical activity and participation in sports are considered to be important components in the overall management of asthma, especially in children and adolescents — this aspect of the link between asthma and exercise has been under-researched.

Laboratory studies have confirmed the clinical impression from both gymnasia and playing fields that intermittent patterns of exercise are less provocative of exercise-induced asthma than continuous exertion. Recent research has revealed that 'running through asthma' may be a misnomer and merely reflect enhanced endurance fitness rather than 'exhaustion of chemical mediators'. Exercise-induced asthma occurs even after long periods of continuous running. Thus pre-exercise prophylactic medication is essential for all who are at risk of developing exercise-induced asthma. Sodium cromoglycate and a beta$_2$-adrenergic drug (fenoterol, salbutamol or terbutaline) should be administered by aerosol, either singly or in combination, immediately before exercise. Beta agonists rapidly reverse exercise-induced asthma in almost every instance and should be always available. All of these drugs have been approved for international sports competitions which are subject to doping controls.

Because it is less likely to induce asthma, swimming is an excellent activity for asthmatics to undertake regularly and thereby develop exertional confidence and competence. With adequate control of asthma and exercise-induced asthma, a normal physical and sporting lifestyle should be the goal. However, between swimming programmes solely for asthmatics and unrestricted participation in sport, those with chronic and severe asthma often require medically supervised programmes of graded physical activity. After a warm-up the major activities should be aerobic and intermittent. They should include basic motor skills, emphasising participation — not competition — and aim to induce pleasure and social interaction — not distress or boredom. Psychological gains often outstrip physical benefits. For those severe asthmatics who are unable to tolerate any land-based activity more intense than walking, water polo is a valuable adjunct to swimming.

Publication of success by asthmatics in international sport is a great boost for those having difficulty with exercise-induced asthma. Even training to world level does not eliminate exercise bronchial hyperreactivity. This fact was once again demonstrated at the XXII Olympiad where each of the three Australian asthmatic medal winners — two gold (swimmers), one silver (track athlete) — required medication before the event.

INTRODUCTION

Asthmatics have a unique relationship to physical activity. On the one hand, exercise will induce bronchoconstriction in most asthmatics — a technique that has been utilised extensively to examine exercise-induced asthma during the past two decades. On the other hand, regular physical activity and participation in sport are considered by most authorities to be significant components in the overall management of asthma, especially in children and adolescents. By comparison with the amount of work that has been done on how and why exercise provokes increased airways resistance, this aspect of the link between asthma and exercise has received relatively little research attention.

HISTORY OF EXERCISE PRESCRIPTION

Biologically man is an animal with an evolutional need for physical activity. People with asthma have an equal, or perhaps greater, need for regular exercise than those without. Regrettably, and too often, because of an inability to compete with their normal contemporaries on account of their exercise-induced asthma — and compounded by frequent absences from school and sport as a result of asthma and periods in hospital — many asthmatics are either unable to participate in sport and physical recreation or are able to do so only to a very limited extent.

Historically, one of the first reports of exercise being prescribed for a patient with asthma was in 1551 when the patient was the 40-year-old

Archibald Hamilton, Archbishop of St Andrew's, and the physician, Professor Cardan from Pavia [1]. Apart from some wise general measures, Cardan ordered a daily ride on horseback for the cleric who had been incapacitated for 10 years. Buchan [2] in 1769 advised asthmatics to take as much daily exercise as they could bear, whether on foot, on horseback or in a carriage, while Cullen [3] in 1784 recommended riding and sailing. A notable of the 19th century who had asthma was Theodore Roosevelt, later president of the USA. Encouraged by his doctor and his father, he embarked on a strenuous programme of walking, swimming, rowing and running and is said to have obtained great benefit [4]. About the same time, Thorogood [5] wrote in the 1873 edition of his *Notes on Asthma* that several patients had related that a steady walk could prevent an attack of asthma "even when it threatens".

Apart from these notable exceptions, the value of exercise in the management of asthma was neither acknowledged nor recommended by most authors. *Physical Exercises for the Asthmatic*, published in 1934 for the Asthma Research Council of Great Britain [6], contained nothing more strenuous than remedial breathing exercises. It appears that a report presented in 1958 by Scherr and Frankel [7] of West Virginia, USA, may have triggered off an era of more vigorous exercise prescription for asthmatics. Labelled the 'Bucking Bronchos' from bucking bronchial asthma, these authors described a physical conditioning programme involving gymnastics, wrestling, basketball and swimming.

ASTHMAGENICITY OF VARIOUS FORMS AND PATTERNS OF EXERCISE

Swimming is now well accepted as the least asthmagenic exercise of any degree of intensity [8] although the reason remains obscure. Suggestions that it can be explained simply by the inspiration of humidified air have been disproved. In a study in Israel, Inbar and his colleagues [9] demonstrated that swimming while breathing either dry or humid air did not provoke exercise-induced asthma in marked contrast to running at similar metabolic and ventilatory rates.

The long-held and often quoted belief that interrupted patterns of physical activity are less asthmagenic than continuous exercise, has been verified. In a recent study Morton and his colleagues [10] reported that continuous treadmill running provoked exercise-induced asthma with significantly greater frequency and severity than any of four different intermittent running regimens (Figure 1). Whether this finding is a consequence of reduced minute ventilation and thus lowered respiratory heat

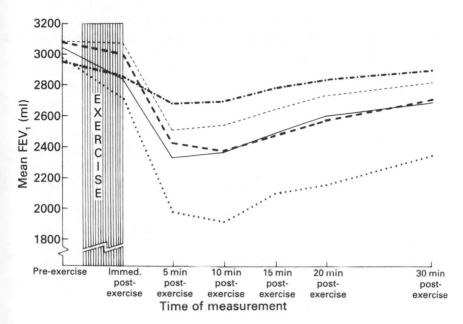

Figure 1. Mean FEV_1 values of 27 subjects before and at various stages after each of five differently organised sessions of treadmill running. . . . – A. Continuous running for 6 minutes (slow); – – – = B. 3 minutes running, 5 minutes rest, 3 minutes running (slow); — · — = C. 36 repetitions of 10 seconds running, 30 seconds rest (slow); —— = D. 20 repetitions of 10 seconds running, 30 seconds rest (fast); - - - - = E. 10 repetitions of 20 seconds running, 60 seconds rest (fast)
(Reproduced by permission of Annals of Allergy)

loss, or is a manifestation of tachyphylaxis is unclear. However, its therapeutic implications are important.

Repeated exercise performed on the same day with short rests (less than an hour) result in a temporary state of refractoriness to further exercise challenge [11]. While this may not be relevant to clinical exercise prescription, a recent re-evaluation of the duration of continuous running on the provocation of exercise-induced asthma is. Morton and his colleagues (unpublished observations) observed little difference in the incidence and severity of exercise-induced asthma after submaximal treadmill running for varying periods of between eight and 32 minutes. 'Running through asthma' may thus be a misnomer and merely reflect enhanced endurance fitness rather than exhaustion of chemical mediators. Of interest was the occurrence of exercise-induced asthma which necessitated a 25-year-old man to stop at the 35km mark of his first marathon. This happened about four hours after his pre-run aerosol salbutamol dose of 200µg. A hand-held salbutamol nebuliser was promptly dispatched to the runner and rapidly reversed his exercise-induced asthma, enabling him to complete the 26 miles 385 yards (42km) in a very modest 4 hours 25 minutes.

Environmental factors can contribute significantly to the provocation or amelioration of exercise-induced asthma. Warming [12] and humidifying [13] the inspired air reduces or abolishes running-induced bronchospasm – which is probably the mechanism whereby wearing a surgical face mask [14] or nasal breathing [15] reduces exercise-induced asthma. Cooling [16] and drying [17] the inspired air aggravates exercise-induced asthma. Air pollutants have attracted little research attention, although sulphur dioxide [18] and ozone [19] appear to have detrimental effects on hyper-responsive airways.

As the XXIII Olympiad is being held in Los Angeles, a city with significant problems of air pollution, there is an urgent need to study the effects of strenuous exercise by asthmatics in environments containing different oxidative and reductive pollutants and the pharmacological modification of any unfavourable consequences.

PRE-EXERCISE MEDICATION

As has been demonstrated in many studies from many countries, sodium cromoglycate as a pre-exercise agent effectively reduces or abolishes exercise-induced asthma in about 70 per cent of asthmatics [20] (Figure 2). The aerosol beta$_2$-agonists, salbutamol, terbutaline and fenoterol, are equally effective in both the prevention and reversal of exercise-induced asthma. The combination of sodium cromoglycate and an aerosol beta$_2$-adrenergic stimulant provides particularly effective protection. However, because of a waning of the protection afforded by these agents [21,22], it is essential to ensure that a dose is administered immediately before exercise either by modifying the timing of regular medication or by giving an additional dose. All persons who are at risk of developing exercise-induced asthma should avail themselves of suitable pre-exercise medication to enable them to participate in physical activity and sport with minimal respiratory disadvantage. Of importance is the fact that the asthmatic athlete subjected to doping control procedures is no longer disadvantaged (Table I).

CURRENT CONCEPTS OF EXERCISE PRESCRIPTION

Although research into exercise-induced asthma has been undertaken by most investigators primarily to elucidate the mechanisms of its occurrence and to evaluate its modification by pharmacological means, the knowledge

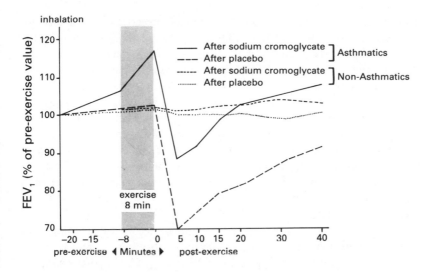

Figure 2. Changes in mean FEV$_1$ after eight minutes of submaximal treadmill running after inhalation of sodium cromoglycate and placebo. ——— = after sodium cromoglycate; − − − = after placebo in asthmatics; - - - - - = after sodium cromoglycate; · · · · · = after placebo in non-asthmatics
(Reproduced by permission of the *Medical Journal of Australia*)

TABLE I. Drugs used to prevent exercise-induced asthma: effectiveness and legal status for competition* (Reprinted by permission of the *Physician and Sportsmedicine*, a McGraw-Hill publication)

Drug	Route of administration	Effectiveness	Legal or banned
Ephedrine	Oral	Uncertain	Banned
Isoprenaline	Oral	Slight	Banned
	Aerosol	Fair	Banned
Orciprenaline	Oral	Fair	Banned
	Aerosol	Good	Banned
Atropine	Aerosol	Slight	Legal
Glucocorticosteroids	Oral	Uncertain	Legal
	Aerosol	Uncertain	Legal
Theophylline	Oral	Good	Legal
Sodium cromoglycate	Aerosol	Good	Legal
Beta$_2$ -agonists			
Salbutamol	Oral	Good	Legal
Terbutaline	Aerosol	Excellent	Legal
Fenoterol			

*According to the Medical Commission of the International Olympic Committee thus gained has provided a sound basis for the prescription of exercise for asthmatics. It is of interest that empirical recommendations, mainly based on experience derived, for example, from swimming, intermittent exercise and a preference for warm humidified environments, have been borne out by laboratory research.

Despite the absence of research evidence [23], it has been suggested [24] that a warm-up period may reduce exercise-induced asthma because of a graduated release of chemical mediators. Warm-up is well known to be advisable before moderate or intense physical activity for a variety of reasons – for example, to reduce the risk of injury, to assist flexibility and to enhance skill and performance. In practice, warming-up activities often alleviate mild wheeze or tightness in the chest, possibly due to the release of catecholamines.

Programmes of physical activities for asthmatics should include warming up for reasons apart from any possible respiratory benefit and is recommended in published examples from Norway [25], Sweden [26], the USA [27] and Australia [28]. Likewise, cooling down [28] should be undertaken for the benefit of the circulatory and musculoskeletal systems whether respiratory gains will be achieved or not. The subject of warming up and cooling down begs further research.

Although the mechanism may remain in dispute, there is little disagreement on the low asthmagenic potential of swimming. This is adequate justification for its being termed the cornerstone of exercise prescription for asthmatics. Extensive experience in many countries has demonstrated the safety and success of swimming for asthmatics of virtually all ages and all degrees of severity [29]. The special problems of teaching children with asthma to swim have been elaborated upon [30]. One noteworthy feature of swimming is that it is an available exercise and will benefit even the most severely afflicted, including those with chronic severe asthma, totally steroid-dependent and with Cushingoid side-effects (S Oseid, personal communication).

While swimming remains the activity through which asthmatics can achieve confidence in exertional activities and attain basic aerobic fitness, the aim of those with mild to moderate asthma should be to lead normal physical and sporting lives. Each individual can be allowed to choose his own activity or sport depending on skill, availability, body build, aspiration and cost. No asthmatic should be excluded from any sport or physical activity for which he or she has the necessary training and skill. Restrictions should be imposed only during a bout of asthma or infection or when exertional asthma cannot be controlled. Scuba diving is an oft-quoted contraindication, presumably because it is believed asthmatics are more prone to pulmonary barotrauma. Since many asthmatics have participated successfully and uneventfully in scuba diving, its exclusion must be questioned.

Selection for a team sport is a major objective for many asthmatics. It is fortunate that intermittent patterns of running, which are part of most ball games, are well tolerated [10]. However, a measure of tolerance by coaches is often necessary. Apart from the need to take medication before and possibly during exercise, special difficulties include the unfavourable nature of prolonged, continuous running, especially in cold, dry weather and the problem of wheeze before a game. Not infrequently asthmatics are erroneously excluded because of a mild wheeze before the event. The resulting disappointment is likely to exacerbate the wheeze, whereas exercise-induced bronchodilatation would probably stop the wheeze if the asthmatic was allowed to take part.

Between the two extremes of participating solely in special swimming classes for asthmatics and participating unrestrictedly in sports, there is a need for medically supervised programmes of graded physical activities for those with chronic and severe asthma. After warming up, the major activities should be aerobic and intermittent. They should include basic motor skills with the emphasis on participation, not competition, and aim to be pleasurable and encourage social interaction, not distress or boredom. Games and physical training programmes of this type are valuable and have been described in depth by Oseid and his colleagues [25].

Teenagers, particularly those who had severe asthma in childhood and have residual chest deformity and poor muscle development, become aware of their physical peculiarities and wish to do something about them. Weight training, rowing, canoeing and the martial arts help in the development of the upper part of the body. For those severe asthmatics who are unable to tolerate any land-based activity more intense than walking, water polo is a valuable sequel to swimming and provides the camaraderie of a team game.

BENEFITS OF REGULAR EXERCISE

The benefits obtained by asthmatics from regular participation in physical activity and sport may be subdivided into physical, psychological and social.

Physical benefits

Physical gains include increased aerobic fitness which will reduce the ventilation rate as well as the heart rate, for any given submaximal load.

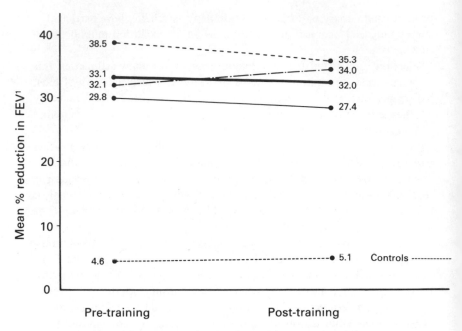

Figure 3. Effect of five months of swimming training on mean maximum percentage reduction of FEV_1 after nine minutes of submaximal treadmill running to attain and maintain heart rates of 170 beats/min. Grouping of asthmatic swimmers based on achieved swimming distance: group 1 (n = 14) swam less than 50km; group 2 (n = 16) swam 50–100km; group 3 (n = 16) swam more than 100km. Control group (n = 16) were free of asthma and swam more than 100km. Group 1 – – –; group 2 – · –; group 3 ——; all asthmatics ▬▬ (Reproduced by permission of University Park Press)

Improvements in breathing mechanics, posture, lean body mass, cardiac output and muscle strength and endurance can be expected [31]. Reductions in the requirements for medication [32], the frequency and severity of asthma [32,33] and absenteeism from school and work have all been reported [33].

Running-induced bronchial reactivity was found to be unchanged after a five months' programme of swimming training by 46 Australian asthmatic children and adolescents [32] (Figure 3). This is not in conflict with evidence from Norway [34]. In the Norwegian study, the same cycling challenge before and after training showed a significant mean reduction of exercise-induced asthma. In the Australian investigation the exercise stress after training was increased (by a mean of 11%) to match each subject's improved aerobic fitness. Thus the running challenges before and after training represented an equal percentage of their $\dot{V}O_{2\,max}$. The effect of a running training programme on running-induced bronchial lability is currently under investigation.

Psychological benefits

Both asthmatics and their parents may gain psychologically. Not only do they achieve a more positive attitude towards exercise, but the improved physique, lessened asthma and superior fitness result in a more confident, less introverted child. The parents are inevitably affected and they react by becoming less protective and imposing fewer restrictions [32]. They develop a better understanding of asthma and a greater confidence in handling their child, when well or ill.

Selection as a member of a sporting team, solely on merit, is a major achievement for both the asthmatic child and his or her parents and gives a significant psychological boost to all concerned.

Social benefits

Social benefits are derived from group programmes of physical activities. The gains achieved as a result of groups meeting regularly have been previously reported [25]. A valuable addition is the summer camp for children with asthma, which has become a major annual event in the lives of many Australian asthmatics [35]. With medical, physiotherapy, nursing and physical education staff to back up group leaders, asthmatic children from completely different social backgrounds and very different geographical locations thrive on camp life. The social and physical environments benefit the introverted, overprotected child whose previous absences from home have solely been in hospital. Each child rapidly discovers that he or she is not unique and the social interaction of fixed groups or teams within the camp evokes positive reactions in all children. The gains for the parents are significant, too; often they sleep easily and uninterruptedly for the first time in many years.

Group activities and camps with other asthmatics often lead to such improvements — physical, psychological and social — that the child becomes more confident and starts to move out from recreation arranged solely for asthmatics to join his or her normal contemporaries in a variety of sporting and social activities.

SUCCESS BY ASTHMATICS IN SPORT

Asthmatics have achieved outstanding success in a variety of sports [30]. Those of us constantly involved in promoting exercise as an integral and essential component of the lifestyle of asthmatics, have observed that publication of sporting successes by asthmatics has been a great boost to others. It is pleasing to note the readiness with which a number of outstanding sportsmen and women with asthma have allowed their condition to be publicised.

Despite the intense training necessary to become a world champion, the bronchial hyperreactivity to exercise does not appear to be obliterated. This fact was once again demonstrated at the 1980 Olympic Games when each of the three Australian asthmatics who won medals – two gold (swimming), one silver (track athletics) – required medication before their events.

References

1   Major RH.
    A note on the history of asthma. In Underwood EA, ed.
    Science, Medicine and History 1953; 2: 522.
    London: Oxford University Press

2   Buchan W.
    Domestic Medicine 1854.
    Philadelphia: W W Leary

3   Cullen W.
    Practice of Physic 1784.
    Edinburgh: W Crech

4   Szanton VL.
    Theodore Roosevelt, the asthmatic.
    Ann Allergy 1969; 27: 485

5   Thorogood JC.
    Notes on Asthma, 2nd edition 1873.
    London: Churchill

6   Hurst A, Livingstone JL, Reed J.
    Physical Exercises for Asthma 1934.
    London: Headley Brothers for the Asthma Research Council

7   Scherr MS, Frankel L.
    Physical conditioning for asthmatic children.
    JAMA 1958; 168: 1996–2000

8   Fitch KD, Morton AR.
    Specificity of exercise in exercise-induced asthma.
    Br Med J 1971; 4: 577–581

9   Inbar O, Dotan R, Dlin RA et al.
    Breathing dry or humid air and exercise-induced asthma during swimming.
    Eur J Appl Physiol 1980; 44: 43–50

10   Morton AR, Hahn AG, Fitch KD.
     Continuous and intermittent running in the provocation of asthma.
     Ann Allergy 1982; 48: 123–129

11   Edmunds AT, Tooley M, Godfrey S.
     The refractory period after exercise-induced asthma.
     Am Rev Respir Dis 1981; 67: 391–397

12   Chen WY, Horton DJ.
     Heat and water loss from the airways and exercise-induced asthma.
     Respiration 1977; 34: 305–313

13   Bar-Or O, Neuman I, Dotan R.
     Effects of dry and humid climates on exercise-induced asthma in children and
     pre-adolescents. *J Allergy Clin Immunol 1977; 60:* 153–168

14   Brenner AM, Weiser PC, Krogh LA, Loren ML.
     Effectiveness of a portable face mask in attenuating exercise-induced asthma.
     JAMA 1980; 244: 2196–2198

15   Shturman-Ellstein R, Zeballos RH, Buckley JM, Souhrada JF.
     The beneficial effect of nasal breathing on exercise-induced bronchoconstriction.
     Am Rev Respir Dis 1978; 118: 65–73

16   Strauss RH, McFadden ER, Ingram RH, Jaeger JJ.
     Enhancement of exercise-induced asthma by cold air.
     N Engl J Med 1977; 297: 743–747

17   Deal EC, McFadden ER, Ingram RH et al.
     Role of respiratory heat exchange in production of exercise-induced asthma.
     J Appl Physiol 1979; 46: 467–475

18   Sheppard D, Saisho A, Nadel JA, Boushey HA.
     Exercise increases sulfur dioxide-induced bronchoconstriction in asthmatic
     subjects. *Am Rev Respir Dis 1981; 123:* 486–491

19   Hackney JD, Linn WS, Mohler JG et al.
     Experimental studies on human health effects of air pollutants II.
     Arch Environ Health 1975; 30: 379–384

20   Morton AR, Fitch KD.
     Sodium cromoglycate in the prevention of exercise-induced asthma.
     Med J Aust 1974; 2: 158–162

21   Anderson SD, Seale JP, Ferris L et al.
     An evaluation of pharmacotherapy for exercise-induced asthma.
     J Allergy Clin Immunol 1979; 64: 612–624

22   Silverman M, Andrea T.
     Time course of effect of disodium cromoglycate on exercise-induced asthma.
     Arch Dis Child 1972; 47: 419–422

23   Morton AR, Fitch KD, Davis T.
     The effect of 'warm-up' on exercise-induced asthma.
     Ann Allergy 1979; 42: 257–260

24   Godfrey S.
     Clinical variables of exercise-induced bronchospasm.
     In Dempsey JA, Reed C, eds. *Muscular Exercise and the Lung 1977:* 247–263.
     Madison: University of Wisconsin Press

25   Oseid S, Kendall M, Larsen RB, Selbekk R.
      Physical activity programs for children with exercise-induced asthma.
      In Eriksson B, Furberg B, eds. *Swimming Medicine IV 1978:* 45–51.
      Baltimore: University Park Press

26   Graff-Lonnevig V, Bevegard S, Eriksson BO et al.
      Two years follow-up of asthmatic boys participating in a physical activity pro-
      gramme. *Acta Paediatr Scand 1980; 69:* 347–352

27   Millman M, Grundon WG, Kasch F et al.
      Controlled exercise in asthmatic children.
      Ann Allergy 1965; 23: 220–225

28   Morton AR.
      Exercise for asthmatics.
      Patient Management 1980; 9: 55–56

29   Fitch KD, Godfrey S.
      Asthma and athletic performance.
      JAMA 1976; 236: 152–157

30   Fitch KD.
      Swimming, medicine and asthma. In Eriksson B, Furberg B, eds.
      Swimming Medicine IV 1978: 16–31.
      Baltimore: University Park Press

31   Morton AR, Fitch KD, Hahn AG.
      Physical activity and the asthmatic.
      Physician Sportsmed 1981; 9: 50–64

32   Fitch KD, Morton AR, Blanksby BA.
      Effects of swimming training on children with asthma.
      Arch Dis Child 1976; 51: 190–194

33   Petersen KH, McElhenney TR.
      Effects of a physical fitness program upon asthmatic boys.
      Pediatrics 1965; 35: 295–299

34   Oseid S, Haaland K.
      Exercise studies on asthmatic children before and after regular physical training.
      In Eriksson B, Furberg B, eds. *Swimming Medicine IV 1978;* 32–41.
      Baltimore: University Park Press

35   Isbister C.
      Summer camp for asthmatic children.
      Med J Aust 1972; 1: 768–770

Chapter 24

TRAINING, PHYSICAL FITNESS, AND HORMONE RESPONSE TO EXERCISE IN CHILDREN WITH BRONCHIAL ASTHMA

M-J Finnilä, E Kiuru, S Leisti

Jorvi Hospital, City of Espoo, Maria Hospital, City of Helsinki, and Children's Hospital, University of Helsinki, Finland

SUMMARY

Training programmes have been evaluated for improving the poor physical fitness of asthmatic children. Exercise stimulates the secretion of several hormones and training may modify the responses. Therefore, we set out to study whether the exercise-induced responses of adrenaline, cortisol and growth hormone would change during a training programme for asthmatic children.

A four-month period of physical training increased the physical working capacity of 16 asthmatic children (aged 9.3–13.6 years) by a mean of 11 per cent. The increase was greater in boys and was negatively correlated with pre-training capacity. Urinary excretion of adrenaline, measured during a submaximal exercise test, decreased during the training period; the decrease was significantly correlated with the increase in working capacity.

Before the training period exercise induced an increase in the plasma cortisol level; no increase was evident after training. In contrast, the training did not affect the exercise-induced increase in the plasma level of growth hormone. Thus, physical training reduced the reactivity of stress hormones to short submaximal exercise.

The training period had some effect on exercise-induced asthma, only two children had a decrease of more than 15 per cent in peak expiratory flow rate (PEFR) in pre-training tests, carried out on the bicycle ergometer. During the training programme we were able to demonstrate exercise-induced asthma in one-third of the children but there was a decrease during the training period.

INTRODUCTION

Children with bronchial asthma are often physically unfit which adds to their disability, especially during the pollen season at the end of the school year. Moreover, the phenomenon of exercise-induced bronchial constriction excludes any traditional approach in the attempt to improve their fitness. Two methods of training have, however, proved useful: swimming [1] and the short, repeated interval type of exercise [2] seem to avoid most of the difficulties encountered. We have reported on a training programme based on the interval type of exercise [3] in which we investigated, in particular, the responses of cortisol, growth hormone and adrenaline to bicycle ergometry tests done before and after a training period that lasted several months.

SUBJECTS AND METHODS

Our methods have already been described [3]. In brief, 16 children aged between 9 years 3 months and 13 years 6 months were offered a total of 31 training sessions on Mondays and Thursdays. All the children had bronchial asthma of several years' duration. Every 60-minute training session consisted of warming up, breathing exercises, skipping, fast jumping, chair stepping, rings, parallel bars and sports (football, table tennis, relay races). Bursts of activity were interspersed with periods of rest or lighter exercises. Working power was determined by a 12-minute bicycle ergometry test. The tests were submaximal and identical loads were used in the tests before and after the training period. Before the exercise tests an indwelling venous catheter was introduced for collecting blood samples. Half-hourly samples for determination of plasma growth hormone and cortisol levels were taken for two hours; a two-hour ACTH test followed. Also, a two-hour specimen of urine was collected for determining the exercise-induced excretion of adrenaline.

RESULTS

Figure 1 shows the effect of basal working capacity as measured in the ergometry tests before the training on the subsequent increase in the working capacity (expressed as percentage of the original capacity). It is readily apparent that only children with a low basal capacity profited from this particular training programme. A significant negative correlation was detected ($r = -0.54$, $p < 0.05$). The low intensity programme was most probably insufficient to affect the capacity in children with good basic fitness.

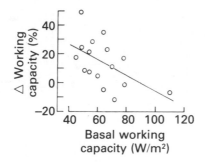

Figure 1. Training induced change (%) in the working capacity in relation to the original untrained capacity in children with bronchial asthma (r = −0.54; p < 0.05)

In Figure 2 the increase in the working capacity induced by training has been plotted against the frequency of attendance at the training sessions. Surprisingly, no difference was detectable between children with a poor attendance rate as compared with children whose attendance rate was good. Moreover, the response of the children with a low basal capacity (less than 60W/m² as indicated in the Figure) was no different to that of those with a good basal capacity. Clearly a programme that contained fewer than our planned 31 sessions may be adequate for increasing physical fitness. A short programme may also improve motivation and lead to a better attendance rate than the one illustrated by Figure 2.

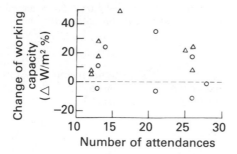

Figure 2. Effect of frequency of attendance at the training sessions on the change of working capacity in children with bronchial asthma (o = basal capacity more than 60W/m² ; △ = basal capacity equal to or less than 60W/m²)

Figure 3 shows the mean plasma cortisol and growth hormone levels as measured in samples taken before and after the bicycle ergometry test. The levels of growth hormone showed no change. The cortisol levels were raised before but not after the training period. The peak cortisol levels did not, however, show a significant difference between the two sets of measurements. The ACTH responses were unchanged.

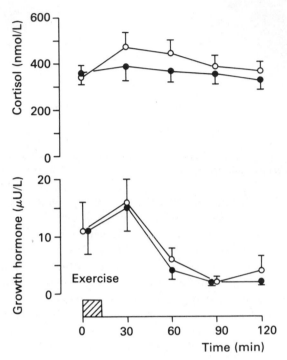

Figure 3. Mean levels of plasma cortisol and growth hormone before and after bicycle ergometry tests in children with bronchial asthma (○ = before training; ● = after training)

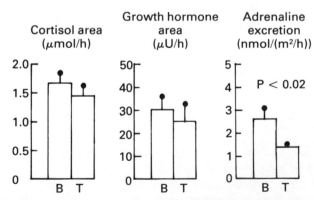

Figure 4. Effect of training on the exercise-induced secretion of cortisol and growth hormone, and excretion of adrenaline in children with bronchial asthma (B = measurements before training; T = measurements after training)

Comparison of the areas under the cortisol and growth hormone curves (Figure 4) shows no significant difference. In contrast, the excretion of adrenaline in the urine was significantly lower after the training period (Figure 4).

In Figure 5 the individual changes in plasma cortisol and growth hormone response areas, and in urinary excretion of adrenaline have been plotted against changes in the physical working capacity. The cortisol area showed no intraindividual correlation. In contrast, the excretion of adrenaline showed a significant negative correlation with the working capacity. The correlation between growth hormone area and working capacity was not significant although the plot suggests an association resembling that between adrenaline and working capacity.

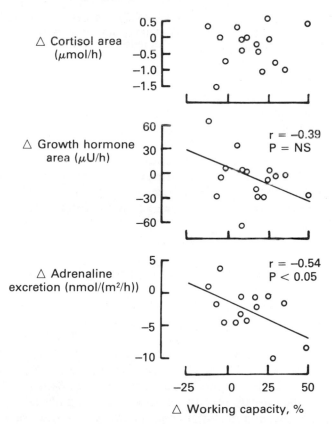

Figure 5.   Changes of the exercise-induced hormone responses in relation to the changes in the working capacity in children with bronchial asthma (intraindividual correlation plots)

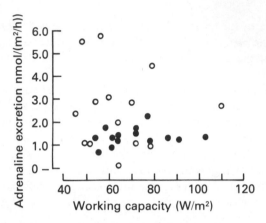

Figure 6. Association between the urinary excretion of adrenaline, as measured during exercise tests in children with bronchial asthma, and the working capacity (○ = excretion before training; ● = excretion after training)

Further analysis between the association of adrenaline and working capacity is shown in Figure 6 in which exercise-induced excretion of adrenaline is plotted against the working capacity. The plot includes both the values measured basally and the values measured after the training period. No significant correlation between individuals is detected even though the values measured before training suggest that a low working capacity may be associated with a high adrenaline response. It may be significant that only low levels of excretion of adrenaline were detected in the trained children over the whole range of working capacities (Figure 6).

DISCUSSION

Our programme was clearly effective in increasing the working capacity of children with bronchial asthma, and the mean increase was comparable to those previously published [1, 3]. However, some comments may be valuable in the planning of further training programmes.

First, only children with a low initial basal working capacity seem to profit from the type of programme described here. Nevertheless, we should not exclude children with a good capacity as their presence in small groups clearly motivates the other children. Second, objective increase in the capacity may be expected relatively early during a programme. Because of the low intensity of the work no further increase seemed to be possible and the patient's enthusiasm possibly suffered as a consequence. Physical working capacity should be tested during the course of a programme and children with a good response in working capacity should be introduced to a more demanding programme. It remains to be seen whether shorter programmes of 10–15 sessions will increase the attendance rate. Third, it was possible to avoid the phenomenon of exercise-induced asthma in our programme [3]. At present we have increased the volume of training among our asthmatic children to see whether the frequency of exercise-induced asthma will decrease in children whose working capacity is increased.

The analysis of the endocrine responses brought no new findings to those published in our original report [3]. A clear decrease in the exercise-induced excretion of adrenaline was demonstrated both in the mean values and in the intraindividual correlation analysis. A similar negative correlation between the decrease in hormone and increase in working capacity was possibly also present in the growth hormone response. The plasma cortisol levels were raised only in tests done before the training. Clearly, a major source of criticism could be our selection of identical working loads in our basal ergometry tests and those carried out after the training period. In an experimental situation such as this, the working load may appear significantly reduced after training even though no major change in working capacity has taken place. In future experimental work a load selected to produce an identical cardiovascular response might provide information of greater value. However, we still interpret our results as showing a significant training-induced decrease in the adrenaline response – a fact that may be relevant to the study of the generation of exercise-induced bronchial asthma.

References

1   Fitch KD, Morton AR, Blanksby BA.
    Effects of swimming training on children with asthma.
    Arch Dis Child 1976; 51: 190–194

2   Strick L.
    Breathing and physical fitness exercises for asthmatic children.
    Pediatr Clin North Am 1969; 16: 31–42

3   Leisti S, Finnilä M-J, Kiuru E.
    Effects of physical training on hormonal responses to exercise in asthmatic
    children. Arch Dis Child 1979; 54: 524–528

Chapter 25

PHYSICAL REHABILITATION OF CHILDREN WITH EXERCISE-INDUCED ASTHMA

J M Henriksen

Aarhus Kommunehospital, Denmark

SUMMARY

A study is reported which shows that physical training twice a week for a period of six weeks is sufficient to improve physical fitness and reduce exercise-induced asthma in asthmatic children.

Premedication is considered to be of importance in obtaining adequate intensities of training in asthmatic children.

The effect of training on exercise-induced asthma depends on the methods used for evaluating the exercise tests.

The reduction in exercise-induced asthma is most probably related to the improvement in work capacity.

INTRODUCTION

Exercise-induced asthma can be prevented or reduced by pretreatment with many anti-asthmatic drugs. Nevertheless, it is a clinical fact that exercise-induced asthma inhibits asthmatic children from taking part in physical activities, which leads to poor physical fitness and inability to keep up in sports and physically related games.

Several physical training programmes have been designed for asthmatic children with the aim of improving physical fitness, neuromuscular co-ordination and self-confidence, but the results have varied and have been difficult to compare on account of the different methods employed [1—4].

The present study — which is part of a more extensive investigation [5] — was undertaken to compare the cardiopulmonary response to exercise before and after six weeks of endurance training. The activities in the training programme followed, to some extent, the principles previously described by Oseid and his colleagues [6] and consisted of premedication, warming up and various physical exercises.

METHODS

Subjects

Seventeen asthmatic children, 7—13 years of age, participated (with the approval of their parents) in the study. All had perennial symptoms and showed a fall in the forced expiratory volume in one second (FEV_1) of at least 15 per cent from base-line after submaximal exercise. All were on maintenance therapy and were taking either sodium cromoglycate, beclomethasone, salbutamol or terbutaline. Two were taking oral theophylline. Medication was not changed during the study.

Exercise testing

Immediately before the training course the children performed an exercise test consisting of five to six minutes' continuous treadmill running with a constant work load adjusted to produce a heart rate of 170—180 beats/min. Loads ranged from 408—1024kpm/min (mean ± SD, 611 ± 166 kpm/min). During exercise the subjects were provided with a nose clip. The heart rates at rest and at end of the exercise were registered by radio-telemetry. After training the tests were repeated using the same work load for each individual as before training. Medication was withheld for at least 12 hours before an exercise test. At each visit body weight and height, room temperature and relative humidity were recorded.

Lung function

FEV_1 was measured with a Vitalograph immediately before exercise (base line) and at 3, 10 and 20 minutes after exercise. The best of three efforts was used in the calculations. Values were expressed as percentages of expected normal values. The exercise-induced changes were expressed in terms of per cent fall from baseline:

$$\frac{\text{base line – lowest post exercise value}}{\text{baseline}} \times 100$$

Training programme

Participants were assigned to 90 minutes of supervised physical training twice a week for a period of six weeks. Each training session was preceded by the recording of the peak expiratory flow rate (PEFR) using a Wright's peak flowmeter and inhalation of sodium cromoglycate or a sympathomimetic to prevent exercise-induced asthma. Then a 15 minute period of warming up was followed by various ball games (15 minutes), running (10 minutes), physical exercises (20 minutes) circuit training (20 minutes) and various team games (10 minutes). The intensity of training was gradually increased during the six weeks.

Statistics

The results were compared by Student's t test for paired data.

RESULTS

Relative humidity (mean ± SD) in the laboratory was 56 ± 8 per cent before and 59 ± 8 per cent after training – a difference that was not significant. Room temperature ranged from 20–22°C.

The heart rates at rest and at the end of exercise were significantly reduced by training. The resting heart rate (mean ± SD) was 93 ± 13 beats/min before and 86 ± 9 beats/min after training ($p < 0.05$), and the maximum heart rate fell from 181 ± 8 beats/min before training to 171 ± 10 beats/min afterwards ($p < 0.001$).

The resting FEV_1 remained unchanged at 70 ± 16 per cent (mean ± SD) both before and after training. However, the magnitude of the exercise-induced asthma was reduced by 39 per cent. Figure 1 shows the individual data for the per cent fall in FEV_1 after submaximal exercise before and

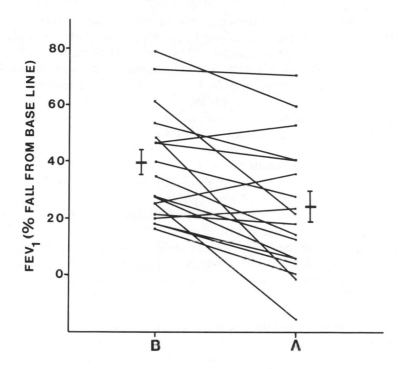

Figure 1. Individual per cent falls in FEV_1 after submaximal exercise in 17 asthmatic children before (B) and after (A) six weeks of physical training (means ± SEM)

after completion of the training course. The mean (± SD) per cent fall in FEV_1 was reduced from 39 ± 19 per cent to 24 ± 23 per cent (p < 0.002).

DISCUSSION

Three of the major issues related to the physical rehabilitation of asthmatic children are: (1) what are the results we are looking for? (2) how intensive should a training course be and how long should it last before an effect can be attained? and (3) which methods should be used to evaluate the effect of training?

Several authors have reported marked psychological gains in asthmatic children after endurance training [1,3,7]. Though such observations are sufficient to justify physical training programmes, more objective — some would say scientific — determinations of the training-effect are necessary if the above questions are to be answered. In the present study the effects of training on physical fitness and exercise-induced asthma were investigated by standardised exercise challenges immediately before and after of six-weeks' training programme. After training, resting and maximum heart rates were significantly reduced, suggesting an improved work capacity. This impression was further supported by the results of our more extensive study [5], which showed a highly significant reduction in post-exercise plasma lactate levels after training. That these results were obtained after just six weeks is in accordance with the finding that the maximal increase in work capacity occurs within three weeks of the start of training in healthy adults [8].

The crucial point in physical training designed to improve fitness is to reach adequate intensities of training. However, that is almost impossible when training children with exercise-induced asthma and failure of pre-medication could, at least partly, explain the lack of improved work capacity found in some other training studies [2, 4]. In the present study the children were treated with sodium cromoglycate or $beta_2$-agonists to prevent troublesome exercise-induced asthma during training.

The effect of physical training on exercise-induced asthma remains controversial. For instance, an effect implies improved physical fitness. The present study and the findings of Oseid and Haaland [1] have shown that when this requirement is fulfilled and the same individual work load is used in the pre- and post-training exercise tests, the degree of exercise-induced asthma is significantly reduced. However, there is no evidence to support the view that physical training decreases bronchial hyperreactivity. Moreover, physical training has never been shown to improve resting pulmonary function and Fitch and his colleagues [3], who used the physical work capacity at a heart rate of 170 beats/min (PWC_{170}) to evaluate the exercise challenges, found exercise-induced asthma to be unchanged after swimming training despite an increase in physical fitness. These results indicate a dose-response relationship between work load and post-exercise bronchoconstriction. This view is further supported by data from the more extensive part of the present study [5] which show a positive correlation between the training-induced reduction in exercise-induced asthma and the plasma lactate levels after exercise.

References

1   Oseid S, Haaland K.
      Exercise studies on asthmatic children before and after regular physical training.
      In Eriksson BO, Furberg B, eds. *Swimming Medicine IV: 32 1978;* 32–41.
      Baltimore: University Park Press

2   Vavra J, Macek M, Mrzena B, Spicak V.
    Intensive physical training in children with bronchial asthma.
    Acta Paediatr Scand 1971; 217: 90–92

3   Fitch KD, Morton AR, Blanksby BA.
    Effects of swimming training on children with asthma.
    Arch Dis Child 1979; 51: 190–194

4   Graff-Lonnevig V, Bevegård S, Eriksson BO et al.
    Two years' follow-up of asthmatic boys participating in a physical activity pro-
    gramme. *Acta Paediatr Scand 1980; 69:* 347–352

5   Henriksen JM, Nielsen TT.
    Effect of physical training on exercise-induced bronchoconstriction.
    Acta Paediatr Scand. In press

6   Oseid S, Kendall M, Larsen RB et al.
    Physical activity programs for children with exercise-induced asthma.
    In Eriksson BO, Furberg B, eds. *Swimming Medicine IV: 32 1978;* 42–51.
    Baltimore: University Park Press

7   Keens TG.
    Exercise training programs for pediatric patients with chronic lung disease.
    Pediatr Clin North Am 1979; 26: 517–524

8   Winder WW, Hickson RC, Hagberg JM et al.
    Training-induced changes in hormonal and metabolic responses to submaximal
    exercise. *J Appl Physiol 1979; 46:* 766–771

DISCUSSION

CAMPBELL   Dr Fitch, is it true that salbutamol is allowed at the
(Cardiff, UK)   Olympics when taken orally but not when inhaled?

FITCH   No, this is not true. However, it might be worth re-
                  peating the history of salbutamol in this context as I
                  have been on record in previous symposia as being
                  critical of the Medical Commission of the Interna-
                  tional Olympic Committee. In 1972, two days before
                  the start of the Munich Olympics, written permission
                  to use salbutamol was received from the Commission.
                  On the opening day this permission was rescinded,
                  although sodium cromoglycate was permitted. In May
                  1975 the Medical Commission approved the use of
                  salbutamol and terbutaline provided written notifica-
                  tion was given of the timing of the dose and its route
                  of administration prior to the event. Since this is not
                  practical, I provided the Medical Commission of the
                  International Olympic Committee in 1976 and again
                  in 1980 with a letter stating that the athletes I listed
                  had asthma and might need pre-exercise medication
                  with certain named $beta_2$-adrenergic stimulants. This
                  was found acceptable. In 1980 in Moscow after dis-
                  cussion with the Chairman and Secretary of the
                  Medical Commission of the International Olympic
                  Committee approval was granted to use fenoterol.
                  Thus at present all three $beta_2$ drugs may be used in
                  both oral and inhalational forms — and, I presume,
                  could be administered by nebuliser if necessary.

AASMUNDTVEIT   How long before exercise should sodium cromoglycate
(Fredrikstad,   and $beta_2$ stimulants be taken to be most effective?
Norway)   How short a time before exercise can these drugs be
                  taken?

FITCH   I think the answer is virtually immediately and the
                  studies on sodium cromoglycate would confirm that.

Oral agents usually do not give protection in much under 45 minutes and I do not choose to use them (with their greater incidence of side effects) when I can obtain superior effects by other routes in 45 seconds. Dr Anderson in Sydney has studied the timed effect of beta$_2$-agonists and Dr Silverman in London that of sodium cromoglycate. These studies would indicate these agents suffer a significant loss in their protective effects after one hour. There is still some protective effect remaining after four hours and I consider that those who allow only four hours between the last medication and the performance of standard physiological exercise testing are not leaving enough time. It is our policy to require 12 hours without medication before testing.

SPEIGHT
(Newcastle upon
Tyne, UK)

Surely there must be a large number of people, already participating keenly in sports activities, who have a very mild degree of *undiagnosed* asthma which prevents them from reaching their full potential?

FITCH

As a sports physician my answer is most certainly yes. Many persons, especially those with a family history of other atopic conditions, are prone to mild exertional asthma. This may take the form of an irritating cough occurring five to ten minutes after exercise. Continuous running, especially in cold dry air is likely to uncover subclinical bronchoconstriction. Those with a history of mild 'wheezing bronchitis' or asthma with an early remission and years of wheeze-free life may also find that their exercise bronchial reactivity can be uncovered by any asthmagenic type of exercise.

One example was the occurrence in an Australian sprint cyclist at the Moscow Olympic Games of subclinical bronchoconstriction after cycling. With the limited testing of pulmonary function available his FEV$_1$ was found to have fallen to 65 per cent. He was placed on pre-exercise medication and recorded a very fast time trial on the following day. That cyclist had been a Commonwealth Games Gold Medallist in 1978.

OSEID

I have already mentioned those children who have stridor regardless of climatic conditions, but we have also seen children with subclinical asthma who have been unaware of their condition and have problems only in the cold part of winter. For the rest of the year they can exercise freely at fairly intensive levels but when it is as cold and windy as we experienced, for example, in December 1981 and in January 1982 they suffered badly. I have also seen many children who have actually competed at a fairly high standard but when tested in the laboratory have shown mild degrees of exercise-induced asthma. I believe there are quite a number of such cases.

MEHROTRA
(Newport, UK)

Does Professor Oseid agree with my opinion and perhaps that of others that the only physical activity *not* to be recommended to asthmatics is non stop cross-country running?

OSEID

I do agree. We have had a few asthmatics who have run and skied cross-country, but they developed asthma after a while and had to take their broncho-dilator — they ran with a bronchodilator in the pocket. In my opinion this is not the right form of exercise to motivate an asthmatic and make the child or adult secure about being able to take exercise. Non stop cross-country running might have a negative psychological impact.

EDWARDS
(Chairman)

In the recent London marathon, in which nearly 17,000 runners took part, there was at least one asthmatic with large letters across his chest saying "Asthmatics Can Run".

STRUNK
(Denver, USA)

Professor Oseid, you noted that many children had a negative reaction to group sessions. How do you approach these children?

OSEID

That is an important question. Although we do give exercises individually or in very small groups, our usual approach is to start out with group treatment.

But individuals differ. In Norway, for instance, we have children from many different parts of the country who have different opinions not only about what we do at Voksentoppen but also about the sports they want or do not want to perform, so they can be difficult to treat in groups. They also may have different dialects and not understand each other or the instructor. That is why we also run individual exercises either in the physiotherapy department or by extra hours in the school.

BAR-OR
(Hamilton, Canada)

Would you speculate on the mechanism by which increase in aerobic capacity helps decrease exercise-induced asthma? My own guess is that once asthmatics are better trained they function at a lower *percentage* of their maximal ventilation when given a standard exercise test. This in itself may reduce their airway response to heat loss.

OSEID

I think that is a very good explanation.

SMITH
(Warwick, UK)

The training programmes appear to have been concentrated on control groups in special establishments. How successful have been the efforts to 'educate' the physical education teachers in schools to cope with asthmatic children in their classes?

OSEID

We are continuously striving to improve our programmes in our Institution. Of course, the children should not be there for prolonged periods. The objective should be to transfer these activity programmes so that they are organised in the child's home surroundings and in the local community.

EDWARDS

In the UK we have been encouraging the development of special training groups and have encouraged three types of people to lead them: physical education teachers, swimming instructors in local swimming baths and physiotherapists in hospitals.

GILLAM

Dr Henriksen, was there a significant correlation

between the decrease in the exercise heart rate after training and the change in the per cent fall indices after training?

HENRIKSEN I have not made that calculation. However, we have shown that the decrease in exercise-induced broncho-constriction and the plasma lactate levels after exercise were not related to work load.

BRENNAN (Sheffield, UK) What happened to the *total* drug usage during these programmes? Are the children simply using more drugs?

HENRIKSEN No, we have investigated that and in the short periods of six to eight weeks we found no change in medication.

EDWARDS In his work at Loughborough University, Dr Monks has shown that over a three-month period the children used less drugs as their training progressed.

INBAR (Netanya, Israel) Would you agree that your findings indicate that the less exercise-induced asthma that occurred after the training programme was due to lower $\dot{V}E$ ventilation caused by the lower plasma lactate levels which, in turn, you showed was a prime cause for reduced respiratory heat exchange and exercise-induced asthma and not due to any significant clinical change from the training programme itself?

HENRIKSEN No, I think that the reduction in post-exercise plasma lactate levels after training was the result of improved physical fitness, which probably resulted in a lower $\dot{V}E$ and heat exchange.

Chapter 26

PHYSIOLOGICAL AND PSYCHOSOCIAL ASPECTS OF THE TRAINING OF ASTHMATIC CHILDREN

A Backman

Helsinki University Central Hospital, Helsinki, Finland

SUMMARY

The asthmatic child often has a special place in the family and it is obvious that many factors besides medical, physical and psychosocial ones play an important role in the development of the disease. In many cases the asthmatic child has been protected and spoiled and has been living within a vicious circle of warnings and prohibitions. It is important to include the whole family in the treatment and rehabilitation programme and, when planning the rehabilitation programme, to realise that all factors used in the programme are of equal importance.

We have investigated these problems in two different studies. The first, performed at the beginning of the 1970s, included 47 children during and after a rehabilitation programme that lasted for a mean period of five years and nine months. The following factors were studied: number of asthmatic attacks per year, drug consumption, results of physical training measured by work capacity and simple mechanical pulmonary function tests, psychosocial factors and family therapy.

The results were very encouraging and showed that all the above factors were equally important for the treatment of a child with chronic asthma.

The second study at the end of the 1970s included 59 asthmatic children in a residential home for chronically ill children. It was carried out mainly along the same lines as the first and the results were similar. A rehabilitation counsellor was used as a link between the treatment team, the home and society.

We conclude that optimal response to a rehabilitation programme for asthmatic children can be obtained with a comprehensive programme which besides medical treatment includes physiotherapy and training, psychotherapy and family therapy together with education and occupational guidance adjusted for each child.

INTRODUCTION

The asthmatic child often has a special place in the family and many factors besides the medical, physical and psychosocial ones play an important role in the development of the disease. The asthmatic child is often protected and spoiled and lives within a vicious circle of warnings and prohibitions.

The psychosocial development of asthma as a chronic disease has been charted by S Oseid and can be summed up as follows: first asthma attack produces anxious parents; symptomatic medication, the child is pacified; attention is turned towards symptoms and their causes (such as allergens, exercise, infection, and so on); the parents restrict their child's activities and prevent him from taking part in play and games; asthma becomes the central topic of conversation ("How is your asthma?"); the child becomes a loser among his friends; the child is treated as a 'sick person' even in asymptomatic phases; the child looks upon himself as being sick even in his good phases; the child becomes a 'sick person'.

It is obvious that the family with an asthmatic child needs outside help if it is to cope with all the different problems that arise over treatment, attitudes and the immediate surroundings. This help can be provided by the hospital staff who take care of asthmatic children. However, it is important to include the whole family in the treatment and rehabilitation programme. We have investigated these problems in two different studies.

FIRST REHABILITATION STUDY

Our first study took place in the early 1970s. Forty-seven children with chronic asthma were selected from the patients at the Children's Hospital, University of Helsinki. They were studied during and after a rehabilitation programme that lasted for a mean of five years and nine months. The investigations covered psychiatric, psychological and social adjustment in addition to physical training and allergy testing. Twenty patients were referred for psychotherapy and family therapy.

Material

The patients were divided into two groups: group I was comprised of the children who were only investigated psychologically and sociologically; group II was comprised of those who, in addition, were referred for psychotherapy and family therapy.

At the follow-up examination, 37 of the original 47 children were

TABLE I. Response to treatment assessed in terms of changes in severity of the degree of asthma

Severity of asthma	At the beginning of the study		At the end of the study	
	Group I	Group II	Group I	Group II
Symptom-free	–	–	3	5
5 attacks per year	–	–	7	6
5–10 attacks per year	3	–	4	7
10 attacks per year	7	7	3	1
10 attacks per year and complications	7	13	–	1
Total number of patients	17	20	17	20
Mean of severity of asthma on a 0–4 scale	3.29	3.75	1.47	1.27
		3.52		1.37

available. Three patients had died, one had left the country and six had defaulted. Thus group I comprises 17 and group II 20 patients: the mean age of the girls was 14 years and that of the boys 13 years 6 months.

The severity of asthma was graded on a 0–4 scale: 1 = fewer than 5 attacks per year, 2 = 5–10 attacks per year, 3 = more than 10 attacks per year, and 4 = more than 10 attacks per year plus complicating factors. At the beginning of the study, the severity of asthma was 3.52 in the whole sample – 3.29 in group I and 3.75 in group II (Table I).

Treatment was based on team work which, in addition to conventional paediatric allergy therapy, included consideration of psychological and social factors and physical training.

Results

The response to treatment was assessed in terms of changes in the degree of severity of the asthma (Table I).

Physical examination of the chest and pulmonary function studies at the beginning of treatment were normal in five patients; minor pathological changes were noted in 22 patients and distinct chest pathology in 10. At the follow-up the results of chest examination and lung function tests were normal in 25 patients, minor pathology was noted in nine and definite pathology in three.

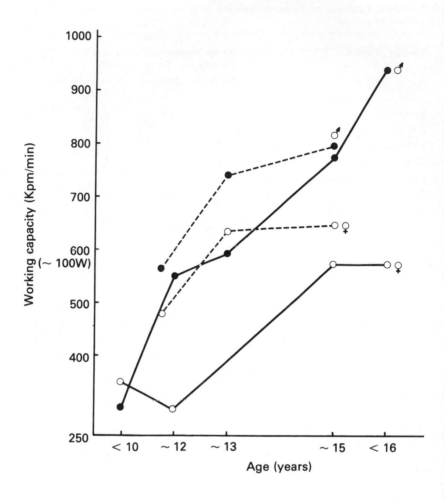

Figure 1. Working capacity (Kpm/min) of children with chronic asthma. The results of bicycle ergometry in different age groups after a rehabilitation programme (unbroken lines = asthmatics (16 girls; 21 boys); broken lines = control children)

Working capacity (Kpm/min) was measured using a bicycle ergometer at the follow-up examination. Healthy school children were used as a control group. The results are shown in Figure 1, which illustrates that after their rehabilitation programme the asthmatic children had an almost normal working capacity.

Psychological aspects

The psychological part of the study aimed at clarifying to what extent psychotherapy, in combination with family counselling, and team work can help the asthmatic child to gain emotional balance and independence. When emotional conflicts can be solved the number of attacks decrease.

Psychotherapy and the solving of emotional conflicts achieved the following results: the conception of the ego was clarified; the need to express aggressions indirectly through asthma was diminished; the mode of relating to the disease became more realistic; fears associated with the attacks of asthma lessened; unrealistic demands for the need of compensation lessened in importance; the ability to establish social contacts was improved.

The study clearly showed that a child's asthma in many ways threatens the family equilibrium, causing problems in relationships and activities both within and outside the family. How grave and extensive these difficulties will be, depends on the family's resources and strength.

The family with an asthmatic child needs outside help and the goals to be set for family therapy can be stated as follows:

to activate both parents to assume responsibility for the care of the asthmatic child

to help the family realise and accept the negative emotions to which the disorder gives rise

to help the family overcome the fears evoked by asthma and reduce overprotective care and limitations on the child's activities

to teach the family to accept occasional wheezing as an integral part of the asthmatic child's personality

to prevent the development of overprotective attitudes

to help with solving emotional conflicts which the child's disorder has already caused in the family life.

The people needed for this kind of team work include nurses, physiotherapists, psychologists, medical social workers and paediatric allergologists. Additional experts who are needed occasionally include child psychiatrists and teachers specially trained in the care of chronically sick children.

The results were most encouraging and our experience was that all the above-mentioned factors were equally important for the treatment of a child with chronic asthma.

SECOND REHABILITATION STUDY

The second study at the end of the 1970s concerned 59 asthmatic children in a residential home for chronically ill children. The study was mainly carried out along the same lines as the first and the results were similar. In this second study, however, we were also able to analyse different 'stress factors' that influenced the prognosis of chronic disease in children. The most important of these were continuing symptoms, bad experiences in hospital, difficulties at school, conflicts within the family, poor economic and housing conditions. The result of the rehabilitation programme depended very much on the extent to which the team was able to change the 'stress factors' or diminish their effect on the progress of the disease.

CONCLUSION

The complete rehabilitation programme for a child with chronic asthma is complex, consisting, as it does, of team work between many different experts. In many cases the team is able to solve the problems. But in some cases the problems are so complex that the addition of a specially trained rehabilitation counsellor is needed to act as a link between the team in the hospital, the home, and society. The rehabilitation counsellor is able to inform the school and the local authorities about the disease, to make the demands on diet, elimination of allergens or other necessary changes in the surroundings more acceptable, and to change false attitudes towards the asthmatic child.

We conclude that the optimal response to a rehabilitation programme for asthmatic children can be obtained with a comprehensive programme which, besides medical treatment, includes physiotherapy and training, psychotherapy and family therapy together with education and occupational guidance adjusted for each child.

Bibliography

Aas K.
The Biochemical and Immunological Basis of Bronchial Asthma 1971.
Springfield: C C Thomas

Backman A, Haikonen P, Hirvonen E, Räsänen E.
Chronic asthma in children: a medicopsychosocial approach.
Allergol Immunopathol (Madr) 1979; Suppl VI: 37

Backman A.
Psychosocial aspects of asthma.
Allergol Immunopathol (Madr) 1979; Suppl VI: 117

Furukava C, Roesler T.
Psychogenic aspects of allergic disease. In Bierman C, Pearlman D, eds.
Allergic Diseases of Infancy, Childhood and Adolescence 1980: 353.
Philadelphia: WB Saunders

Chapter 27

RECREATION THERAPY IN THE REHABILITATION OF ASTHMATIC CHILDREN. Making the most of leisure

R C Strunk, Laura J Kelly, Diane L Rubin

National Jewish Hospital and Research Center/National Asthma Center, Denver, Colorado, USA

SUMMARY

The recreational therapy programme is designed to encourage both normal attitudes towards, and the practice of, leisure activities in children with chronic asthma. Emphasis is placed on physical aspects of recreation, but the programme includes all aspects of leisure including cognitive pastimes, spectator events, outdoor education and free play, in addition to individual, single opponent and team sports.

One of the most frequent problems observed in children with chronic asthma is lack of exposure to, or experience in, activities appropriate to their stage of development. The comprehensive approach used in the recreational therapy programme guarantees that all children have the opportunity to be exposed to and to acquire skills in these activities.

Another problem that is seen frequently is a negative concept of self. This can be manifested in unwillingness to explore the development of new skills, anticipation of failure, and inability to relate productively with peers. The negative self-concept is often accompanied by a lack of motivation to succeed, which results from having gained from being ill. The training in specific skills provided by the recreational therapists is designed to enable the children to join in with their peers. In addition, recreational therapy focuses on wellness and ability rather than on illness and disability. Positive responses are given for appropriate participation, initiative, independence and accomplishment. The greatest rewards go to those who try hardest, not necessarily to those who are best.

Play is a natural mechanism for change in children and it is important that they use play productively. It provides an opportunity to experiment with new ideas, to express feelings safely, to try out different roles, to develop necessary internal controls and to enhance physical functioning. Through play, chronically ill children learn what they can do – how hard they can play, friends they can make, feelings they can express and independence they can achieve. Many children with chronic asthma have accepted sickness as a way of life. We maintain that exposure to play in a manner that provides the optimum chances of success will open their minds to the possible rewards of being well.

INTRODUCTION

Almost all asthmatic children are restricted to some degree in their ability to take part in physical activities. There are two main reasons why this is so: the first is the occurrence of bronchospasm during exercise (exercise-induced bronchospasm). This can be especially troublesome if the physician does not thoroughly investigate the degree of exercise-induced broncho-spasm and design a therapeutic regimen for its control. However, even with optimum therapy, there are some asthmatics who may not be able to exercise under certain conditions without wheezing. The second reason is the attempt by parents to protect their child from wheezing episodes. Since one of the primary methods of treatment for asthma is to identify precipitating factors and then avoid them, this protection is often useful or even necessary – for example, in the case of children who are allergic to animals or who wheeze when exposed to irritants, such as tobacco smoke or paint fumes. Unfortunately many parents (and even some physicians) often interpret the concept of avoidance to include avoidance of exercise. Instead of using a medication that will limit exercise-induced bronchospasm and then encouraging a child to exercise, they limit the exercise. This results in overprotection and unnecessary restrictions.

Whatever their basis, restrictions can severely limit the asthmatic child's ability to participate in normal play and activities. Instead of being given the space and encouragement to explore his or her universe, challenge budding skills and test social competence, the asthmatic child, from an early age, gets the message that he or she is different and that what is available to most other children, is taboo for them.

Play is fundamental to the process of arriving at a productive adulthood. In fact, according to many social scientists, including Freud, Erikson and Piaget, the process starts in the play of the very young. Through play, children explore their surroundings, test their physical, cognitive and social skills, and attempt to master increasingly complex tasks to be ready to meet the challenges of adult life. They must therefore grow up in an environment conducive to play. When the external environment inhibits progression through the natural stages of play, the child's growth and development are blocked — and the environment of a child with severe asthma contains many of these inhibiting factors, in particular parental fear and anxiety, social isolation and pain. A child with chronic severe asthma is often denied an atmosphere conducive to normal play and consequently becomes unable or unwilling to engage in productive play. This increases the likelihood of underdeveloped motor proficiency, social and cultural isolation, underlying or overt depression, negative concept of self, generalised anxiety and fear of failure and over-dependency. Thus, the asthmatic child can enter into a vicious cycle of failure. In some children failure can become the major problem, and can continue even if the asthma is resolved.

RECREATION THERAPY

To tackle these problems, the National Jewish Hospital/National Asthma Center turned to a discipline relatively new in the field of health services: recreation therapy. Recreation therapy emerged during World Wars I and II to provide diversional activities for American soldiers in hospital. During the ensuing years, as the amount of time for leisure and play increased among the general population of the USA, recreation therapy became recognised as a vital and necessary part of the rehabilitation of the ill and disabled.

The object of recreation therapy is to ensure the best use of leisure for the ill and the disabled so that they may enjoy a lifestyle that promotes physical, mental and emotional well-being, allows for creativity and self-expression, gives the individual a sense of control and mastery over some portion of his or her environment, and is, for the most part, motivated from within. Our purpose here is to describe the recreation therapy programme at the National Jewish Hospital/National Asthma Center and show how it can contribute to the rehabilitation of the child with chronic asthma.

Gunn and Peterson [1] provided a systematic framework of recreation therapy services, suggesting that the techniques and programme could be designed as a continuum. Figure 1 illustrates the nature of the interactions between therapist and patient. At the left of the continuum, noted as recreation therapy, activities are prescribed with specific objectives for rehabilitation in mind. The patient has little control over the activities chosen. At the centre of the continuum, noted as leisure education, the patient possesses some skills and the therapist's role is to explore possible ways to use these in leisure. The patient and therapist plan the activities together, sharing in the final decision. At the right side of the continuum, noted as special recreation, the patient possesses the skills and knowledge

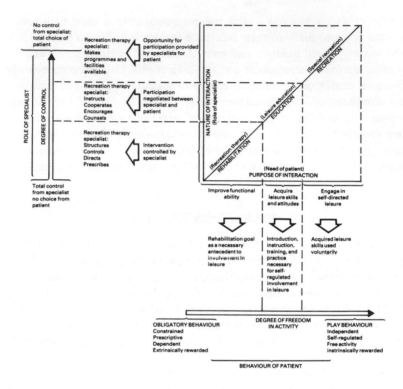

Figure 1. A recreation therapy service model (from Gunn and Peterson [1] by courtesy of the authors and Prentice-Hall, Inc.)

necessary to enjoy their leisure. Here the patient has the freedom to choose activities; the therapist relinquishes control and acts instead as an advocate.

The focus of the interactions between therapist and patient is determined by the latter's need. While the services and interactions appear to be placed rigidly along this continuum, Gunn and Peterson recognised that, in the normal course of treatment, many occurred simultaneously. The ultimate objective is to alter the individual's method of play; to move the patient from dependent, extrinsically motivated behaviour to independent, intrinsically motivated behaviour.

RECREATION THERAPY AT NATIONAL JEWISH HOSPITAL/ NATIONAL ASTHMA CENTER

National Jewish Hospital/National Asthma Center has, over the past three years, expanded its services for chronically asthmatic children to include comprehensive recreation therapy programmes. Based on the principles and guidelines suggested by Gunn and Peterson [1], the recreation therapy department established the following objectives to make the most of each child's leisure by (1) increasing the repertoire of skills; (2) expanding the awareness of resources available both within themselves and outside; and (3) altering the perceptions of self-competence and, thereby, increasing the motivation to engage in satisfying, productive leisure activities. One of the major premises at National Jewish Hospital/National Asthma Center is that, in addition to teaching fundamental play skills and providing opportunities for their use, the programmes must also be designed to alter the children's attitudes towards themselves, their play, and their perceptions of personal competence to play successfully, thus removing them from the cycle of failure. It is this change in attitude and direction, combined with the reduction in restrictions, that will have the greatest impact on the child's ability and motivation to lead a more normal, fulfilling life when he or she returns home.

The multifaceted assessment starts with separate interviews with the parents and the child. These interviews are designed to give the therapist a picture of the child's strengths, weaknesses, interests and leisure activities. The child is then given a number of tasks to assess gross motor, fine motor, cognitive and social skills and to determine his or her ability to participate in a wide variety of leisure activities. Subsequently, the child is observed participating in a large number of structured and unstructured play situations to see whether the results of the tests correspond with actual daily performance. Once this information is gathered, areas in which there might be difficulties are identified and an approach to treatment is designed to build on the child's apparent or latent strengths, and to minimise the deleterious effects of real or imagined weaknesses.

Having used and refined this method of assessment on hundreds of children over the past two years, the recreation therapy department has arrived at the following picture of the leisure skills and attitudes of children with severe chronic asthma:

1) they lack exposure to, or experience in, activities appropriate to their development

2) they display functional deficiencies in the skills necessary to take part successfully in recreational activities appropriate to their age

3) they are in generally poor physical condition and are often obese

4) they have negative perceptions of their own worth and competence manifested in an unwillingness to explore the development of new

skills, anticipation of failure, inability to relate productively with their contemporaries, and underlying anger and/or depression

5) they have developed compensatory patterns of receiving secondary gains from their illness and often lack the motivation to be well or successful

6) they have home and school environments that often foster their perceptions of incompetence and reinforce negative patterns and characteristics

7) they are unaware of, or cannot make suitable use of, available recreational resources.

Case report

To illustrate the issues that children present when referred to the National Jewish Hospital/National Asthma Center, the following case study is given.

Steven, a 13½-year-old white boy, with severe asthma, lived at home with his mother and father in a metropolitan area. He appeared to have a very close relationship with his parents, particularly his mother.

He was of average height and mildly obese. Many of his mannerisms were effeminate. He avoided any type of physical labour or exercise, even chores, with an attitude of "I don't have to do that". His muscle tone was noticeably poor. He appeared totally dependent on adults, and seemed to expect them to meet his needs, both physical and emotional.

Steven seemed to lack the ability to interact with his contemporaries. His mother reported that, at home, he preferred to read or occupy himself in his room, he rarely joined in neighbourhood games or had friends in to visit. This was consistent with what was observed on the unit: Steven continually avoided interaction with his fellows unless absolutely necessary. He spent his free time in his room doing homework, reading, and/or crying. He appeared to be a needy child seeking almost constant contact with adults and even requiring special times with his primary nurse when he could have her undivided attention.

The initial recreation therapy assessment pointed out that except for physical stature, Steven appeared as a much younger child. Many of his skills were far inferior to those necessary for successful participation in the activity programme for his age group. His basic gross motor skills at such exercises as running, jumping, and throwing and catching a ball were minimal. However, Steven could not integrate even such skills as he possessed in a useful manner: he could not play or keep up with his fellows in any organised games or sports. He had little understanding of the rules of games or the strategies of play. His lack of skills, his mannerisms, and the fact that he expended little effort in games quickly made Steven a scapecoat among his contemporaries. He had no interest in these types of activities saying "they are boring" and "I don't like them".

Both cognitive and fine motor skills appeared at least average. There were no problems noted that would hinder his participation in recreation therapy programmes.

There was, however, something appealing about this young adolescent. He was able to engage adults in his affairs, although in a somewhat manipulative manner. The staff were often annoyed by his whining and his constant seeking of attention, yet they liked him. This, plus his ability to learn, made Steven seem a workable prospect.

Changing Steven's pattern of leisure behaviour from one that was dependent and extrinsically motivated into one that was independent and intrinsically motivated (as outlined in the recreation therapy service model) required a comprehensive and creative effort on the part of the recreation therapy staff.

In common with other patients at the National Jewish Hospital/National Asthma Center, Steven was assigned to an activity programme according to his age and level of functioning. Each age group has several activities that fall into the rehabilitation category in the recreation therapy service model, with the object of increasing a child's functional ability. These include activities to increase physical conditioning, basic fine and gross motor skills, and social aptitude. The programme includes physical recreation, arts and crafts, use of a games room and kitchen, and outside trips. Generally, these are group activities; attendance is mandatory and the activities are usually decided by the therapist. However, if learning is inhibited by being with a group, as was the case with Steven, individual therapy is also provided.

Steven simply did not attend the group activities for which he was scheduled. He used excuses such as having "too much homework" or "needing a treatment" to avoid involvement in any activities that required social contact and/or physical exertion. Staff believed that the harassment Steven sustained was probably a contributory factor.

An individual recreation therapy session was scheduled for Steven five times a week. Two therapists, one man and one woman, alternated spending time alone with him. The therapists decided to centre on improving Steven's games and sports skills because (1) therein lay his greatest weakness, (2) he was most likely to be made a scapegoat during games and (3) he was in serious need of some form of physical conditioning. Each week sessions focused on the skills and rules for one game, alternating between individual sports (such as tennis and bowling) and team sports (such as softball and basketball). Every few weeks Steven was encouraged to choose the game or sport for that week.

Concurrently with rehabilitation programmes, the recreation therapy programme at the National Jewish Hospital/National Asthma Center provides patients with a variety of leisure educational activities so that the child, with the support of the therapist, can broaden his or her recreational experiences while continuing to practise and improve basic skills. Usually, this is done during the group activities. For example, after a basketball drill, a game is organised and played. Or the group may take a trip to the community roller skating rink. Options are introduced so that children can experiment with making their own decisions and begin to realise that they can choose what they do with their leisure time.

To engage Steven in this process, the individual therapy sessions were designed to include playing one-on-one basketball, learning to keep score in bowling, and other such activities, so that his skills would become closer to those of his fellows and help him feel more confident when with the group. But, as Steven still refused to attend group activities, the hospital staff decided to draw up a contract with him. If he agreed to attend individual recreational therapy daily and attended one of the two group activities that evening he would be allowed to go on outside trips and be given weekend passes.

The recreation therapy staff as a whole focuses on *wellness* and *ability*, seeking to help children discover what they can do, the games they can play, the friends they can make and the feelings they can express. Participation, initiative, perseverance and independence are positively rewarded in the belief that as a child experiences success and fun in leisure, the motivation for further involvement becomes inbuilt. The therapists who looked after Steven played many roles in achieving this goal. They taught basic skills and they created a safe atmosphere in which he could try new skills and discover new abilities. They encouraged him. They talked about making friends and being a friend. One of the therapists discussed his contract with him every day, helping him learn to make decisions about how it should be fulfilled.

Initially, Steven resisted individual therapy. However, progress notes indicated that his attitude toward the sessions began to change even during the first week. As the level of his skills slowly improved, his interest and enthusiasm increased. The therapists' progress notes indicated that he began to take pride in his accomplishments during individual therapy. These sessions continued throughout his stay in hospital. Steven discovered a preference for individual sports and even enjoyed a few team sports. The contract was dropped when Steven became more willing to attend group activities. His excuses about homework decreased. On the unit, he continued to prefer being alone rather than fraternising, but there was a noticeable increase of interaction during formal activities. Steven was more accepted among his fellows and he was subjected to less teasing and harassment.

After discharge, Steven maintained informal contact with his individual recreation therapist by mail. He reported to the therapist that he had joined a bowling league almost immediately after leaving hospital and had convinced his family to buy the equipment for badminton, which he enjoyed playing. In later correspondence, he mentioned playing some softball as well.

Steven's case is one in which a child, caught in the cycle of failure, was given the opportunity and support to break out successfully. The recreation therapy department at the National Jewish Hospital/National Asthma Center does not pretend to make athletes, artisans or chess masters out of asthmatic children, but we do contend that it is possible to move a child along the path toward a more satisfying, well-rounded use of leisure.

CONCLUSIONS

There are several principles that can be drawn from Steven's experience at the National Jewish Hospital/National Asthma Center and applied to children with asthma in other settings. First, the real and the unnecessary restrictions placed on each asthmatic child must be recognised and differentiated. Second, there must be more education for parents, teachers, community workers and the asthmatic children themselves, concerning the nature, the symptoms and the treatment of asthma, so that the children will not be unnecessarily restricted at home. Unnecessary restrictions are kept to a minimum at the National Jewish Hospital/National Asthma Center by having a recreation therapy staff that is medically trained to understand the disease, to recognise the symptoms and to take the proper steps when treatment is necessary. We believe that such education prevents the staff from being overprotective with these children. In addition, the patients feel more secure, knowing that they can explore their abilities more fully because a knowledgeable adult is on hand to assist them should they exceed their limits.

Third, practitioners need to focus on wellness, ability and 'can-do'. Steven's success was due, in part, to tackling the activities and interactions in sequence and by continually encouraging him. Recreation therapy gave him a chance to learn that he had latent abilities that, when used, could give him pleasure.

Finally, practitioners need to be constantly aware of the level at which the child is functioning and of what has to be done to ensure an independent, satisfying use of leisure. Certainly, the facilities available and the content of the programme can contribute significantly in this respect. For example, if a child fears or dislikes physical recreation, a therapist can make an approach through a familiar avenue, such as crafts projects, and use that gradually to persuade the patient to try physical recreation. But still, it is the process, and not simply the content of a programme that fosters self-confidence and motivation.

We feel that limitations in the skills of play and leisure have a major impact on the development of chronically ill asthmatic children. Recreation therapy can help overcome these limitations and can contribute to the overall success of a rehabilitation programme for asthmatic children.

Reference

1   Gunn SL, Peterson CA.
      Therapeutic Recreation Program Design: Principles and Procedures 1978.
      Englewood Cliffs, NJ: Prentice-Hall, Inc

Chapter 28

THE USE OF TRAINING PROGRAMMES IN THE REHABILITATION OF ASTHMATIC CHILDREN

R H Andrasch

Hochgebirgsklinik Davos-Wolfgang, Davos-Wolfgang, Switzerland

SUMMARY

The respiratory capacity of many asthmatic children is severely impaired and frequently deteriorates during exertion. Fear of exercise-induced asthma and undue overprotection often leads to physical inactivity and loss of condition, which further complicates not only their respiratory problems, but also their emotional and social development.

Numerous studies have shown the importance of exercise programmes in the rehabilitation of asthmatic children. Although reports on improvement in cardiovascular and pulmonary functions are not always in agreement there is a consensus that exercise programmes can exert significant beneficial changes in general health, exercise tolerance, independence, emotional and social adjustment. Many of the children need less medication, develop fewer asthmatic attacks and are able to control their breathing better during exercise and wheezing episodes.

The training programmes should be individually designed after careful evaluation of each child, and should offer a broad variety of physical and breathing exercises, taking place in a happy and playful atmosphere. Simple, easily achievable exercises should be followed by more challenging tasks as the programme goes on. The response to training depends on the intensity, duration and frequency of the effort. Emphasis should be placed on group activities and interval training. Three to five training sessions of approximately 60 minutes preceded by a prolonged warm-up period should be undertaken each week. It is convenient to start the programme in a rehabilitation centre, but thereafter instructions should be given for continuing the programme at home preferably for several years so as to maintain or even improve the many beneficial effects for the asthmatic child.

INTRODUCTION

Bronchial asthma is a common disorder with a prevalence of 3–5 per cent among children in the USA. As many as 75 per cent of these affected children eventually develop exercise-induced asthma [1]. Fear of exercise-induced asthma, the low level of respiratory and cardiovascular fitness of many asthmatic children and parental overprotection frequently lead to a severe restriction of physical activities even if the children are free of symptoms. It has been shown that 60 per cent of asthmatic children do not participate regularly in physical education at school or in physical activities during their leisure time [2]. The lack of physical exercise and active play leads to further deterioration in exercise tolerance. Consequently, many asthmatic children become isolated from their contemporaries, miss important social events and contacts, lose self-confidence and develop emotional problems. Since approximately 30 per cent of these children will continue to have asthma during their adult life [3] every effort must be made to improve their outlook early in the course of the disease.

RESULTS OF PHYSICAL EXERCISE PROGRAMMES

One of the first of the more systematic conditioning programmes for asthmatic children was described by Scherr and Frankel in 1958 [4]. Twenty-five children met twice weekly at a local YMCA for a general programme of breathing and postural exercises, gymnastics, swimming and activities such as judo and boxing designed to build their self-confidence. All but three children tolerated the programme well and showed gratifying improvement in general physical condition, pulmonary function, school attendance and in the number of asthmatic attacks and admissions to hospital.

A few years later Petersen and McElhenney [5] reported that 20 asthmatic boys participating in an eight-month programme of physical fitness training of calisthenics, relays, team sports and self-testing activities developed a significant increase in vital capacity. The programme also led to improvement in physical competence, self-confidence, acceptance by their contemporaries, intelligence scores and number of days absence from school. It was felt that the personal attention given to the children may have contributed considerably to their improvement.

Millman and his colleagues [6] evaluated the use of progressive and interval training methods in nine asthmatic children. The programme consisted of warm-up exercises, cardiovascular conditioning and vigorous 'rough and tumble' exercises. The maximal breathing capacity increased significantly while vital capacity and forced expiratory volume in one second (FEV_1) remained unchanged. It was thought that physical conditioning improved the cardiovascular efficiency and general physical state of these children.

Itkin and Nacman [7] studied 39 adolescents and young adults with asthma. After a control period of three months they conducted a three-month programme of specific conditioning exercises and athletics lasting two hours on five days a week. Two-thirds of the patients showed improvement in athletic ability and in three-quarters the maximum oxygen uptake after the exercise period was increased.

No improvement in cardiovascular fitness and maximum oxygen uptake was noted by Vavra and his colleagues [8] in a study of 16 asthmatic children after a vigorous three-month training programme.

Sly and his colleagues [9] carried out a controlled study of 12 asthmatic children participating in a three-month programme of physical conditioning and breathing exercises. Physical training resulted in a highly significant decrease in wheezing episodes, but there were no changes in pulmonary function or response to treadmill exercise. Most parents reported improved exercise tolerance, better co-ordination and breathing control and an increase in cheerfulness and co-operation in their children.

In another controlled study Findeisen [10] reported on 37 asthmatic children and adolescents participating in a programme lasting five to 11 months which consisted of very intensive competitive swimming, bicycling, cross-country skiing and long-distance running. Exercises were geared to increase the resting heart rate to a level between 160 and 180 beats/min, and were performed for 45 minutes two to three times a week. Asthmatic attacks decreased or even disappeared after an average of eight weeks. Improvements were also noted in pulmonary function, physical performance, somatic development and attendance at school. Medications could be decreased significantly and corticosteroids were discontinued in all children after an average training period of 3.2 months. Exercise-induced asthma developed only at the beginning of training and subsided with improving physical condition. The asthmatic state of the patients had, however, deteriorated three to five months after the end of the programme.

Fitch and his colleagues [11] examined the effects of five months' swimming training in 45 asthmatic children and reported improvement in physical condition, fitness, posture, swimming performance and number of asthma attacks and medications required. The frequency of exercise-induced asthma after running was not, however, changed by the programme.

Graff-Lonnevig and his colleagues [12] conducted a 20-month programme of increasing physical intensity in 20 asthmatic boys. All adapted well, even to heavy physical work without taking any premedication, although no significant improvement in cardiovascular fitness could be demonstrated.

Summer camps

In recent years several summer camps have been established for asthmatic children to provide comprehensive therapy and physical rehabilitation in a scenic area away from home and hospital. One of the best known is the Bronco Junction Camp, founded by Scherr in 1968 [13], where asthmatic children can spend eight weeks in a rebuilt railroad camp and participate in a diversified programme of physical and social activities. Emphasis is placed on breathing exercises, gymnastics, swimming, team sports and various camp activities. Analysis of the experience of the first two camps revealed that in all 54 children the severity and frequency of the asthmatic attacks and the amount of medication were reduced and that all showed significant improvement in both physical condition and psychosocial adjustment. These improvements persisted in most of the children with continuing exercise during a 10-month follow-up period.

Similar results have been reported by Götz and his colleagues [14] who conducted three camps for 118 asthmatic children in the Austrian Alps.

A more objective study of physical training was that of Geubelle and his colleagues [15] on 11 asthmatic children during a three-month stay in a mountain camp. Despite organising a strenuous programme of extensive hikes in the mountains, swimming, boxing and other physical exercise, they were unable to demonstrate any improvement in the working capacity of these children.

RECOMMENDATIONS FOR PHYSICAL TRAINING PROGRAMMES

Physical rehabilitation programmes for asthmatic children should be designed to improve physical health, exercise tolerance, participation in recreational activities, self-esteem, independence and emotional stability. These ambitious aims can only be achieved with the help of a multidisciplinary team of physicians, physical educators, physiotherapists, health instructors, psychologists and social workers [16]. Thorough medical knowledge of the complex nature and management of asthma have to be combined with scientifically approved techniques of physical and psychosocial rehabilitation.

The training should preferably be started at a rehabilitation centre or a summer camp and continued at home for several years. The atmosphere should be enjoyable and light-hearted, with attractive equipment, suitably decorated facilities, and the frequent use of music. Exposure to allergens and irritants and temperature and humidity should be controlled.

Continued health education at an appropriate level should be part of each programme. The children should learn as much as possible about asthma and exercise-induced asthma and should be instructed in self-monitoring and self-help techniques such as breathing exercises, progressive relaxation and the use, whenever possible, of warm drinks to prevent imminent wheezing episodes without the use of medications [17]. It is important to explain that exercise-induced shortness of breath without wheezing is a physiological event, which does not demand that the exercise should be stopped. Monthly conferences with children and parents should be conducted to discuss fresh problems or to consolidate the progress achieved. The more debilitated children will need continuous support and encouragement to stay in the programme and to perform the training with adequate effort.

Before joining the programme each child should be carefully evaluated with regard to severity of asthmatic symptoms, exercise-induced asthma, precipitating factors and defects of motor function and psychosocial behaviour. The exercise has to be prescribed individually and depends on current health and fitness as determined by a graded exercise stress test. The effectiveness of the programme depends on the intensity, duration, frequency, type and regularity of the physical effort. A heart rate of 60—70 per cent of the predicted maximal heart rate is the generally recommended target for effective training [18]; however, over-exertion or exhaustion has to be avoided.

Initially a work load should be chosen that can be tolerated for 10—15 minutes. With improving tolerance the stress should be gradually increased and prolonged to approximately 60 minutes, three to five times per week. Interval training consisting of short periods of exercise for five to seven minutes with intervening periods of relaxation or rest but without complete recovery is usually preferred to endurance training. Each session should start with a warm-up period of 15 minutes of easy calisthenics and stretching exercises and should end with a similar period of 10 minutes. When an adequate warm-up period is followed by interval training of gradually increasing intensity, exercise-induced asthma seldom becomes a problem and usually disappears after five to 10 minutes of rest without the use of medications [12]. Only a few children with more severe exercise-induced asthma require prophylactic treatment with sodium cromoglycate or beta$_2$-adrenergic agents before exercise. The training programme should be realistic and achievable within a relatively short period by most of the children. Each child should set his own pace and should compete against himself rather than against other members of the group who may have already achieved a higher level of fitness.

The training programme should offer a broad range of activities to allow the training of different muscle groups, since the training effect is mainly limited to the trained muscle. Exercises that strengthen the upper body musculature and swimming have an excellent conditioning effect and the least asthmagenic potential [19] and are particularly useful. Active children may engage in calisthenics, gymnastics, walking, hiking, bicycling, ball-games, cross-country skiing and free-range running, which have a greater training effect but are more liable to cause exercise-induced asthma. The more incapacitated children should perform less strenuous exercises built around the special needs of their daily living until they can progress to more challenging activities.

Breathing exercises should be part of any physical rehabilitation programme, but cannot replace aerobic fitness training [20]. During exercise, attention should be paid to the achievement of a controlled, slow, deep and rhythmic breathing pattern with a gradual decrease in the respiratory rate during the rest periods. Shallow hyperventilation and breath-holding must be avoided. Breathing through the nose should be encouraged whenever possible because of the filtering and warming effects and the consequent lower risk of exercise-induced asthma [21], but with an increasing aerobic work load mouth breathing will have to take over to meet the metabolic requirements of the body.

CONCLUSIONS

The results of physical training programmes in the rehabilitation of asthmatic children have been very encouraging, although several aspects of respiratory and cardiovascular reconditioning still remain to be resolved in larger, controlled studies. During exercise training most children develop marked improvement in general health, exercise tolerance, self-esteem, independence and number of asthmatic attacks, are better able to control their breathing pattern during exercise and wheezing episodes, use less medication and lose fewer days from school. Participation in individualised training programmes of progressive intensity and in physical education at school is therefore strongly advocated for all asthmatic children so that they may eventually overcome the negative impact of asthma on their development. Training should be continued almost indefinitely to maintain or even improve the beneficial effects of physical exercise.

Acknowledgments

The kind assistance of Dr Robert C Strunk and Warren Dennis, National Jewish Hospital and Research Center, Denver, Colorado, USA, and of Ms R Müller, Hochgebirgsklinik Davos-Wolfgang, is gratefully appreciated.

References

1 Cropp GJA.
   Exercise-induced asthma.
   Pediatr Clin North Am 1975; 22: 63–76

2 Findeisen DGR.
   Sporttherapie bei Asthma bronchiale im Kindes- und Jugendalter.
   Dtsch Gesundh-Wes 1974; 29, 44: 2075–2080

3 Rackemann FM, Edwards MC.
   Asthma in children: A follow-up study of 688 patients after an interval of twenty years. *N Engl J Med 1952; 246:* 21, 815–822

4 Scherr MS, Frankel L.
   Physical conditioning program for asthmatic children.
   JAMA 1958; 168, 15: 1996–2000

5 Petersen KH, McElhenney TR.
   Effects of a physical fitness program upon asthmatic boys.
   Pediatrics 1965; 35: 295–299

6 Millman M, Grundon WG, Kasch F et al.
   Controlled exercise in asthmatic children.
   Ann Allergy 1965; 23: 220–225

7 Itkin JH, Nacman M.
   The effect of exercise on the hospitalized asthmatic patient.
   J Allergy 1966; 37: 253–263

8 Vavra J, Macek M, Mrzena B, Spicak V.
   Intensive physical training in children with bronchial asthma.
   Acta Paediatr Scand Suppl 1971; 217: 90–92

9 Sly RM, Harper RT, Rosselot J.
   The effect of physical conditioning upon asthmatic children.
   Ann Allergy 1972; 30: 86–94

10 Findeisen DGR.
   The role of non-drug related treatment of asthma relying on sports ("sports therapy"). *Allergol Immunopathol (Madr) 1975; 3:* 145–148

11 Fitch KD, Morton AR, Blanksby BA.
   Effects of swimming training on children with asthma.
   Arch Dis Child 1976; 51: 190–194

12 Graff-Lonnevig V, Bevegard S, Eriksson BO et al.
   Two year's follow-up of asthmatic boys participating in a physical activity programme. *Acta Paediatr Scand 1980; 69:* 347–352

13   Scherr MS.
     Camp Bronco Junction – second year of experience.
     Ann Allergy 1970; 28: 423–433

14   Götz M, Deutsch J, Singer P.
     Therapielager für asthmakranke Kinder – Versuch einer Analyse.
     Wien Klin Wochenschr 1978; 19: 699–702

15   Geubelle F, Ernould C, Jovanovic M.
     Working capacity and physical training in asthmatic children at 1800m altitude.
     Acta Paediatr Scand Suppl 1971; 217: 93–98

16   Chester EH, Belman MJ, Bahler RC et al.
     Multidisciplinary treatment of chronic pulmonary insufficiency. 3. The effect
     of physical training on cardiopulmonary performance in patients with chronic
     obstructive pulmonary disease. *Chest 1977; 72:* 695–702

17   Staudenmayer H, Harris PS, Selner JC.
     Evaluation of a self-help education-exercise program for asthmatic children and
     their parents: Six-month follow-up. *J Asthma 1981; 18:* 1–5

18   Pollock ML.
     How much exercise is enough?
     Physician Sportsmed 1978; June: 50–64

19   Fitch KD, Morton AR.
     Specificity of exercise in exercise-induced asthma.
     Br Med J 1971; 4: 577–581

20   Keens TG.
     Exercise training program for pediatric patients with chronic lung disease.
     Pediatr Clin North Am 1979; 26, 3: 517–524

21   Shturman-Ellstein R, Zeballos RJ, Buckley JM, Souhrada JF.
     The beneficial effect of nasal breathing on exercise-induced bronchoconstriction.
     Am Rev Respir Dis 1978; 118: 65–73

DISCUSSION

HAIDER (Bury, UK)	Dr Backman, how long have the first group of children been followed after the withdrawal of active medical and psychosocial support? In other words, how successful are you in 'stabilising' them and their families in the long term, i.e. into adult life?
BACKMAN	We followed the children until they reached adulthood when we transferred them to the chest physicians; by that time their condition was generally fairly stable though in some cases there was variation. In the second group of children the follow-up has been such that we know exactly by counting absences from school and numbers of asthma attacks that three years after treatment the condition is completely stable.
STRUNK	It seems that there is evidence that physical training programmes can result in physical conditioning of asthmatic children and that the children can then take more exercise without precipitating exercise-induced bronchospasm. Is this true? Can an ideal programme be defined?
ANDRASCH	This is a general impression that we all have and one that we would like to see substantiated. It has been referred to in several studies but we still desperately need larger groups. In reviewing the literature the numbers of patients evaluated range from three to 39 or 40 patients and this is just not sufficient for making a firm statement.
FITCH (Nedlands, Australia)	Inferior motor skills have been observed in our group (and in others) in asthmatic children. We have been appalled at the poor running ability of many Australian asthmatic children. Our experience leads us to believe that we should attempt to rectify this motor inability

before the age of 11 or 12 years since co-ordination skills, especially hand-eye, are difficult for older children to achieve. Does the National Jewish Hospital /National Asthma Center recreational therapy department have any experience or comments?

STRUNK

We have an occupational therapy department at our institution as well where they deal more with those kinds of problems. It is our impression, however, that physical incoordination is no more frequent in the asthmatic population than in the general population. However, abnormalities that would be insignificant in a child without asthma may tend to be more of a problem and need to be attended to in the asthmatic child.

EDWARDS
(Chairman)

What measurements should be made in trying to prove that physical activity programmes are beneficial to asthmatic children?

BACKMAN

I do not think that we are able to make direct measurements, only indirect ones, by counting the symptoms, by counting the absences from school, by comparing the child's success in school or in occupational training afterwards and by showing that a child who has been in a rehabilitation programme is able to learn a skill and not be dependent on pensions and suchlike when he reaches adult life. In our research we have shown that there was a mathematical difference between the group who had family therapy and psychotherapy and the group who did not. So at least if you can use as simple a way as counting asthma days and show a difference between the two groups you have achieved something which might impress the authorities.

PART VI
PRACTICAL ASPECTS OF PHYSICAL ACTIVITY PROGRAMMES IN ASTHMATIC CHILDREN

Chairmen: Dr K Fitch, Nedlands, Western Australia
Professor S Oseid, Norway

Chapter 29

THE BENEFITS OF WARM-UP FOR ASTHMATIC CHILDREN

D Lindsay

Royal Prince Alfred Hospital, Camperdown, NSW, Australia

SUMMARY

'Warm-up' is a much misused term. In all publications concerning asthma and warm-up, the effect on body temperature of the prescribed exercise programmes has either not been noted or has not been measured. It has been assumed that warm-up — an increase in body core temperature — had been achieved. The rate of intracellular metabolic processes is dependent on temperature and increases by about 13 per cent for each degree of centigrade of increase; work capacity is increased by warm-up, thus defined.

Astrand has suggested that adequate warm-up for vigorous exercise is achieved by running at 12km/h for 15–30 minutes and has stated: "for ordinary exercise five minutes of light to moderate exercise is usually adequate." Högberg and Ljunggren have suggested that warm-up is achieved by 15–30 minutes of exercise at a relatively high rate of energy expenditure (3.0–3.4 litres oxygen uptake per min). Variation in environmental temperature and clothing means that the recommendations for warm-up have to be modified — the warmer the climate and the clothes the less the time required. Whatever the limitations of published studies it is clear that preceding exercise does *not worsen* exercise-induced asthma.

Unfortunately whilst it is true that brief exercise (less than two minutes' duration) of moderate intensity (less than 70 per cent maximum capacity) provokes less asthma than more prolonged, more intense exercise, in some patients even brief moderate exercise provokes asthma. Nevertheless, the fact that brief exercise of moderate intensity produces bronchodilatation in most asthmatics, makes proper warm-up potentially more beneficial to them than to non-asthmatics.

INTRODUCTION

As muscle temperature increases from 37 to 40°C the capacity for physical work is enhanced (Figure 1). This probably arises from the combined effects of increases in (1) cellular metabolic rate, (2) neural transmission rate, (3) the 'unloading' of oxygen from haemoglobin (Figure 2), and (4) muscle blood flow [1].

Cellular metabolic rate increases by about 13 per cent for each degree centigrade rise of temperature up to 40°C. Neural transmission rate is also temperature-dependent and the oxyhaemoglobin dissociation curve shifts to the right, thus favouring the off-loading of oxygen at tissue level at higher temperatures (Figure 2).

If one accepts the desired or optimal muscle temperature for most effective work to be 39°C, up to 30 minutes of exercise at a quite high rate of energy expenditure (3.0–3.4L O_2 uptake per minute) may be required in athletes to achieve warm-up [2]. The duration and intensity of warm-up (thus defined) would need to be varied to suit the environmental conditions and the type and amount of clothing worn and, presumably, the level of fitness of the subject.

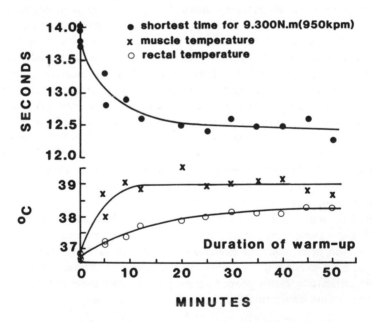

Figure 1. As body temperature increases with warm-up, so does the capacity for physical work (from Asmussen & Böye, 1945)

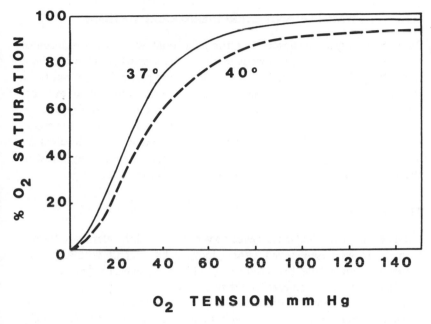

Figure 2. The shift to the right of the oxyhaemoglobin dissociation curve with increase in temperature

If warm-up is defined as exercise sufficient to produce a temperature of 39°C in the muscle groups that are subsequently to be used by the subject in the performance of work (or recreational activity) data are available which clearly shows its beneficial effects. Högberg and Ljunggren [2] showed that active warm-up significantly improved times for 100, 400 and 800 metre runs (by 2.5–6 per cent). This effect has been confirmed in swimmers [3] and some type of warm-up procedure is virtually universally accepted as being beneficial to participants in most sports.

There is no published study of the particular effects of warm-up on patients with asthma before their participation in exercise which might otherwise have provoked asthma. Despite this Fitch has stated "close observation of exercising asthmatics and extensive exercise history-compilation leads to the conclusion that hard exercise (e.g. 75 per cent or greater of VO_2 max) is more liable to produce exercise induced asthma (EIA) if not preceded by 'warm-up'." He recommended "that all asthmatics should 'warm-up' prior to athletic competition and exercise participation" [4]. Thus we may well still ask whether warm-up is of particular benefit to asthmatics – and if so, why?

WARM-UP AND EXERCISE-INDUCED ASTHMA

Since there appear to be no scientific data to allow precise resolution of the questions we can only speculate on the basis of what is known about the provocation of asthma by exercise and, more particularly, about those factors which reduce the asthmatic response to a given quantity of exercise.

The amount of exercise-induced asthma is determined by the type, duration and intensity of exercise, the interval since the last attack of exercise-induced asthma, the temperature and water content of the inspired air during exercise, and the immediately preceding exercise history. Most of these factors are discussed in detail elsewhere in these proceedings.

The refractory period

What seems of particular relevance to warm-up are data relating to 'refractoriness' to exercise-induced asthma induced by exercise within the previous two hours, the bronchodilating effects of exercise [5], and the 'protective effects of repeated short sprints' [6].

Some 50 per cent of asthmatic patients, both children and adults, who recover spontaneously from exercise-induced asthma are at least partially refractory to the effects of a subsequent matched exercise challenge within one hour. When the repeat exercise test is delayed a further one or two hours (that is, two or three hours after the initial test) the exercise-induced asthma does not differ significantly from the initial response. In these patients exercise of sufficient duration and intensity to evoke exercise-induced asthma used as warm-up, even if insufficient to produce a genuine and significant increase in core temperature, might be seen to be 'beneficial' by reducing the exercise-induced asthma provoked by subsequent competitive or recreational exercise begun after recovery from the initial exercise-induced asthma! 'Treating fire with fire' would be one way to interpret and describe such a phenomenon.

Effect of short sprints

Schnall and Landau [6] have identified an effect of short sprints before a standard six-minute running exercise test which gives credence to the observation of the beneficial effects of warm-up in asthmatics. Seven 30-second periods of running separated from each other by 2.5 minutes and by 20 minutes from the standard running test appeared to protect their six patients (aged 12–31 years) from exercise-induced asthma. The mean percentage fall in FEV_1 which followed the standard test not preceded by sprints was 22.3 per cent (mild exercise-induced asthma) whilst it was only 6.9 per cent after the run preceded by the seven sprints. Whether similar protection can be effected by sprints in patients with more severe exercise-induced asthma requires further study, and whether the seven sprints produced warm-up was, unfortunately, not measured. More recent unpublished data from their laboratory have demonstrated protection from subsequent exercise-induced asthma in some patients even if the short sprints were not followed by exercise-induced asthma. They speculate that whatever produces the frequently observed bronchodilatation during exercise might remain to protect against the exercise-induced asthma-producing mechanisms triggered by subsequent more prolonged exercise (personal communication).

Speculation on mechanisms

Since neither temperature changes nor ventilation were measured in their experiments they could only hypothesise that "a warm-up effect of short runs may help improve circulation to the appropriate muscles and reduce anaerobic respiration during the run that provoked asthma". They went on to speculate further that "these short sprints may also have provided sufficient warm-up for the subjects to exercise more efficiently with greater oxygen extraction and therefore lower ventilation during subsequent runs".

If indeed ventilation was lower at the same workload during the subsequent runs, and the ambient environmental conditions (of temperature and relative humidity) were the same, loss of heat and water would have been less and thus, accepting the observations relating loss of heat and water to exercise-induced asthma, there would have been less exercise-induced asthma.

The question nevertheless remains: is the improvement in oxygen transport in the muscles, neural transmission rate and muscle blood flow sufficient to reduce the loss of heat and water, and thus exercise-induced asthma, as based on the data of Deal and his colleagues [7]? To reduce exercise-induced asthma from a 50 per cent fall in FEV_1 to a zero per cent fall would require 2kcal/min (8.4kJ/min) less heat loss. This in turn would necessitate a reduction in ventilation of many litres per minute — a tall order for warm-up alone!

CONCLUSION

In the absence of data clearly demonstrating the benefits of warm-up, *particularly* for asthmatic children, one is tempted to say that there may

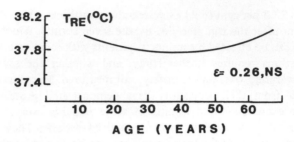

Figure 3. Children dissipate heat less rapidly than adults (NS=not significant)
(modified from Drinkwater & Horvath *Medicine and Science in Sports 1979*)

in fact not be any. And this despite the "close observations" mentioned by
Fitch [4] , the presence of a refractory period after exercise-induced asthma
and also, perhaps, exercise which does not provoke a fall in flow rates [6]
and the well-known bronchodilating effect of exercise in asthmatics [5] .

Children may require less prolonged and less intense exercise to warm-up
adequately because they dissipate heat less rapidly than adults (Figure 3).
However, it still seems unlikely that the types of warm-up calisthenics and
exercise of low intensity for relatively brief periods indulged in by asthmatic children in many, if not all, exercise programmes would effect other
than minimal increase in core temperature.

It might then be fairer to say that the effects of proper warm-up on the
asthmatic response to exercise in asthmatic children have not yet been
properly evaluated. Observations supporting the hypothesis that the
effects, if any, are beneficial [4] appear to justify a properly controlled
study of the phenomenon.

References

1   Astrand PO, Rodahl K.
     Textbook of Work Physiology 2nd Edition 1977: 562–563
     New York: McGraw Hill

2   Högberg P, Ljunggren O.
     Uppvärmningens inverkan pa löpprestationerna.
     Svensk Idrott 1947; 40

3   Muido L.
     The influence of body temperature on performances in swimming.
     Acta Physiol Scand 1946; 12: 102

4   Fitch KD.
     Exercise-induced asthma and competitive athletics.
     Paediatrics (Suppl) 1975; 56 No 5 Part 2: 942–943

5   Joseph J, Bandler L, Anderson SD.
     Exercise as a bronchodilator.
     Aust J Physiother 1976: 47–50

6   Schnall RP, Landau LI.
     Protective effects of repeated short sprints in exercise-induced asthma.
     Thorax 1980; 35: 828–832

7   Deal EC, McFadden ER Jr, Ingram RH Jr et al.
     Role of respiratory heat exchange in production of exercise induced asthma.
     J Appl Physiol 1979; 46: 467–475

Chapter 30

THE USE OF TRAINING PROGRAMMES IN ASTHMATIC CHILDREN

R Verrier Jones, H Williams, V Zarabbi, Beverley Roberts

University Hospital of Wales, Cardiff, United Kingdom

SUMMARY

Most asthmatic children show evidence of exercise-induced asthma. The fact that exercise is the triggering factor often goes unrecognised with the result that these children often stop, or are stopped by others, from doing any kind of strenuous activity and grow up in an atmosphere in which ordinary physical activity, and in particular games, is denied them. Training programmes can promote an interest in games and can help the children and their parents to overcome this non-playing attitude.

Ten children attending an asthma clinic were selected for the programme; all had exercise-induced asthma. It was explained to the children and their parents that a three-month course consisting of weekly sessions of gymnastics and swimming was about to start. Each session was attended by a doctor, premedication was given and the activities were supervised by physiotherapists.

After three months the children were assessed. Not surprisingly their level of physical fitness had improved, but more important was the fact that they (and their parents) felt more confident in their ability to enter into sports activities at school. A further assessment at six months showed that this improvement had been maintained: all were now taking part in sports, several had started new sports and their asthma had improved as shown by fewer school absences, fewer visits to the doctor and less medication taken. The training programmes thus encouraged the children to take exercise and gave them and their parents confidence in their ability. The programme should be supervised by doctors or physiotherapists if possible, due attention being paid to premedication and the role that exercise-induced asthma plays in these children.

INTRODUCTION

Most asthmatic children have exercise-induced asthma [1]. In the pre-school child this is usually manifested as bouts of coughing after exercise and is not usually a serious problem. The older child, however, takes part in more serious games and exercise and will therefore show the more typical features of exercise-induced asthma with bronchoconstriction and consequent shortness of breath and wheezing. These symptoms restrict the ability to participate in games and activities and a pattern may be set up whereby the child stops playing games and loses confidence in his ability to indulge in any strenuous physical activity. His parents and teachers, because they have seen him becoming distressed after games, readily cooperate in this life-style of non-activity and the child is liable to grow up with neither the desire nor the confidence to play games.

With the realisation by the asthmatic child himself, his parents, teachers and especially his doctors, that exercise is such a potent factor in his asthma, a rational programme of management can be undertaken. This includes identifying the most appropriate medications and the correct time to use them, and the giving of encouragement and advice about the amount and type of exercise that is best for that child. The most suitable way to achieve these ideals is to enrol the child in a physical training programme.

Physical activity programmes have been advocated for many years in the overall management of asthmatic children, notably in Norway, Australia and the USA [2], possibly because in these countries there is a greater awareness of the benefits of physical fitness in the population at large. In the UK such programmes have been less popular, the emphasis being on good 'medical' management and it is only recently that physical activity programmes have been described and advocated, though there has been controversy that they do little more than improve the child's physical fitness and do not improve his asthma [3].

In order to look at these hypotheses, a physical activity programme was set up in Cardiff in 1981.

METHODS

Ten children attending an asthma clinic were selected on the basis that they had had asthma for at least three years and had direct evidence of exercise-induced asthma and that consequently both they and their parents would be motivated to participate in and complete the three-month course. A preliminary meeting was held to explain to the children and their parents what the programme entailed and what was hoped would be achieved.

The intention was to gather objective and subjective proof that such a programme of physical activity would not only improve the children's asthma and improve their attitude to exercise and games, but also convince their parents, teachers and general practitioners. A programme was designed so that the children were subjected to two contrasting types of exercise. One, gymnastics, was deemed 'asthmagenic' and the other, swimming, was not.

The programme lasted for three months. It was conducted by two physiotherapists and consisted of weekly hour-long sessions of either swimming or gymnastics. A doctor was always in attendance. Before the start of every session, each child was medically assessed by the doctor, a peak expiratory flow reading (PEFR) obtained and premedication with either sodium cromoglycate or salbutamol or both given. The activity work load was gradually increased throughout the course. Each session began with a warm-up period of five minutes during which the children were encouraged to play and have fun before the middle period of fairly hard and structured exercises were performed. Each session ended with some sort of competitive game between two teams. Afterwards the children would relax and calm down, be medically assessed and have their PEFRs recorded again.

RESULTS

Objective and subjective evidence was sought in order to assess whether the course had improved the children's asthma and also whether their attitude to sports had been changed by the three-month training programme.

Objective assessment

PEFRs were performed before and after each weekly session throughout the three month period. The PEFR of each child tended to improve after each session, but overall the improvement between beginning and end of the course was not significant.

As stated, all ten children had evidence of exercise-induced asthma. Six had repeat exercise tests after the course, but although it was evident that they were physically fitter than before, without premedication they still showed the same degree of fall in PEFR after exercise that they had shown before the course started.

Subjective assessment

A questionnaire (Figure 1) was given to each family after completion of the programme. It was stressed to them that they should make their answers as accurate as possible and not try and 'please' the doctors by exaggerating the improvements they thought had been made. The answers are given in Table I — all 10 families returned their questionnaires.

QUESTIONNAIRE

	Yes	No	Don't know
Did the 3-month course have the effect of			
improving asthma	. . . .	. . . .	. . . .
reducing the number of attacks	. . . .	. . . .	. . . .
increasing activity	. . . .	. . . .	. . . .

Has your child started any new physical activities since the course? YES/NO

If yes, which are they? . . . .

Has there been any change in his/her attitude to games at school? YES/NO

	Improved	Not improved	Become worse
Has your child's attitude to his asthma	. . . .	. . . .	. . . .
Has your (i.e. parent's) attitude	. . . .	. . . .	. . . .
Has the teacher's attitude	. . . .	. . . .	. . . .

	Yes	No	Don't know
Has there been any change in your child's			
mood	. . . .	. . . .	. . . .
attitude	. . . .	. . . .	. . . .
need for medication	. . . .	. . . .	. . . .
school attendance	. . . .	. . . .	. . . .

Figure 1. The questionnaire given to each family to complete at the end of the programme

TABLE I. Answers to questionnaire

Question	Number giving positive response (out of 10)
The three month course	
improved the asthma	9
reduced the number of attacks	8
increased the child's activity	8
New physical activities started	9
Improved attitude to games	10
Improved attitude to asthma	
children's	9
parents'	8
teacher's	6

DISCUSSION

Physical activity programmes have been advocated for asthmatic children for many years [4]. Most workers have shown that although there has been good evidence that the child's physical fitness has improved, there is little evidence to show that these programmes actually improve the asthma according to the normally accepted measures of lung function – that is, PEFR, forced expiratory volume in one second (FEV_1) and forced vital capacity (FVC). Nevertheless there is clinical evidence that the programmes do improve the child's asthma; for instance, the children use less medication, have fewer attacks and better school attendance records and their attitude to games is improved, as is that of their parents and teachers [5, 6].

This present study indicates that 'hard' objective data to show that a programme of physical activity is beneficial to a child with asthma is difficult to come by, but that 'soft' objective data – such as school attendance, amount of medication taken and the reduction in number of asthmatic attacks – can be taken as good proof that such a programme can actually improve a child's asthma.

Equally important is the definite improvement in the children's attitude to their asthma and to sports in general. In addition we found that the parents' attitudes improved as they saw and realised what their children were achieving in athletic terms – in fact, the whole group of children and parents became noticeably more enthusiastic about physical activities and games than they had been before.

The one-year follow-up of these 10 children indicates that the level of physical activity achieved after the initial course has been maintained, and several are now indulging in competitive sports in a way they would not have attempted a year before.

References

1   Cropp GJA.
     Exercise-induced asthma.
     Pediatr Clin N Am 1975; 22: 63–76

2   Scherr MS, Frankel L.
     Physical conditioning program for asthmatic children.
     JAMA 1958; 168: 1996–2000

3   Fitch KD, Morton AR, Blanksby BA.
     Effects of swimming training on children with asthma.
     Arch Dis Child 1976; 51: 190–194

4   Monks AW, Edwards AM.
     Asthma and Exercise. Simple activity programmes for asthmatic groups 1981.
     Loughborough: Fisons

5   Verma S, Hyde JS.
     Physical education programs and exercise-induced asthma.
     Clin Pediatr (Phila) 1976; 15: 697–705

6   Petersen KH, McElhenney TR.
     Effects of a physical fitness program upon asthmatic boys.
     Pediatrics 1965; 35: 295–299

Chapter 31

DOUBLE-BLIND PROSPECTIVE STUDY OF THE EFFECT OF PHYSICAL TRAINING ON CHILDHOOD ASTHMA

I L Swann, Cheryl Anita Hanson

Burnley General Hospital, United Kingdom

SUMMARY

Twenty-seven children, attending an asthma clinic with confirmed exercise-induced bronchospasm, were the subjects of a prospective study of the effect of physical training on asthma. They were randomly allocated to a physical training schedule or to a schedule of relaxation classes, twice weekly for a period of three months. On induction the child performed a free-running exercise test, and this was repeated at monthly intervals during the trial. Each child was supplied with a Wright Mini Peak Flow Meter and recorded the peak expiratory flow rate (PEFR) morning and night. Diary record cards of respiratory symptom scores were kept by all the children during the trial.

Physical training and relaxation schedules were designed and supervised by one paediatric physiotherapist and exercise testing was independently assessed by a doctor. The medication the children were receiving for their asthma was not varied during the study.

There was no significant change in the PEFRs during the study, nor was there significant variation between the two groups. The same applied to the diary symptom scores. There was, however, a significantly smaller percentage fall in the PEFR after exercise and an increase in the minimum PEFR after exercise as the trial proceeded. This effect was seen both in the physical training and relaxation groups. At the end of the study, children in the activity group could accomplish 100 per cent more physical training than at the beginning.

INTRODUCTION

Exercise-induced bronchoconstriction is extremely common in children with asthma [1]. It may result in the child's withdrawal from normal sporting activity, leading to loss of self-confidence, introspection, loss of physical fitness and occasionally isolation. A prospective double-blind study was performed to assess the effect of a physical training programme on asthmatic children known to have exercise-induced bronchoconstriction.

METHODS

Children attending the asthma clinic with proven exercise-induced broncho-spasm (> 20% fall in peak expiratory flow rate (PEFR) after exercise) were, with consent, randomly allocated to one of two groups. The first underwent a graduated physical training programme, designed and super-vised by a paediatric physiotherapist. The second took part in relaxation classes supervised by the same physiotherapist.

Physical training group

The physical training programme began with a warming-up period of exer-cises interspersed with short rests in positions suitable for controlling wheeze. This was followed by an intensive programme of exercise compris-ing step-ups, squat thrusts, star jumps, sit-ups and press-ups. These exercises were performed in the same order at each session and were repeated daily, at home. Each child's exercise tolerance was individually assessed before entry to the group and the exercise programme determined from the result. The sessions were held twice weekly for three months and the exercise load increased at each session. Children received premedication with sodium cromoglycate by Spinhaler, 15 minutes before the exercise.

Relaxation group

Children in the relaxation group attended once weekly for three months and repeated the programme daily at home. Their routine comprised contrast relaxation in various positions appropriate for use during an episode of wheezing and controlled diaphragmatic breathing. Sessions began and ended with a short period of activity selected by the children themselves — relay games were the most popular choice.

Both groups

On introduction to the project and at monthly intervals for three months each child underwent a free-running exercise test [2]. This consisted of running along a level corridor for six minutes at sufficient speed to achieve a pulse rate of 170 beats/min or more. After the exercise the PEFR was measured at 0, 1, 3, 5, 10 and 15 minutes.

Each child was supplied with a Wright Mini Peak Flow Meter and performed daily PEFR measurements in the morning and at night for the duration of the study. A daily diary score of asthmatic symptoms was recorded. Symptoms of wheeze, breathlessness, cough, chest tightness and sputum production were scored from one to 10 according to severity, both by day and by night.

RESULTS

The study started with 27 children and ended with 21 (five children dropped out of the relaxation group). The children's ages ranged from seven to 14 years and in all cases the severity of their asthma was assessed clinically as moderate.

TABLE I. The characteristics of the patients in the two groups

Characteristic	Relaxation group	Graduated exercise group
Number	7	14
Age (years)		
Mean	10.3	11.1
Range	7–14	8–13
Height (cm)		
Mean	137.4	135.6*
Range	130–154	125–150
Predicted PEFR (L/min)		
Mean	292.8	304.6
Range	260–375	225–380
Actual PEFR (L/min)		
Mean	235.7	218.8
Range	200–310	110–360
Per cent predicted PEFR		
Mean	80.4	71.7
Range	73–95	30–96
Medication		
Intal	6	11
Becotide	1	2
Ventolin	4	9
Phyllocontin	1	0

* Mean of 10 patients

Seven children completed the relaxation course and 14 the physical training. The characteristics of the patients were similar in both groups (Table I) — normal values were taken from the date of Godfrey and his colleagues [3].

Daily PEFR measurements did not vary significantly between the groups during the study, nor was there any significant variation within the groups. Analysis of the diary card data similarly showed no difference between groups and no variation during the study.

As the study progressed there was a significant increase in the minimum PEFR recorded after the exercise test (p < 0.01) (exercise tests 2, 3 and 4 > test 1). Similarly there was a decrease in the maximum percentage fall

TABLE II. Minimum PEFR after the free-running exercise tests in the two groups (SD_1 = standard deviation for comparison of therapy; SD_2 = standard deviation for comparison of exercise tests)

| Exercise test | Minimum PEFR (L/min) | |
	Relaxation group	Graduated exercise group
On entry	200.0	178.2
At month 1	262.8	197.5
At month 2	250.7	232.8
At month 3	238.6	225.0
SD_1 (19 df)	93.12	
SD_2 (57 df)	45.96	
Significant effects	Exercise test (p < 0.01)	

TABLE III. Maximum percentage fall in PEFR after the free-running exercise tests in the two groups (SD_1 = standard deviation for comparison of therapy; SD_2 = standard deviation for comparison of exercise tests)

| Exercise test | Maximum percentage fall in PEFR | |
	Relaxation group	Graduated exercise group
On entry	28.4	38.0
At month 1	14.3	33.7
At month 2	13.5	23.3
At month 3	19.2	21.8
SD_1 (19 df)	20.94	
SD_2 (57 df)	13.10	
Significant effects	Therapy (p = 0.045) Exercise test (p < 0.01)	

TABLE IV. PEFRs (L/min) after the free-running exercise tests in the two groups (R = relaxation group. GE = graduated exercise group)

Exercise test	Group	Before exercise	Time after exercise (min)					
			0	1	3	5	10	15
On entry	R	275	272.8	222.1	217.8	218.6	217.8	230.7
	GE	277.5	245.4	215.7	195	196.8	207.5	227.5
At month 1	R	310	301.4	285.7	275.7	274.3	279.3	280
	GE	295.4	277.8	247.1	211.1	216.8	226.8	242.8
At month 2	R	290	311.4	274.3	259.3	260	263.6	264.3
	GE	303.2	295	284.3	248.6	240.4	248.6	256.8
At month 3	R	297.1	289.3	254.3	252.8	250	262.8	282.1
	GE	289.6	296.1	262.1	239.3	245.7	251.4	248.6

in PEFR after exercise (p < 0.01) (exercise test 2 > test 1 and tests 3 and 4 > test 2). This effect was seen, however, in both the relaxation and the exercise groups, suggesting the influence of factors other than exercise (Tables II–IV). The children in the physical training group increased their exercise capacity by about 100 per cent by the end of the study.

DISCUSSION

The trend to a reduction in exercise-induced bronchoconstriction during the study may be explained in several ways. Involvement in the trial tended to increase the general knowledge and understanding of asthma of both parents and children. It may be that routine asthma medication was taken more regularly and effectively. Psychological influences may also have been at work, but we would stress that the numbers involved in the project were small and the results should therefore be interpreted with caution.

The improved exercise capacity in these children would seem to be a highly desirable outcome, and this was achieved with apparent complete safety.

References

1   Editorial.
     Exercise induced asthma.
     Br Med J 1980; 280: 271

2   Day G, Mearns MB.
     Bronchial lability in cystic fibrosis.
     Arch Dis Child 1973; 48: 355–359

3   Godfrey S, Kamburoff PL, Nairn JR et al.
     Spirometry, lung volumes and airway resistance in normal children aged 5–18 years. Br J Dis Chest 1970; 64: 15–24

DISCUSSION

GILLAM (Victoria, Australia)	Is it possible that the warm-up period could result in improved ventilation/perfusion ratios in the lung, and thus, in patients with severe exercise-induced asthma, prevent any fall in the arterial pO_2? This may be important in ensuring that children can continue in the exercise session. Would Dr Lindsay please comment?
LINDSAY	I think what Dr Gillam means is that an increase in pulmonary blood flow might improve ventilation/perfusion ratios. It might also make them worse. It depends on the distribution of ventilation as well as the distribution of perfusion and so to say that you could consistently produce an improvement in arterial oxygen tension by a warm-up procedure is not valid. A warm-up does improve efficiency, can improve performance, and would reduce ventilation at the given work load but, as I said, the reduction in ventilation at the given work load that would be produced by a proper warm-up is very unlikely to have the suggested effect on exercise-induced asthma.
FITCH (Chairman)	We did attempt to evaluate exercise-induced asthma. Seventeen subjects undertook a three-minute warm-up period. This was chosen because we did not want to induce asthma before we gave them the standard challenge on the running treadmill. This three minutes of exercise consisted of either jogging or walking to develop heart rates up to 60 per cent of predicted maxima. The resultant falls of between 37 and 38 per cent in FEV_1 were identical in the 17 subjects whether or not they had had this three minute warm-up.
LINDSAY	I am concerned that the term is being used when in fact nobody is measuring core temperature or muscle temperature. Those who are involved in sports medi-

cine recognise the value of warm-up. If you send a sprinter out into a competition cold, apart from the fact that he might damage a muscle, he will perform three to six per cent worse than if his muscles were 2°C hotter than at rest. That fact has been known for 25 years. The problem is that we are using the term for three minutes of gentle exercise. *That* will not warm the muscles at all! If we are going to use the term warm-up and not be confusing, we have to measure temperature and show that what we say is a warm-up is indeed warming the subject up.

SMITH
(Warwick, UK)

The UK lacks the multidisciplinary approach advocated by Dr Andrasch. Which 'disciplines' do you consider contribute the least at the moment?

VERRIER JONES

It has been very interesting to us from the UK to hear about the superb exercise and training programmes practised in Australia, Scandinavia and Switzerland. In the United Kingdom, as Mr Smith said, the multidisciplinary approach to this subject is sadly lagging behind that in other countries and if I had to say which people were the most important yet contributed the least, I would have to say the teachers — but general practitioners are not blameless, either. Paediatricians should know about exercise-induced asthma and its effect on physical activity, but then only 20 per cent of asthmatic children come to paediatricians. Eighty per cent are seen either by their general practitioners or, perhaps, not at all. Therefore the only group of people in some authority who see these children are teachers and they do not know about exercise-induced asthma. So it is teachers, particularly physical education teachers, who should be educated about asthma and exercise.

IIKURA
(Tokyo, Japan)

Do you supervise the group activities every week?

VERRIER JONES   Yes. During the three-month course I saw my patients every week, whereas normally I would not see my patients anything like as frequently. But it is only a very small proportion of my patients who are actually attending courses — 10 out of a possible 300 or 400 patients.

VÄLIMÄKI
(Turku, Finland)   How reproducible are the benefits of a rehabilitation programme?

VERRIER JONES   I think they are reproducible.

Chapter 32

BRONCHIAL HYPERREACTIVITY IN CHILDREN WITH PERENNIAL EXTRINSIC ASTHMA

P Aa Østergaard, S Pedersen

Aalborg Hospital North, Denmark

SUMMARY

Using a 20 per cent fall in peak expiratory flow rate (PEFR) and in forced expiratory volume in one second (FEV_1) from the base-line values as the criteria, we found exercise-induced asthma in 48 per cent of a total of 75 children with perennial IgE-mediated asthma on testing on a bicycle ergometer.

Compared to 39 children without evidence of exercise-induced asthma the 36 patients who exhibited this symptom were found to have elevated levels of blood eosinophil leucocytes and considerably higher serum IgE levels. Furthermore, allergy to moulds and house-dust mites, increased serum IgE levels and elevated levels of blood eosinophil leucocytes were more significant in 13 of 24 patients with exercise-induced asthma who did not improve after a physical training programme, compared to the remaining 11 children who did. Finally, in the former patients, base-line PEFR and FEV_1 levels were extremely low before as well as after the training programme. Thus, these results indicate that in children with perennial IgE-mediated asthma complicated by exercise-induced asthma, the latter may be greatly influenced by a continuous release of chemical mediators, probably in the bronchial wall from mast cells and eosinophil leucocytes.

INTRODUCTION

Asthma can be regarded as a complex syndrome of reversible airway obstruction characterised by bronchial hyperreactivity to a variety of stimuli, such as physical exercise. However, the threshold for exercise-induced asthma varies considerably among asthmatic children and also in the same individual at different times [1].

It has been shown that the fall in pulmonary function after exercise can be reduced by physical training of the interval type [2]. It is, however, our experience that some children with extrinsic asthma do not respond satisfactorily to physical training, in particular those with a very high serum IgE and/or blood eosinophil level.

We therefore decided to investigate whether factors such as the levels of serum IgE and blood eosinophils, as well as the nature of the allergy in children with perennial, extrinsic asthma could influence the incidence of exercise-induced asthma and the base-line levels of peak expiratory flow rate (PEFR) and forced expiratory volume in one second (FEV_1). We also studied the effect of physical training in these children.

MATERIALS AND METHODS

Our series consisted of 75 children, six to 15 years of age, with perennial, extrinsic asthma. All were tested for the presence of exercise-induced asthma on a bicycle ergometer for six minutes, aiming to achieve a constant pulse rate of 170 beats/min or more for the last four minutes of the ride. All medication was stopped at least 48 hours before challenge. We used a 20 per cent or greater fall in PEFR and/or FEV_1 from the base-line values as the criterion of exercise-induced asthma. Those children who were found to have exercise-induced asthma were selected to take part in a programme of interval training lasting 1½ hours per week over a period of four months.

Serum IgE and blood eosinophil levels were checked twice and the average taken as the value for that individual. Furthermore, prick tests and radioallergosorbent tests (RAST) to several commercial allergens were carried out, and if there was inconsistency between the results of the two tests, a bronchial provocation test was performed.

The criterion for a successful outcome of the physical training was that the PEFR or FEV_1 after exercise should not fall more than 20 per cent below base-line values at two to four weeks after the end of the training in a child who had taken no medication for at least two weeks.

RESULTS

In our original series of 75 children, 36 (48%) were found to have exercise-induced asthma; they also had serum IgE levels and blood eosinophil levels that were significantly higher than those of the 39 children without evidence of exercise-induced asthma (p <0.005 and <0.05, respectively). Furthermore, allergies to moulds and house-dust mites were more common in the patients with exercise-induced asthma than in those without (p <0.02 and <0.002, respectively). Finally, base-line FEV_1 levels were considerably reduced in the children with exercise-induced asthma, a finding that did not apply to the children without exercise-induced asthma (p <0.005).

So far, 24 of the 36 children with exercise-induced asthma have participated in our physical training programme: 11 have benefited, 13 have not.

TABLE I. Blood eosinophil levels in the 24 patients who participated in the physical training programme

| | No. | Blood eosinophil level $(x\ 10^6/L)$ | | |
		Range	Median	p value
Patients who benefited	11	93–1040	510	
				<0.02
Patients who did not benefit	13	104–5080	990	

Table I shows that blood eosinophil levels were raised in the 13 children who failed to benefit from the training, as compared to the 11 who did. Moreover, extremely high serum IgE concentrations were found in those who did not benefit (Table II). In addition, allergy to moulds – and

TABLE II. Serum IgE levels in the 24 patients who participated in the physical training programme

| | No. | Serum IgE level (IU/ml) | | |
		Range	Median	p value
Patients who benefited	11	88–1480	450	
				<0.01
Patients who did not benefit	13	140–4090	1240	

specifically to house-dust mites — was far more common among them than among the children who had no obvious signs of exercise-induced asthma after completing the training programme (Table III). Lastly, the base-line

TABLE III. The nature of the allergies in the 24 patients who participated in the physical training programme

Allergen	Patients who benefited (11)	Patients who did not benefit (13)
Pollen	7 (65.5%)	5 (38.4%)
Animal danders	5 (45.4%)	5 (38.4%)
House-dust mites	3 (27.2%)	10 (80%)
Moulds	2 (18.2%)	5 (38.4%)

PEFR levels, and, more significantly, the base-line FEV_1 levels before the start of training were low in the 13 patients in whom exercise-induced asthma was still demonstrated afterwards (Table IV), and they were even lower after completion of the training programme (Table V).

TABLE IV. Base-line PEFR and FEV_1 levels (per cent of predicted normal levels) in the 24 patients before they entered the training programme

	No.	PEFR			FEV_1		
		Range	Median	p value	Range	Median	p value
Patients who benefited	11	87–130%	115%		70–110%	95%	
				>0.05			<0.05
Patients who did not benefit	13	61–118%	95%		55–95%	68.5%	

TABLE V. Base-line PEFR and FEV_1 levels (per cent of predicted normal levels) in the 24 patients after completing the training programme

	No.	PEFR			FEV_1		
		Range	Median	p value	Range	Median	p value
Patients who benefited	11	88–145%	130%		74–120%	98%	
				<0.05			<0.02
Patients who did not benefit	13	64–112%	82%		52–88%	54.5%	

It must be emphasised that the 24 patients who took part in the physical training programme also were participators in a double-blind study in which sodium cromoglycate or placebo, both provided as a spray, was given to the patients to investigate whether or not sodium cromoglycate could improve the results of physical training. In five of the 13 children who did not benefit from training, exercise-induced asthma was blocked by the inhalation of sodium cromoglycate 15 minutes before challenge.

DISCUSSION

Despite all the work that has been done on exercise-induced asthma, we still have no definite explanation of its pathogenesis. Hypotheses that invoke hyperventilation, hypocapnia or acidosis cannot explain differences in asthmagenicity between various kinds of exercise [3]. Furthermore, although they are obvious candidates, neither histamine nor acetylcholine has yet been shown to be the mediator of exercise-induced asthma. On the other hand, in most patients with exercise-induced asthma, the full constrictor effect of the physical exercise does not occur till some two to five minutes or more after stopping the run; moreover, the refractory period of one hour or more after an initial episode of exercise-induced asthma points to the release of a mediator being an important factor in the development of exercise-induced asthma [4] – once mast cells have been degranulated, an hour or more is required for them to resynthesise their mediators. This observation favours the theory that mast cells, to some extent, participate in the development of exercise-induced asthma.

The findings that our children with perennial, extrinsic asthma complicated by exercise-induced asthma have far higher levels of serum IgE and blood eosinophils, as well as being more allergic to moulds and house-dust mites than those whose asthma is not complicated in this manner, point to the mast cell and its release of chemical mediators as important factors in the pathogenesis of exercise-induced asthma. Of possible significance is the fact that moulds and, in particular, house-dust mites are allergens known to be operating throughout the year as compared to allergens such as pollen and animal danders, which are more seasonal and occupationally-related allergens.

It has been shown that children with extrinsic asthma are more liable to the spontaneous release of histamine as a result of triggering by nonspecific stimuli, such as exercise, than are normal children [3]. Furthermore, Neijens and his colleagues [3] found that the histamine threshold was considerably lower in children with extrinsic asthma who suffered from exercise-induced asthma than in asthmatic children who did not. Thus, in our patients with exercise-induced asthma who obtained no benefit from physical training, the extremely high serum IgE and blood eosinophil levels may reflect a hypersensitivity state with a low threshold for the release of chemical mediators from the mast cells which makes them more vulnerable to non-specific stimuli such as exercise.

References

1   Anderson SD, Silverman M et al.
    Exercise-induced asthma.
    Br J Dis Chest 1975; 69: 1–39

2   Oseid S.
    Exercise-induced asthma — its importance in childhood asthma and its management. In Pepys J, Edwards AM, eds.
    The Mast Cell: its Role in Health and Disease 1979: 265.
    Tunbridge Wells: Pitman Medical

3   Neijens HJ, Degenhart HJ, Raatgeep R et al.
    Spontaneous release of histamine in asthmatic children sensitive to non-specific stimuli. In Pepys J, Edwards AM, eds.
    The Mast Cell: its Role in Health and Disease 1979: 322.
    Tunbridge Wells: Pitman Medical

4   Godfrey S.
    Exercise-induced asthma.
    Asthma 1977; 3: 56–78

Chapter 33

TRAINING OF CHILDREN WITH EXERCISE-INDUCED ASTHMA IN HALLAND, SWEDEN

H Hildebrand, E Sundstén*

Children's Hospital, and *Habilitation Unit, Halmstad, Sweden

SUMMARY

The county of Halland in Sweden has 56,000 children; those with asthma attend four outpatient departments. During the past three years all children who had problems with exercise-induced asthma or were in poor physical condition secondary to asthma were referred to a habilitation programme that included education and physical training.

Most of the 179 referred children attended school; only 25 were four to six years old. The education consisted of information about asthma, drugs, technique of administering medication and the importance of regular physical training. The training was swimming, gymnastics or both arranged once or twice a week in groups of two to 12 children. The groups were led by one physiotherapist and one physical training instructor. Each term 19 groups were trained in six different places.

All the children had exercise-induced asthma. Regular medication before exercise was often not taken as prescribed or was regarded by the children as ineffective. The majority of the children were in poor physical condition.

After one to five terms, most children still had exercise-induced asthma, but it was usually much better controlled. Prescribed premedication was taken and with an improved technique. Half of the children had fewer asthmatic symptoms. Physical condition as judged by the children and their parents was improved in 75 per cent. Parallel to the physical improvement many children were improved psychically and were better socially adapted.

Habilitation of asthmatic children, including education and physical training, leads to better control of exercise-induced asthma and improved physical condition. Partly this improvement is due to more regular premedication with an improved technique. Education and physical training are important aspects of the treatment of children with asthma.

INTRODUCTION

Exercise-induced asthma is found in about 80 per cent of children with asthma [1]. Many of these children are in poor physical condition, have problems with gymnastics at school and their relationships with other children are difficult. Anxiety on the part of their parents leads to over-protection and avoidance of physical activities. Three years ago we started a programme to identify these children and offer them regular training. Our goal was a child with asthma who could cope with his or her exercise-induced asthma, be in normal physical condition and have normal relationships with schoolmates and parents.

Halland is a county council area on the west coast of Sweden with 230,000 inhabitants (Figure 1). There are 21,000 pre-school children under 6 years old, and 35,000 schoolchildren between 7 and 16 years old. The expected number of asthmatics among the children of school age is 560 [2]. The

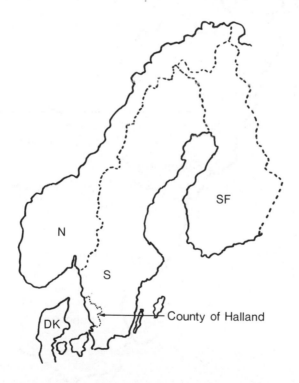

Figure 1. Halland County Council in Sweden marked on a map of the Scandinavian countries (N = Norway, S = Sweden, SF = Finland, DK = Denmark)

area has one hospital for children and three paediatric outpatient clinics. Close co-operation between child, school and district health services and the paediatric clinics, combined with the reasonably short distances that have to be travelled to these clinics, ensures that all children suffering from asthma are supervised by a paediatrician.

HABILITATION IN HALLAND AND SWEDEN

The habilitation clinics in Sweden had previously only worked with children with neuromuscular diseases. During the past three years, however,

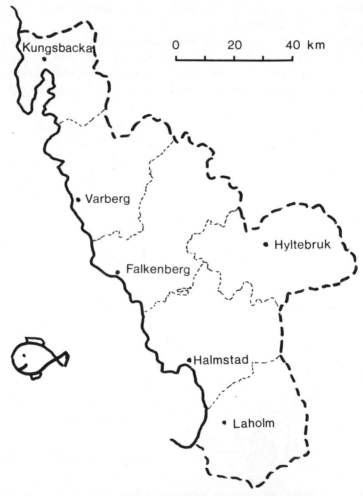

Figure 2. The habilitation clinics in Halland, Sweden

children with other chronic diseases have been incorporated into the programme. By incorporating the asthmatic children into the existing habilitation organisation it was possible to start training them in those six places
where physiotherapists were already working (Figure 2).

MATERIAL

All schoolchildren with exercise-induced asthma who found the condition
a handicap were referred to a habilitation programme. The criteria for
inclusion in the habilitation training programme are shown in Table I.
During the past year a pilot programme for younger children, aged four to
six years, has been started. Children whose exercise-induced asthma was
easily controlled by premedication and was of no problem to them were
not referred.

TABLE I. Criteria for inclusion in a habilitation programme

Exercise-induced asthma combined with
Poor physical condition
Inadequacy of premedication
Poor technique with aerosols
Psychosocial problems
Parental overprotection

A fall in peak expiratory flow rate of more than 20 per cent after exercise
was used as the diagnostic criterion of exercise-induced asthma [3]. A
treadmill was used to provoke exercise-induced asthma. Some patients
with a typical history of exercise-induced asthma were included in the
programme without a treadmill test. All patients in whom the diagnosis
of exercise-induced asthma was uncertain and all patients with asthma who
denied having exercise-induced asthma, were tested on the treadmill. A
total of 179 children started the habilitation programme: 154 were attending school and aged between 7 and 16 years; 25 were between 4 and 6 years
old. The boys outnumbered the girls by 112 to 67.

Ten children did not complete the two terms of training as this either
interfered with school work or they found that travelling from home to
the training places took too much time. Two found the programme boring.

ASTHMA HABILITATION PROGRAMME

Training groups were started in six different places in Halland (Figure 2).
Each group contained four to 10 children. As far as possible the members
of a group were of the same age. Each group had two leaders, one a physio-

therapist and the other a physical training teacher. The training took place once or twice a week and lasted for 60 minutes. We planned that each child should train for at least two terms.

At start of the programme, the mechanism of exercise-induced asthma and the importance of premedication were discussed in the group. Two of the groups also ran a more detailed education programme of four lessons covering asthma, drugs and the techniques of their administration and the importance of regular training.

The three basic principles for training of asthmatic children proposed by Oseid [3] were adopted: namely, premedication, a long warm-up period of mild intensity, and interval training with submaximal work.

All the children took their premedication under the supervision of a physiotherapist. Special emphasis was put on the inhalation technique. The effect of premedication was, if necessary, tested on the treadmill in order to find the best premedication for the individual child (Table II).

TABLE II. Choices of pre-exercise medication

1. Terbutaline or salbutamol
2. Sodium cromoglycate
3. Ipratropium
4. Terbutaline or salbutamol + sodium cromoglycate
5. Terbutaline or salbutamol + ipratropium

The training activities, gymnastics and swimming, were carried out in groups. There were two groups of pre-school children and six groups of schoolchildren doing gymnastics, two groups of children doing school swimming and nine groups doing competition swimming. As the gymnastics for pre-school children and the training for competition swimming differ from traditional programmes of training, they are described in more detail.

Gymnastics for pre-school children

The pre-school programme must contain more play than gymnastics. Pre-medication must be given in calm surroundings and individually – not all together as in the school groups. The long warm-up period of mild intensity is difficult with these small children, who run around as fast as possible as soon as they enter a large room. Activities such as relay-races, games of 'follow-my-leader' and 'acting out stories' are examples of how to reach submaximal work load in this age group. There can be difficulties in getting them to take advantage of the breaks in the interval training, but telling fairy-stories is one way of handling the situation.

Competition swimming

The swimming takes the form of instruction for the younger non-swimmers and more advanced competition for the older children. The habilitation unit in Halland has the advantage of having two former competitive swimmers as leaders in the team. They teach the four different swimming strokes, using exactly the same methods as do the swimming clubs in training children for competition. These methods are considered the most ergonomically efficient way of utilising the muscles. This form of training in technique allows the children to learn a competitive sport whereby they get the chance to join other swimmers in competition when their physical condition improves.

FOLLOW-UP

After two to five terms of training, many of the children had achieved the goal set by the habilitation programme — that is a child with asthma who is in normal physical condition and is well adapted to family, school and friends.

Seventy-seven children answered a questionnaire in which they evaluated their condition before and after their terms of training. Asthma, apart from exercise-induced asthma, had improved in 47 children, was unchanged in 26 and had deteriorated in four. Parallel with this improvement the need for daily asthma medication had diminished. Most children still had exercise-induced asthma but it was easier to control The exercise-induced asthma in four children had disappeared. Of the 25 children who had always had asthma during exercise before the training period, only five still had it after the training had ended.

The physical condition of 55 children was improved; it remained unchanged in the other 22. In no child was there a worsening of physical condition. Sixty-seven of the children regarded the habilitation programme to be an important part of the overall treatment of asthma.

DISCUSSION

The organisation of training groups of asthmatic children in places near their homes made it possible for most of our children to follow the training programme for at least two terms. We believe that all school children with handicapping exercise-induced asthma in our county council area were referred to a training group. If this is true, every third school child with asthma is a candidate for habilitation.

We found the training to be an excellent way of showing the asthmatic children and their parents that they could perform a hard exercise programme without producing symptoms. This was especially important for the parents of the youngest children as it forestalls overprotection at an early stage. Their improved physical condition also increased the children's self-confidence.

The improvement in the asthma, the more easily controlled exercise-induced asthma and the better physical condition could admittedly, in some of the children, have other explanations than the training, such as better medication or improvement with age.

CONCLUSIONS

In a county council in Sweden with 230,000 inhabitants, 179 children with exercise-induced asthma were referred to a habilitation programme that included education, controlled medication and physical training. After a minimum of two terms most of the children found that their asthma and general physical condition improved and that their exercise-induced asthma was easier to control. From these findings we regard habilitation to be an important part of management of these children. 'Habilitation of children with asthma is a profitable investment' (Figure 3).

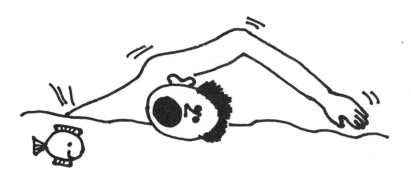

Figure 3. Habilitation of children with asthma is a profitable investment

References

1   Oseid S, Haaland K.
     Exercise studies on asthmatic children before and after regular physical training.
     In Eriksson BO, Furberg B, eds. *International Series on Sport Sciences. Vol 6: Swimming Medicine IV 1978;* 42–51. Baltimore: University Park Press

2   Foucard T.
     Prophylaxis against allergies in childhood.
     Lakartidningen 1980; 77: 3485–3490

3   Oseid S.
     Exercise-induced asthma: a review. In Berg K, Eriksson BO, eds.
     International Series on Sport Sciences. Vol 10: Children and Exercise IX 1980;
     277–288. Baltimore: University Park Press

Chapter 34

EXPERIENCES IN TRAINING OF ASTHMATIC CHILDREN IN A NORTH NORWEGIAN POPULATION

R Bolle

University Hospital of Tromsø, Norway

SUMMARY

Training of asthmatic children in arctic areas poses problems additional to those usually encountered. The scattered population makes it more difficult to compose a homogeneous training group and to organise and to finance the transport of the participants. A cold dry climate is supposed to present a special problem. Ten children (boys between 9—14 years of age) have been trained twice a week for six months (November 1981—May 1982). The method of training by a specialist teacher of gymnastics and her students from a teacher-training college has had positive physical, psychological and social effects.

INTRODUCTION

In asthma, an environmentally-related disease, factors such as the climate, the biology of the atmosphere and the social conditions of the actual area should be taken into consideration when physical training programmes are being prepared. The arctic regions are special in all these respects.

MATERIAL AND METHODS

The study area and the study population

The first organised training-group of asthmatics in the arctic area shown in Figure 1 were chosen from patients being treated at the Department of Pediatrics, University Hospital of Tromsø. This hospital, in the northern-most university city of the world, serves as the university hospital of North Norway. Fewer than half a million inhabitants are spread over an area of

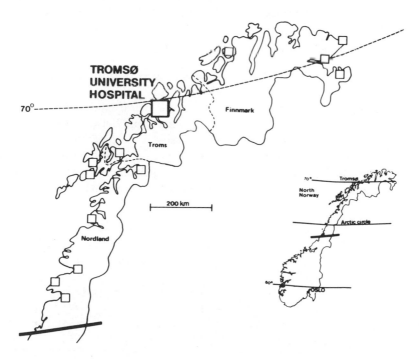

Figure 1. North Norway has a population of 463,000 persons, with a population density of 4.1 inhabitants per km²

113,000 km^2 or three times the size of Denmark. This scattered population makes it difficult to compose homogeneous training-groups out of the estimated 1–2 per cent of children suffering from asthma, many of whom are in need of physical training. Transport to the training centre is the limiting factor. So, in order not to make the travelling too strenuous for the children or their parents, a group was formed of children living not more than 12km from the training centre in the city of Tromsφ (46,000 inhabitants). The responsibility for transporting the children by car rotated among the parents, no one driving more than four times a month. Transport back to their homes by taxi was sponsored by collected funds.

Due to problems with changing-rooms in the much-used training centre, the group had to consist of just one sex and since there are more boys than girls with asthma, the group was made up of 10 boys between 9 and 14 years of age. The mean duration of their asthmatic disease was 9.8 years (range 7–14 years). The nine who suffered from exercise-induced asthma also had a history of bronchial obstruction when exposed to cold. Moreover all 10 patients had an asthmatic reaction when provoked with one or more allergen. Three of the patients were using steroids by inhalation.

The climate of the study area

The influence of the climate on asthma is a controversial subject [1], though recent studies (as reported in these proceedings) have added to our understanding of some of the pathophysiological mechanisms involved.

In North Norway the difference in temperature between the coast and the inland area — that is, from west to east — is greater than from north to south. Therefore it is usual to consider three different temperature zones, namely the coastal area, the fiord region (including Tromsφ) and the inland area. Table I shows the main meteorological data of these zones.

TABLE I. Meteorological conditions in representative areas of the main temperature zones in the central part of North Norway (Troms County, 1931–1960)

Zone	Mean		Temperature (°C) Minimum	Maximum	Relative humidity (per cent)	
	January	July			January	July
Coastal	−0.4	11.3	−15.1	27.2	74	81
Fiord	−3.7	13.4	−19.5	29.4	81	80
Inland	−8.8	14.2	−35.3	31.7	84	76

However, because the regions are close together, it is not uncommon for patients living in one area to visit another region, and, consequently, to be exposed to the climate of that region. Furthermore, the temperature may vary considerably from one year to another. When the deviation from the mean temperature exceeds 2–3°C in the coastal area, the conditions influence the outdoor activities and well-being of the people. There is, indeed, reason to believe that bad weather influences the emigration from this region [2] and also has psychological effects on asthmatic patients.

The ground is usually snow-covered from October to April, but before Christmas the skiing conditions are seldom good. Thus, the months at the end of the year are poorly suited for outdoor activities.

The aerobiology and social conditions of the study area

Natural airborne allergens known to cause asthma, such as pollens and fungus spores, were considered to present no special problems for the patients in the study area during the period of the study (H Hoegh, R Bolle, unpublished observations). However, airborne allergens or irritants related to human activities, such as products from the fishing industry concentrated in this area could be of importance. Yet so far we have been unable to demonstrate any relation between the heavier effluents from this industry and worsening of the bronchial obstruction or reduction in exercise tolerance in asthmatic children.

The influences of the special social conditions of an arctic milieu on asthma have not been extensively studied [World Health Organisation Workshop on Environmental Health Problems in Arctic and Sub-arctic areas, Copenhagen, 3–7 August, 1981]. However, there is no reason to believe that the social conditions of the study population described here are very different from those of an average Norwegian population.

The mode of training

The training programme was carried out for one hour twice a week for six months (November 1981 — May 1982), alternately in a gymnasium and a swimming-pool. In the gymnasium circuit-training, different ball games (basketball, volleyball, soccer, indoor hockey) and play activities were performed. In the swimming-pool the children devoted themselves to different kinds of training and play activities.

The training was led by a special gymnastics teacher and four of her students from a teacher-training college, so at least two coaches were present at each session, together with a doctor and/or a nurse. (Beforehand the leaders were given a lecture on asthma and allergy, including the use of medicines.) Before and after training auscultation, spirography and measurements of peak expiratory flow rate (PEFR) were performed on all children. Prophylactic medication was given in the form of sodium cromoglycate and/or a beta$_2$ stimulant in either aerosol or powder form. Some of the patients preferred to take their medicines at home immediately before coming to the training centre. When the examinations before the training session indicated the presence of bronchial obstruction, additional broncholytic therapy (a beta$_2$ stimulant) was given.

Interviews

After finishing the training programme I interviewed the children, their parents and the coaches.

RESULTS AND DISCUSSION

Experiences of the children

All the children wanted to continue the training in the asthma group. It is interesting to note that the five who had previously been training regularly (soccer, basketball, table-tennis, skiing), wanted to continue with both kinds of activities. If not given the opportunity to continue with group training, two were uncertain whether they would want to join an athletics club, whereas eight wanted to do so.

Nine children preferred training twice a week. Only one boy wanted to continue training just once a week, and the reason he gave was that travel was so time-consuming – he was the only child travelling by bus and had to leave his home more than one hour before the start of training.

When asked about the greatest benefit of the training period, eight of the children answered fun and learning new skills (swimming) and two said physical fitness (endurance training). One of these last two is a very good table-tennis player who had not participated in endurance-training before; the other is probably the most handicapped asthmatic child in the group and often gives expression to his feeling of improved physical fitness.

So far as the dislikes were concerned, four children listed special details concerning the swimming programme or the gymnastics, two the relatively great age-differences in the group which influenced the training especially during the first two months, and one (as mentioned above) drew attention to the time-consuming nature of his transport.

Experiences of the parents

The advantages of the training programme were reported by the parents to be as follows.

(1) Physical training under medical supervision gave them a feeling of security, since they were often in doubt as to how much exercise their child could tolerate.

(2) The regularity of a training programme ensured that the training was carried out.

(3) The medical control twice a week ensured that their child received optimal medication.

(4) The children motivated each other not only in physical training but also for taking their medicines.

(5) The improved physical fitness (that the parents of seven of the children said they noticed) gave their children greater self-confidence and a sense of improved performance.

(6) Being together with other children and adults had positive psychosocial effects.

(7) There was a loosening of the overprotective role of the parents.

(8) The parents had more time for themselves.

The only disadvantage listed by the parents was related to the transport. Two of the parents described the contact with other parents in co-ordinating the transport as something of a strain. One found the transport too time-consuming for the child.

Experiences of the coaches

The coaches reported the following advantages of the training programme.

(1) As the training proceeded, the children seemed to become 'tougher', tolerating more in both the physical and the mental sense.

(2) The children's motor skills were increased. At the beginning of the training period, only four children were able to swim more than 200m, and two could only swim 25m. At the end of the period all 10 boys succeeded in taking the 'seahorse' medal — breaststroke, 400m; backstroke, 200m; swimming with clothes on 200m followed by undressing in the water; freestyle swimming 100m in 2 min 40 sec; floating on the back, 50m; swimming under water, 8m, diving and life-saving. They were also able to swim further than 1000m.

(3) In spite of the age-differences the children in the group worked very well together. The comradeship between the participants was described as exceptional.

(4) The coaches themselves gained a better insight into asthma as a disease and achieved an understanding of the special problems of the patients and their parents. This was thought to be important for their future work as teachers and coaches. All of them were willing to serve as 'contact-persons' and connecting links between hospital and school.

The relatively great age-differences in the group, which initially was mentioned as a disadvantage, turned out not to be a significant problem, since the programme was adjusted during the first few weeks to meet the demands of the different participants. This was the only negative factor mentioned by the coaches.

Experiences of the physician and the nurse

The frequency of attendance of the children at the training programmes varied between 71 and 100 per cent (Figure 2). About two-thirds of the

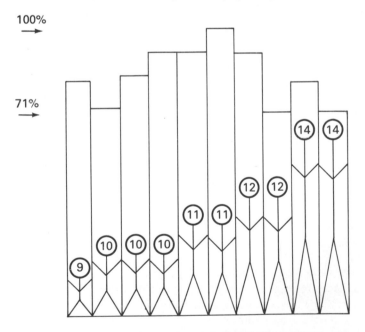

Figure 2. Frequency of attendance in a six-month physical training programme of 10 asthmatic boys from an arctic population (their ages are shown in the circles)

absences from training were due to intercurrent diseases (respiratory infections with or without asthma; varicella).

Detailed analysis was made of all training periods in which the PEFRs either on arrival in the training centre or after finishing the training were reduced to more than 15 per cent of the patient's normal PEFR and the clinical examination and/or the spirogram indicated bronchial obstruction. These criteria were fulfilled in 34 per cent of all training periods, ranging from 60 per cent of training periods in one patient to none in two patients.

TABLE II. Mean PEFR (in per cent of normal PEFR) in eight boys before and after training during periods of bronchial obstruction

Age (years)	No. of observations	Mean PEFR (per cent of normal) Before training	After training
9	16	78	91
10	10	80	91
10	3	83	82
10	20	74	93
12	18	86	73
12	5	92	79
14	9	93	77
14	6	84	79

In 13 per cent of all training periods the initial PEFR was reduced to $\geqslant 20$ per cent of the patient's normal PEFR, in 9 per cent to $\geqslant 25$ per cent, in 5 per cent to $\geqslant 3$ per cent, in 1.6 per cent to $\geqslant 35$ per cent and in a single period (or 0.3 per cent) the initial PEFR was reduced to as much as 45 per cent of the patient's normal PEFR (Table II). In spite of this considerable bronchial obstruction the training was started after premedication as described. One child always had to take two inhalations of a beta$_2$ stimulant and two inhalations of sodium cromoglycate.

Extra medicines during the training were given in seven per cent of all training periods. Only in one case was it necessary to stop the training – when the patient became clearly obstructed eight minutes after starting the training and his PEFR fell from an initial 71 per cent to 41 per cent of his normal PEFR.

Three of the children who thought they were becoming obstructed were misinterpreting dyspnoea on effort. This was registered between two and five times during the first four months of the training. We considered that as the training proceeded the children became able to distinguish between asthmatic obstruction and the normal dyspnoea of effort.

One great advantage that I must emphasise is that the children did not need to visit the hospital during the training period. Apart from achieving clinical control, the necessary prescriptions were given in the course of the training. This contributed to the children's feeling of being healthier and was, in our opinion, an important element in the rehabilitation of these asthmatic children.

References

1   Lopez M, Salvaggio IE.
    Climate – weather – air pollution. In Middleton E Jr, Reed CE, Ellis EF, eds.
    Allergy. Principles and Practice 1978: 965.
    St Louis: Mosby

2   Wilhelmsen K.
    Klima og vær. In Kristoffersen L, ed.
    Troms 1979: 73.
    Oslo: Gyldendal

Chapter 35

THE TREATMENT OF EXERCISE-INDUCED ASTHMA IN A PHYSIOTHERAPY DEPARTMENT

Barbara M Mallinson

Booth Hall Children's Hospital, Manchester,
United Kingdom

SUMMARY

The Asthma Training Group at Booth Hall Children's Hospital, Manchester, adopts the principles of training used at Voksentoppen. The group, which is for outpatients only, is held twice weekly in the Physiotherapy Department and is run by three physiotherapists. One session each week is for exercises, carrying out a programme of muscle building exercises, games, group activities and the use of equipment such as the treadmill. The second session is for swimming which is an ideal sport for children with asthma as it takes place in a warm, humid atmosphere. The swimming session is very popular with all the children.

The principles of pre-exercise medication, a warm-up period and interval training are observed both in the exercise session and in the swimming session. Time is also spent teaching the children how to take their anti-asthma drugs more effectively and also how to control an attack of asthma. This is an important function of the group.

One of the main aims of the group is to enable the children to live normal active lives at home and school and therefore much time is spent in teaching the parents how to cope more effectively with their children's condition. We also liaise with the teacher of physical education at each child's school.

Fifty children have attended the group during the past three-and-a-half years with very good results. Although it is time-consuming work to incorporate an asthma training group into the normal routine of a hospital physiotherapy department, to see anxious withdrawn asthmatics change into healthy outgoing children gives tremendous satisfaction.

INTRODUCTION

After a visit to Voksentoppen Institute for Children with Asthma and Allergy four years ago, we started an asthma training group at Booth Hall Children's Hospital, Manchester. Our aim was to use the principles of controlled training used so successfully at Voksentoppen.

FORMATION OF THE ASTHMA TRAINING GROUP

The training group meets in the hospital physiotherapy department and makes use of the gymnasium, the swimming-pool and a field conveniently placed behind the department. It is run by three physiotherapists. All the children are outpatients of the hospital and are referred by their paediatricians. We hope that it will soon be possible to accept direct referrals from general practitioners.

There are about eight children in the group at any one time aged between eight and twelve years, although a few younger and several older children have attended. The training group meets twice a week from 4.00 pm until 5.00 pm so that the children do not miss school and evening activities are not interfered with. One session is for exercises and one for swimming.

The aims of the group are to teach better use of anti-asthmatic drugs, to improve muscle power, to increase exercise tolerance, to improve cardiovascular performance, to improve the patient's self-confidence, to liaise with the school, and to give family support and instruction.

THE ACTIVITIES OF THE ASTHMA TRAINING GROUP

Exercise session

The exercise session begins with the taking of a short history from each child paying particular attention to the amount of exercise the child is taking part in at home and at school. A peak flow reading should be taken to determine the child's asthmatic status at that particular session. This is followed by pre-exercise medication and it is most important to watch the children take their drugs. Many children take their medication very badly and it is important to teach them the correct method.

The session continues with a warm-up period lasting about 10 minutes and taking the form of a game, relay races or a group activity. All the children should be encouraged to take part. The rest of the session includes muscle strengthening exercises, activities to improve cardiovascular performance and exercises using equipment – namely the static bicycle (Figure 1), the rowing machine (Figure 2) and the treadmill.

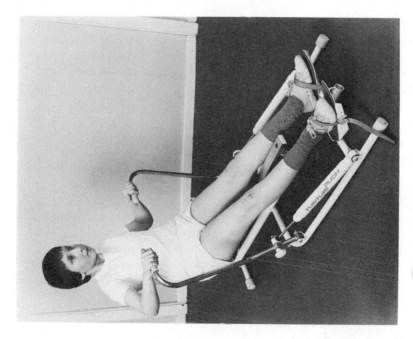

Figure 2. Exercising on the rowing machine

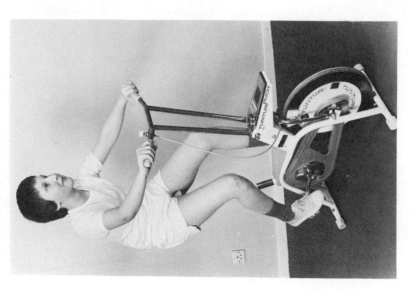

Figure 1. Exercising on the static bicycle

The principle underlying the training of children with exercise-induced asthma is to begin with a small amount of exercise and gradually, over a variable length of time depending on the child's condition, build up to normal or above-normal activities. The principles of training in the Booth Hall training group are similar to those recommended and used at Voksentoppen.

Swimming session

The swimming session follows the same principles of controlled training – namely pre-exercise medication, a warm-up period, interval training, swimming and games.

Many of the children come to the group as non-swimmers or reluctant swimmers and they must begin by learning to swim. Rings, arm bands and neck floats are used to help (Figure 3). Once the children can swim it is important to encourage them to improve their strokes, to develop better breathing control and to become more powerful swimmers. The children

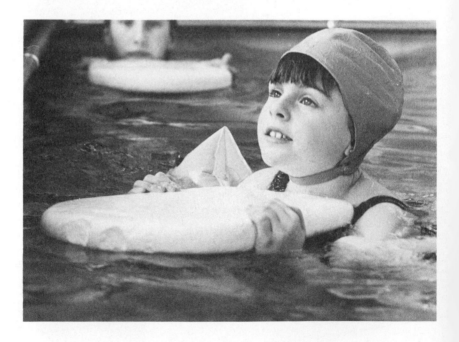

Figure 3. Arm bands and floats help the non-swimmers learn to swim

are encouraged to attend their own local swimming-baths each week as swimming is one of the best activities for children with exercise-induced asthma.

Home and school

One of the main aims of the group is to teach the child to live a normal life in his normal environment — that is at home and at school. To this end teach-ins are held within the group at which the children and the parents learn about the use of anti-asthmatic drugs, the control of attacks and the correct methods of taking part in exercise at home. The children's schools are also contacted and visited, to liaise with the physical education teachers. It is hoped that these teachers will continue to help and encourage the children to take an active part in sport once they have left the asthma training group.

The children continue to attend the asthma training group until they fulfil the following criteria: they are able to run with ease for six minutes on the treadmill; they are taking part in a full programme of physical education and games at school; it appears to the physiotherapists that they have achieved their highest potential within the group's activities; the parents are satisfied with their child's achievements; and the child, himself, feels happy and confident to take part in all activities.

The progress of almost all the children has been followed at their visits to the hospital doctor. Only one child has been referred back to the group as he was failing to make satisfactory progress.

RESULTS

It is difficult to evaluate the results achieved by a group of this type as they range from increased physical fitness, through increased pulmonary function to increased self-confidence. However, during the past three years 50 children have attended the group for an average of six months each, although some children have attended for as long as one year.

It is obviously quite demanding on the parents to bring the children twice weekly, but despite this only four children have dropped out for various reasons.

Eleven children came to the group as complete non-swimmers and 10 of these have learnt to swim. Twenty-five children came as severe or very severe asthmatics taking part in little or no sport and all have gone on to normal or above normal activity, as have the remaining 21.

For the physiotherapists involved with the group, the most exciting results have been to see the children develop confidence in themselves and in their own abilities. To see withdrawn, anxious children change into fit, healthy confident youngsters gives tremendous satisfaction. It is also exciting to see the change that takes place in the parents as they realise that it is actually possible for their child to take part in normal activities. To quote one mother: "it's a miracle".

CONCLUSION

The incorporation of an asthma training group within the normal running of a hospital physiotherapy department is an eminently feasible proposition.

At the end of one training session one boy quite nonchalantly remarked, "I don't know whether you are interested or not but I can now do the cross-country run at school". That *is* just what the physiotherapists are interested in and what the Booth Hall asthma training group aims to achieve. Many children have already been treated with good success and it is hoped that as more knowledge and experience is gained this will continue.

Acknowledgments

My acknowledgments are due to the staff of Voksentoppen Institute for Children with Asthma and Allergy, Oslo; to the staff of the Department of Physiotherapy, Booth Hall Children's Hospital, Manchester, and to the Medical Staff, Booth Hall Children's Hospital, Manchester. I am also grateful to the Editor of *Physiotherapy* for permission to reproduce Figures 1 and 3 which have previously appeared in the April 1981 issue of that journal.

DISCUSSION

HAIDER (Bury, UK)	Dr Østergaard, did your study take any account of the presence or absence of associated symptomatic nasal allergy — in particular nasal obstruction — which could have an affect on exercise-induced asthma and the training programme? When did you do the study: during or outside the pollen season? If it was outside the pollen season the relative importance of increased pollen sensitivity in your 'benefit' group becomes less significant.
ØSTERGAARD	We have been studying the problem for the past two years and this particular group of 24 children for one and a half years. We know that it is important to investigate exercise-induced asthma outside the pollen season, but I do not have the answer to that part of the question. But to answer the first part: about 60 per cent of these patients had nasal allergy.
FITCH (Chairman)	Dr Østergaard, your definition of benefit seems to me to be whether or not there were changes in exercise-induced bronchial reactivity. Is that so?
ØSTERGAARD	Yes.
FITCH	I am questioning whether that is a wise way of evaluating benefit. Certainly in my studies we have found that people even up to world championship standard will have persistent and significant bronchial hyperreactivity and yet be able to swim 100m in less than 50 sec.
ØSTERGAARD	Our criterion of benefit was the inability to demonstrate a fall of 20 per cent or more in FEV_1 and PEFR after completing the training.
FITCH	I think all would agree that that is the only measurable benefit likely to come from a training programme. We

have demonstrated that even after a lot of training and with immense apparent benefit children and adolescents still have identical exercise bronchial reactivity after the training programme, if they are challenged at the same percentage of their maximum working capacity. I am suggesting that some of the other benefits that may have come from this study have been overlooked and may be worthwhile investigating.

ØSTERGAARD   We have, in fact, investigated them.

PATRUNO   Does anybody have experience of long-term exercise
(Bari, Italy) rehabilitation without premedication?

FITCH   I am not aware that anybody has studied this aspect, although I do know that some training studies have been carried out without the use of premedication (for instance, the Swedish study of Graff-Lonnevig et al, reference [26] in my paper). Generally, most of us feel there is no point in running the risk of inducing exercise asthma when the prime objective is to permit the patient to complete an exercise training session.

GEMMELL   Does Miss Mallinson feel that a policy of taking
(Mansfield, UK) groups of children at say five years instead of predominantly eight years and older would help to improve their general life style before too many problems become established?

MALLINSON   We feel that between eight and 12 years is quite a good age to train children. They enjoy the training; they love getting their track suits on and actually training rather than playing. The youngest we have ever taken was six years old and he only joined the group because his older sister was a member but we decided that if he was just going to mess around and be disruptive we would no longer take him. In fact he took the training very seriously. So I think it partly depends on the child. I doubt if four and five year old would take part in serious training, but I think you could organise quite a nice group for them but it would have to be specially adapted and taken separately from the older ones.

HAIDER

It is good to know that a physiotherapist is doing such a programme independently. Would Miss Mallinson include exercise therapy for asthma in the training of physiotherapists?

MALLINSON

We are doing our best. We take students at our hospital and I have taught quite a number of physiotherapy and physical education students. We have a training college near the hospital and I have been to speak to the physical education students there. I think that is important. Nevertheless, it seems that physiotherapy students are still only doing breathing exercises so we do try and educate those who come to our hospital.

YOUNG
(Oxford, UK)

Physical training is an expensive form of treatment to organise and supervise. Many speakers have advocated physical training as therapy for children with asthma. But only *one* of the trials reported to this meeting was scientifically acceptable. Why have there been so few adequate studies? Are we not being irresponsible when we advocate an expensive form of treatment without even attempting to obtain adequate proof of its efficacy? The evaluation of exercise training must be just as rigorous as the evaluation of a drug.

FITCH

I am reminded of Professor P-O Åstrand who some years ago said that he did not know why it was necessary to have a medical examination to take exercise; rather he believed it was necessary for those people who choose not to exercise to have a medical examination. I would suggest to Dr Young that perhaps we should be asking ourselves can we afford *not* to exercise our asthmatics? I put this for a number of reasons. Firstly, it is very difficult to evaluate any exercise programme in a double-blind nature as we would do with drug therapy. I would be surprised if anybody has ever done such an evaluation in a truly double-blind manner. Secondly, I admit freely that most of the studies which have come from eight countries and have been described to this meeting have produced more subjective than objective benefits. But, I ask, has there been any single case in which the asthma has been aggravated or any disadvantage has resulted from the training? Has there been any single paper published which has indicated that exercise-training programmes for asthmatics have worsened their condition? If there has, I am unaware of it. Thirdly, I would question the word expensive. I will give an example from my own city of Perth, where we have 500 asthmatics who exercise once a week, every week for nine months of the year in eight heated indoor swimming pools. It costs them about 20 pence a time. All the instructors and administrators are volunteers and work without remuneration. This has been happening for nine years. We also run an asthma camp for 70 or 80 children. This, too, is conducted by volunteers who cost nobody but themselves money, and it is inexpensive. I do not believe that it is expensive — not when compared with the cost of drugs, and most of all not when it is compared with the cost of admission to hospital. Most of the studies that have been reported to this meeting and that I am aware of have shown that the number of admissions to hospital has been reduced. Admissions to hospital are expensive, exercise programmes are relatively inexpensive. Yes, I do think there is a cost benefit.

Chapter 36

THE TRAINING PROGRAMME AT A SPECIAL SCHOOL FOR ASTHMATIC CHILDREN

Wenche Nystad Lid

Children's Asthma and Allergy Institute, Voksentoppen, Oslo, Norway

SUMMARY

Voksentoppen School, part of Voksentoppen Asthma and Allergy Institute, has 40 pupils from 7–16 years of age. Twenty are children with chronic asthma from the Oslo area who receive part or all of their schooling at Voksentoppen. The remainder are inpatients at the Institute who come from various parts of Norway and receive their obligatory schooling while they are in hospital.

The pupils have two hours of physical education plus two hours of health care per week. Certain children are in addition taken out of other lessons to participate in more individualised physical activity sessions when this is required. Emphasis is placed upon the physical environment of the school. Teaching aims to give the children the opportunity and experience of succeeding in play and sport activities, and we try to give them a sense of security that allows them to expand and explore their physical limits. It is our experience that through this programme we are able to exert a positive influence on their social development. A full-time school nurse is in close contact with the children's own doctors and the parents.

At a weekly team meeting the activity programmes for the individual children are planned and there is close co-operation between the staff at the School and at the Institute. Of particular importance is the establishing of contact and close co-operation between Voksentoppen and the children's home school. Relevant information is distributed by means of teaching reports, by telephone discussions and by personal contact. Special emphasis is placed upon encouraging the pupils to participate actively in leisure activities and physical education in their home school environment.

INTRODUCTION

Voksentoppen School, which is part of Voksentoppen Asthma and Allergy Institute, has 40 pupils between the ages of 7–16 years. Twenty are children with chronic asthma who live in the Oslo area and who receive all or part of their schooling at Voksentoppen. The remainder are inpatients who receive schooling while at the Institute – they come from any part of Norway.

PHYSICAL EDUCATION AND HEALTH CARE

In Norway pupils normally have two hours of physical education per week. At Voksentoppen all the pupils are given two hours' physical education plus two hours' health care per week. Classes in health care are integrated into the physical education programme and include theory, play and practical training. In addition, individual children are selected for special physical training whenever this is found necessary. The experiment with lessons in health care at Voksentoppen School has been part of the school curriculum since 1981 and the subject is to be given high priority in the coming years. Our experiences are also of interest to other schools in Norway.

The subjects that are taught are as follows: basic anatomy and physiology; exercise physiology; asthma and physical activity; ergometry; playground and sport activities; traffic safety; nutrition; alcohol – drugs – tobacco; and common diseases.

The philosophy behind this health-care programme is to give the child a knowledge of his own body, to help him discover how best to use it, and to let him experience the fact that he can take part in and succeed in physical activity. By allowing the children to take responsibility for their own health we hope they may be able to influence and improve their lives. Emphasis is laid on trying to create positive experiences for the children in the natural environment of the Institute.

Voksentoppen is in an area surrounded by a coniferous forest. Despite the fact that the indoor training facilities with a gymnasium and a heated pool are more than adequate, we try to make as much use of the outdoor facilities as possible. By doing so we hope that the children will then participate in physical activities in circumstances when special equipment or training areas are not available.

PUPILS' BACKGROUNDS – TEACHING METHODS

In order to achieve a balance that is closer to that found in the ordinary school, the children are divided into two groups (7–11 years and 11–16 years) for teaching both physical activity and health care. This often creates a group in which the individuals function at different levels and may complicate the choice of activities and the intensity of the training sessions. However, teaching the children to accept and show consideration for each other has overshadowed minor problems of organisation and provides more of a challenge.

The physiotherapists at Voksentoppen may take part in these lessons to observe the child in natural play and sport activities.

During play and training we take into consideration the individual qualifications for participating in physical activity. These are dependent upon several factors such as the pupil's geographical background; climatic and social factors; the parents' attitude towards physical activity, and the circumstances of the home environment. All these factors must be viewed in the light of the individual child and his asthma.

Our teaching is therefore as individualised as possible and no-one is forced into taking part in activities that are beyond their ability. Emphasis is also placed on co-operation during play and sport as a form of social training. In addition activities that the individual child can participate in at home with his friends are practised as much as possible.

Coping is an important aspect in relation to physical activity and the asthmatic child. To succeed in overcoming individual problems creates a sense of security in the child. It also builds up motivation and makes play and sport fun. To start with, untraditional activities are important and may motivate a child who has been unable to use his body properly — you must learn to catch a ball in order to take part in the game.

Some pupils have gross motor problems and function well below the level of their healthy fellows. Many have gaps in their motor development which are difficult to fill in a normal school environment. Other children in our care have to learn what it means to be naturally out of breath after strenuous activity and how this differs from being wheezy. When heart rates were measured during an hour of physical activity it was found that some children's subjective feeling of being exhausted did not correlate with their heart rate. They were unable to achieve any objective effect from endurance training. We all become breathless if we are active enough but the child has to learn not to be afraid of it. Some of our pupils are extremely active and refuse to accept their asthma; they have to be taught to function within the limits imposed by their asthma and not in spite of it. This may demand understanding, will power and self-discipline on the part of these children.

THE PHYSICAL ENVIRONMENT OF THE SCHOOL

To stimulate the children to take part in play activities outside organised lessons emphasis has been placed upon the immediate physical surroundings. This creates opportunities for spontaneous play and sport outside school hours. The planning and completion of these surroundings has been made possible through the help of the hospital staff, teachers and parents. The activities that we are able to offer are under constant development and revision. By increasing the normal level of physical activity of the pupils we found that some became wheezy.

Our summer activities include athletic track (soccer, volleyball, handball, basketball, etc); tennis; orienteering; obstacle course; and playground activities (chess giant, sandbox ballgames, climbing frame). Our winter activities include ski-play activity areas; floodlit country ski trail; ski jump; toboggan run; and alpine skiing.

THE SCHOOL NURSE

The school nurse is in full-time employment at the school and is responsible for the medication of the permanent pupils. The inpatients are cared for by one of the nurses employed at the Institute during school hours. The school nurse is in close contact with the patient's own doctor and with the parents. In the fixed routine that precedes the activity sessions these nurses have an important part to play in connection with premedication. Our routine is as follows:

(1) premedication – a relaxed atmosphere is important
(2) the pupils change into clothes (training suits) appropriate for the activity. This allows time for the premedication to take effect quite naturally
(3) all the pupils start the chosen activity together.

The school nurse is often an active participant in the physical education lessons (for example, skiing). This creates a feeling of security for both the pupils and the teacher especially under difficult circumstances. There is close co-operation between the school and the Institute and individual and group activities are planned at weekly multidisciplinary meetings when the children's individual problems and requirements are discussed.

COMMUNICATION WITH THE HOME SCHOOL

An important aspect of our work at Voksentoppen is keeping the teachers at the pupils' home schools informed through special teaching reports,

telephone contact and personal communication. This is especially important since many physical education teachers feel worried and insecure when
confronted with an asthmatic pupil. They may adopt an attitude which
can lead to the child's becoming inactive and isolated. The home school
therefore needs help to solve the problems that affect the asthmatic child —
and these are highly individualised depending on local resources and the
child's special difficulties. It is important that the information given to the
school is felt by the child to be positive and not an embarrassment to him.
In the classroom, the pupil must not feel that too much attention is being
focused upon his asthma. You do not warm-up only because you have
asthma — a warming-up period is a natural part of any training session and
is closely connected with the chosen activity. Constructive advice and
suggestions with regard to equipment, choice of activity, organisation and
teaching methods are necessary and useful.

To succeed in helping the asthmatic child to function to the best of his
abilities, communication and co-operation between the teacher and the
parents is essential. They will also need support from the school health
system and the child's own doctor.

Our aim is to integrate the pupil in the physical education classes in his
home school and in the leisure activities in his home environment. The
psychosocial effects of this work are equally as important as the physical
effects of training.

We know that children profit from training. But what happens afterwards? What I do with the children during a training period is one thing,
but what the child does afterwards is more important.

CONCLUSION

Voksentoppen School has among its pupils the most severe chronic asthmatics in Norway who show various degrees of disability. Emphasis has
been placed on play and sport activities during the school-day. By physically
building up the asthmatic child and teaching him various physical skills, we
believe that we are able to improve the child's daily life. This belief is based
on clinical experience. The key words for the asthmatic child are to promote
security, *positive experience* and lasting motivation for physical activity.

An important aspect of our work is communication with the teachers at
the pupil's home school. Adequate information is essential and depends on
close co-operation with the child's parents and the school health system.

In the light of our work and our positive experiences we feel that play
and sport activities may be used more directly in the habilitation and
rehabilitation of asthmatic children — and this is something that applies
also to children with other chronic diseases.

Chapter 37

INTEGRATION OF ASTHMATIC CHILDREN IN TRAINING GROUPS AT BEITOSTØLEN HEALTH SPORTS CENTER

I Morisbak

The Norwegian College of Physical Education and Sports, Oslo, and The Beitostølen Health Sports Center, Beitostølen, Norway

SUMMARY

The objective of the Beitostølen Health Sports Center is to increase the capacity of disabled people to take part in normal activities, both at work and in recreation. The centre has three main areas of activity: rehabilitation, scientific research and evaluation and education.

In co-operation with the school authorities in two Norwegian counties the sports centre has a special project known as "Adapted Physical Education". Groups of school children come to the centre for two weeks to train and learn activities they can utilise in their local community. They are accompanied by a teacher from their school. The children have different handicaps — some of them are asthmatic. The integration of these asthmatic children with other children and adults with other disabling conditions is emphasised.

INTRODUCTION

Beitostølen Health Sports Center has from its start in 1970 been receiving asthmatic patients. Until 1973 it was mostly asthmatic adults on their own who came to the centre, but from 1973 groups of children have come from Voksentoppen Asthma and Allergy Institute since Dr Oseid and his staff use the centre as one of the resources in their extensive programme. This collaboration has provided Beitostølen Health Sports Center with the experience and knowledge of how best to use the centre's facilities, programmes and staff to help asthmatic children overcome some of their handicaps related to physical activity.

Beitostølen Health Sports Center is a place where the physically handicapped of all ages from 7 to 75 years can come to improve their health in the broadest sense of the term, by means of sports, exercises and other recreational activities. It is all paid for by the Norwegian social security system. In addition to the daily training (adults usually stay for four weeks and children in groups usually for two weeks) the centre does some research and evaluation work and has an educational function. There are also some other services which are provided as supplements to these basic functions. All are carried out under medical supervision [1].

Asthmatic children who come to stay at Beitostølen Health Sports Center fall into three main categories.

(1) Groups of six to 12 asthmatic children who have been selected by the staff at Voksentoppen Asthma and Allergy Institute come for a stay of two weeks, as a part of the systematic programme conducted by Voksentoppen.

(2) The Norwegian Asthma and Allergy Association has sent one group of eight asthmatic children/youths to Beitostølen Health Sports Center every year for the past four years. These groups have come, respectively, from the south-east, south-west, middle and northern regions of the country, and the participants have been selected by physicians working with asthmatic children in the different regions. The ages of these children have varied between 13 and 17 years. They have stayed for three to four weeks.

(3) Individual asthmatic children have been sent to Beitostølen Health Sports Center as members of school groups consisting of children with different handicaps. These children have been selected by physical education teachers, or sometimes by school physiotherapists, because of their difficulties with the physical education curriculum in the school. The applications and selections are approved by the school's health service personnel and the school administration as well as by the parents. Beitostølen Health Sports Center has the right to, and indeed must, evaluate each application in relation to the activities provided by the centre, and also to

the surroundings, especially with regard to the possibility of allergic reactions. Some asthmatic children have had problems with allergic reactions during their stay, probably in most cases caused by hairs from horses and dogs, but in some from cigarette smoke and food.

The number of children in a group has varied between three and eight, with the children coming either from one school or from different schools in the same community. They have stayed at the centre for two weeks. In the past 13 months there have been 17 groups: eight contained one asthmatic child each and one contained two. Thus there has been a total of 10 asthmatic children in these school groups.

"ADAPTED PHYSICAL EDUCATION"

The stay at the centre for the school groups is part of a project called "Adapted Physical Education" which is a collaborative project between the school directors in two Norwegian counties and the Beitostølen Health Sports Center [2]. The goal of this project is to improve the provision of physical education in school and in leisure for those children with disabling conditions who are integrated in the general school system. The stay at Beitostølen Health Sports Center is important in that it acts as an initiating stimulus for local programmes.

The school directors in the two involved counties have in the period of the project (1979–1982) appointed part-time consultants. Two or three seminars are held each year for the so-called contact-persons in each community at which they can exchange practical ideas and experiences related to activity, and talk with the professionals. The seminars also have an educational function – for example, literature, films and practical demonstrations of physical education programmes suitable for asthmatic children.

There is one contact-person for the project in each community. This person co-ordinates the local activities which include:

the registration of children who need adapted physical education

the eventual organisation of applications for some children to come to Beitostølen Health Sports Center

the organisation of local programmes for the registered children

the co-ordination of collaboration between relevant professions in the community regarding adapted physical education.

Some characteristics of the project

The asthmatic children are registered as having problems with the physical education curriculum in the general school he or she attends.

The children are registered in most cases by their physical education teachers as having problems.

The registration and the application process for a stay at Beitostølen Health Sports Center encourages collaboration between physical education teachers, the local school authorities, the health service personnel and the parents.

The stay at Beitostølen Health Sports Center means new experiences for the children related to physical activity, sports and recreation not only through participation in new activities, but also through new ways of participating in known activities.

The stay at Beitostølen Health Sports Center necessarily means that handicapped children can compare their situations in life — and in a practical manner through participation in common physical activities.

The stay at Beitostølen Health Sports Center allows the teacher, and eventually the parents, to learn through practical experience what is the child's real physical potential and also to discover what are the real restrictions imposed by the disability. They also learn the correct methods for exercising their particular child and asthmatic children in general. (Some theoretical instruction is given to teachers and parents.)

The stay gives the teachers and the parents the chance to discuss matters of interest with various professionals who have expertise in using physical activities as one means of habilitation and rehabilitation.

The stay creates the basis for a locally adapted physical activity programme (follow-up). A report is written at the end of the stay, which will help in making the most use of the experiences at Beitostølen Health Sports Center in the local programmes. The report is prepared in collaboration with the staff at Beitostølen Health Sports Center and the local representative. This means that the report can be adapted to local circumstances and therefore be more useful. (The local representatives have, in fact, been asked to investigate the local resources for activity programmes before they come to the centre, so that they are better prepared for planning a permanent programme in the local school.)

THE ASTHMATIC 'PROJECT-CHILDREN'

Some facts derived from the information sent to the centre before the stay

All 10 children had had difficulties with the physical education curriculum in their schools. The difficulties were described as "cannot follow", "withdrawal", "exemption" and so forth.

About half of them were said to be generally motivated for physical education.

Overprotection by the child's family, especially the mother, was mentioned in three cases.

Four of the children had not swum at school at all. One was excused because he did not want to swim, one because of allergy to chlorine, one because he was in the second class and swimming did not enter the curriculum until the third class, and one because swimming was not on the curriculum that year. One was said to have had very little motivation for swimming and poor skills.

One child had used one of two weekly physical education lessons throughout the entire year for physical therapy.

Some facts derived from the activity reports

The children participated in from four to six programmed physical activities during the stay.

Four stayed during the winter. All participated in skiing. Four stayed during the summer. All participated in kayak/canoe paddling. Two stayed in the spring period when neither paddling nor skiing was available.

All 10 took part in gymnastics and swimming. Four went horseback riding, despite the fact that some were allergic to hair. Other activities that some of the children took part in included table-tennis, archery, ballgames, bicycling, soccer, athletics and orienteering. Each child participated in four or five different activities a day.

The most outstanding aspect of the activity reports was that all participated in swimming in spite of the excuses given by four of them in the applications, and they all made very good progress in the pool. Two of the four non-swimmers learned to swim very well, the other two adjusted to the water and learned the basic skills of swimming. These four also became highly motivated for further training in the pool.

Progress in skills was also frequently mentioned in the reports on the other activities.

The level of activity and self-confidence increased during the stay. Only one child made no special progress in this regard. Most achieved more than they thought would be possible.

They all enjoyed their stay at the centre and would like to come back some time.

A change in the preliminary programme from that planned at the beginning of the stay took place in three cases. These changes were decided in collaboration between the staff, the child and the teacher from the school.

Motivation for physical activity generally increased according to both the school teachers' statements and the instructors' observations.

In addition to the physical activity programme, the children took part in other recreational activities such as music, stone polishing, weaving, dancing, games and so on. Most of them also joined in physical activities such as table-tennis, bicycling, ballgames and swimming outside their programmed activities. They all received one to two hours theoretical school education during the day.

Some information from follow-up after four months

At present we have information on only seven of the 10 children. Two of the other three are still working to establish new routines, but these will not come into effect before the next school year. In the case of the third child the physical education teacher has for some reason not yet received the report on the child's stay at the centre.

In six of the seven cases there have been meetings and discussions between the involved parties in the community. As a result two children have been granted extra hours to pursue their swimming.

Three children have started regular physical activity outside school (one handball, one gymnastics and one swimming).

Some of the other pupils in the schools who have special needs have also been granted extra hours for swimming during school-time and have become involved in swimming and gymnastics outside school hours.

Teachers who came with the children to the centre have sometimes held courses for other teachers in the community centred around their experiences at Beitostølen Health and Sports Center in general, including physical training and asthma.

CONCLUSIONS

Valid conclusions cannot be drawn from our experience with the 10 children referred to here as they are too small a group. However, in the following general comments we have also drawn to some extent on our experiences with other groups of asthmatic children and other individual asthmatic children who have stayed at the centre during the past years.

(1) Teachers who have asthmatic children in their physical education classes in ordinary schools need both theoretical education and, more importantly, practical experience in the provision of physical education for these children.

(2) Beitostølen Health Sports Center is well suited to give the teachers the necessary education and practical experience.

(3) Generally the children have derived positive benefit from their stay at Beitostølen Health Sports Center. Most have increased their skills and their motivation for physical activity, and have acquired a more realistic appreciation of their own capacities and abilities.

(4) The follow-up in the local community seems to be dependent on the contact-person's initiative and the extent to which this person is given the time and resources to make the necessary adaptations to physical education of children with special needs.

(5) Only through education of the local physical education teacher is it possible to integrate the asthmatic child in physical education. Such education must include practical experience.

(6) In most cases it is only through practical experience and direct personal communication that it is possible to instil the necessary understanding of the value of these activities in the local authorities and the parents.

(7) The experience of having taken part in the Adapted Physical Education project has had a beneficial effect on children, teachers and other professionals who have not been to Beitostølen Health Sports Center.

(8) The formalities of the application process to come to Beitostølen Health Sports Center, the accomplishments during the stay, and the follow-up procedures all necessarily enhance collaboration in the community between the professionals to the ultimate benefit of the child.

Some relevant questions

Can a project like this be carried out without a Beitostølen Health Sports Center? Is it possible to create in other places a model with an input similar to that given by Beitostølen Health Sports Center? Would some of the early practical lessons learned from this project be helpful for initiating strategies for improved physical education for asthmatic children elsewhere? If the answer is yes, or at least a conditional yes, to one or more of these questions, I feel that the input given by Beitostølen Health Sports Center has been worthwhile.

References

1   Morisbak I, Nilsson S, Tufto A.
    Funksjonsanalyse for Beitostølen Helsesportsenter. Beitostølen 1976

2   Skoledirektørene i Hedmark og Oppland.
    Tilpasset fysisk opplæring. Prosjektmelding nr.3/82

Chapter 38

REFLECTIONS ON PHYSICAL TRAINING PROGRAMMES FOR THE ASTHMATIC CHILD

Myra Kendall

Children's Asthma and Allergy Institute, Voksentoppen, Oslo, Norway

SUMMARY

Physical training programmes developed for the asthmatic child vary considerably from hospital to hospital and from country to country. Although the aims of these programmes are often similar the methods and activities employed are extremely diverse, as are the criteria for inclusion. Many are orientated towards traditional therapeutic breathing and thorax mobilising exercises while others concentrate on intense endurance training — some even rely upon unsupervised exercises at home. The results are extremely varied and difficult to compare.

The long-term aim of any exercise programme should be the ultimate integration of the asthmatic child into his own environment, taking part in the same activities as his peers. Much of the published literature seems to be more concerned with establishing hard data rather than observing the software — that is, the effect of a training programme on the complete life of the child.

Two secondary gains that are less documented are the effects of physical activity on the mobilising of secretions and on medical compliance.

One of the Voksentoppen models based on a twice-weekly group activity programme over a period of three to six months culminating in 14 days of mountain activity has shown increased general physical performance and secondary gains of improved social and coping abilities.

The instigation and success of any programme is dependent upon full co-operation between the physician and the therapist responsible. There seems in many institutions to be a distinct lack of co-operation between various members of the medical team with many divergent attitudes towards the use of physical activity as part of the total approach to the child in the treatment of asthma.

INTRODUCTION

These reflections are based upon a study trip made in 1980–1981 to various centres responsible for the treatment and care of the asthmatic child in the USA, Australia, New Zealand and Scandinavia. I also visited large general hospitals where patients with asthma were treated.

At Voksentoppen Allergy Institute the use of physical activity has played a major role in the total approach to the treatment and care of asthmatic children. It was important therefore to discover whether or not our approach was the one generally accepted, what other methods and techniques were being used elsewhere, and to what extent physiotherapy was being employed in the total picture. A comparison of methods would then allow us to adjust or alter our programmes in order to make the best of our approach.

ARE PHYSICAL TRAINING PROGRAMMES WORTHWHILE?

Before taking this trip I wondered if the widespread cultural emphasis on physical activity in Norway influenced our approach to patients. The Norwegians are an extremely sports-orientated nation – it seems that most people between the ages of three and 70 years take part in cross-country skiing. So was our emphasis on physical activity in this institute really necessary? Was it relevant only in Norway and similar countries or was it relevant throughout the world?

The therapeutic use of physical activity varies considerably from hospital to hospital and the activities employed are often culturally determined. Teaching an asthmatic in Australia to ski is hardly practical! The aims of the various programmes may be similar but the methods used are extremely diverse. Despite different cultural, social and geographical backgrounds, however, it was obvious to me that children with asthma have much in common. For any child, physical activity is an integral part of daily life. The entire life of a child who cannot take part in the normal activities of childhood is adversely affected.

THE PLACE OF PHYSICAL ACTIVITY PROGRAMMES

Most hospital staff appear to be concerned mainly with the asthmatic's immediate response to his disease. Few observe the patient outside the acute setting for any length of time and are often unaware as to how he copes in other phases of the disease and in particular how he functions physically. The physician is generally the only member of the team to have regular outpatient contact and consequently he is the only one in a position to assess the degree to which asthma represents a handicap; the other members of the team have to rely on his assessment and evaluation.

Very few doctors are sports-orientated and their attitudes may well influence the patient's response. The asthmatic often has no-one with whom to compare himself, as his frame of reference is often extremely limited. He is used to accepting the fact that he is unable to participate as actively as his friends, and adjusts his life accordingly. It may be difficult for the busy physician sitting behind his office desk to discover and often even to appreciate just how much of a functional handicap exercise-induced asthma is for the affected individual. It requires more than the time spent in the surgery to gain any real insight into the problems. A child will seldom admit or even be aware that he is in poor physical condition. Nevertheless many physicians are aware of the problem of exercise-induced asthma and do advise patients to exercise, stressing its importance. For many asthmatics this advice together with advice on premedication is sufficient. But for the child who is unable to cope it may only add to his sense of inadequacy and lead to feelings of guilt because he cannot live up to the doctor's expectations. Fortunately, most asthmatics are able to cope independently, but because they can, the smaller group of children who do experience problems are overlooked in many hospitals. These children who are unable to cope without special help should be our major concern.

The advances in medical treatment with the wider use of sodium cromoglycate and improved bronchodilator therapy also have a negative aspect in that they have led to the attitude that medication eliminates the need for other forms of treatment. Despite better drug therapy it is important to recognise that there are still a number of chronic asthmatics who remain physically passive and require our help.

TRADITIONAL/CONVENTIONAL PHYSIOTHERAPY

Traditionally the physical therapist has used therapeutic breathing and thorax mobilising exercises in the hope of being able to influence the disease or the secondary changes due to inadequate medical therapy. Despite the paucity of evidence to support this form of therapy – which would seem often to be contraindicated in that it accentuates the 'sick child' attitude – there are still many hospitals and institutions in which this is the only form of physical therapy available. Traditional physiotherapy in this context seems to be based on the attitude that at least something is being done.

THE ULTIMATE GOAL

The ultimate goal of any therapeutic exercise programme should be the integration of the asthmatic child into a normal home environment with the ability to take part in any activity that he wishes and is otherwise fit for.

Different approaches

For a physical training programme to be successful a multidisciplinary approach is essential. Co-operation and communication between the members of the team is often the deciding factor. Yet one so frequently meets with an almost total lack of communication in many institutions. Time and time again I encountered physical therapy practised in the traditional form of outdated exercises and correction of posture. Assessment of the patient's level of physical function should be part of the physiotherapists' or physical educators' role in the total care of these patients, but without referrals from the physician, this is impossible. A great many of the physical therapists whom I met had never had an asthmatic patient referred to them by a physician and were unaware of the problems faced by these patients and therefore of their role in treatment.

It is therefore vital that we listen to one another, discuss possible problems, and above all learn to use the resources available in the hospital and in each other.

SELECTION OF PATIENTS FOR A GIVEN PROGRAMME

The criteria for including a child in a training programme appear to be variable. Some authors have selected patients on the grade of involvement and severity of the underlying disease. Others have selected those patients with defined asthma irrespective of severity. Often, little information is available as to the patient's level of daily activity before the training programme — and since many of these children have a normal physical working capacity despite their exercise-induced asthma, it seems unlikely that the results of a conditioning programme would result in an increase in their exercise tolerance level. In a Swedish study on the effects of physical training on 11 boys, no significant increase was shown in the maximal oxygen uptake [1]: In the conclusion, however, the authors stated that the failure to demonstrate the positive effects of physical training on the variables studied was related to the degree of intensity of the programme. In this report the intensity of training during the one-week winter camp was considered to be high, the children completing an average of 22km of cross-country skiing during the week. In comparison, our asthmatics completed 180km in a two-week period in winter camp and this did produce an increase in the oxygen uptake. Obviously, failure to demonstrate positive effects of physical activity can be directly related to the degree of intensity and is influenced by the pre-exercise fitness level of the participants.

It is perhaps for these reasons that reports vary so much in their findings and are often so contradictory. In one recent report the results showed no positive effect of training on levels of physical fitness. The types of activities were unspecified and upon further investigation it was discovered that the entire programme was based upon self-training. The children were given an exercise programme that they were expected to complete at home over a period of months. As physiotherapists we know only too well that this type of training is doomed to failure as it seems highly unlikely that the children were able to complete the training at the required intensity or that the frequency and duration were sufficient to elicit the necessary response.

Swimming training

Since reports on the asthmagenicity of different types of activities have appeared, the use of swimming for the asthmatic patient has been widely recommended and accepted. In Canada the development of an exercise programme PIPE (prone immersion physical activity – L W Jankowski, paper presented at the 23rd Annual Meeting of the American College of Sports Medicine, 1976), allowed the effects of physical reconditioning in water to be compared with those of a bicycle ergometer programme and with a control group. The results showed significant increases in physical working capacity in both active groups, but they were greater for the swimming group. Other studies have demonstrated similar positive results. Swimming is used in many therapeutic programmes and seems often to be the only form of training available for the asthmatic. But though its use is justifiable for aerobic training of the asthmatic, it is important to remember that at least 20 per cent of chronic asthmatics have eczema, which may be considerably aggravated by exposure to water. Some allergic patients may be unable to use swimming as a form of training in their home environment as public swimming-pools may contain unwelcome allergens.

Although swimming allows these children to take part in an activity with less fear of bronchospasm it is also important to teach them how to cope with land activities in which bronchoconstriction is more of a problem. If the ultimate aim is integration of the asthmatic in a normal environment, then the use of all-round activities would seem most suitable. The asthmatic child does not require exercises designed especially for him but he must be assisted in coping with and succeeding in the types of activities enjoyed by his fellows.

PSYCHOSOCIAL EFFECTS

Since the asthmatic child has problems in joining in activities with his contemporaries, the use of group training would seem the most applicable. He is often an onlooker standing on the outside of a group wanting to join in; consequently individual treatment should be designed as a stepping stone to these group activities. One of the centres I visited had a programme that was advanced in its use of physical activity and all the children were treated on a one-to-one basis under the leadership of students. In the long run a programme such as this gives the child little feedback in regard to his performance and interaction with his fellows, something he so badly needs. The social contact he receives through the adult does not prepare him for the realities and competitiveness of a child's world. The economic implications of such an experiment also loom large.

One of the greatest problems encountered in training the chronic asthmatic is lack of motivation, often the result of failure to keep up with others. Consequently training sessions must be made as much fun for the child as possible. Many of the training sessions that I observed — whether led by physiotherapists or physical educators — appeared very one-sided in their concentration on intense endurance training with the object of achieving the necessary heart rate at all costs — a pure blood, sweat and tears regime. The children often appeared to be far from enjoying the session and many tried to avoid taking part by forgetting their medication or simulating an attack. Enjoyment of the training sessions is one of the golden rules of any programme.

One of the outpatient models that we have used for a number of years at Voksentoppen has been based on a twice-weekly group training session for 12 patients (between the ages of 10 and 15 years) over a period of three to nine months culminating in 14 days of activity in the mountains. The children are, moreover, encouraged to take part in activities of their own choice during the weekend. The criterion for participation was initially the demonstration of exercise-induced asthma and less consideration was given to other factors. Our results showed, however, that in addition to an increase in physical working capacity and an increased tolerance to the same workload that originally had induced asthma the programme had a considerable effect on psychological factors. The children who benefited most from this programme were those with poor images of themselves, underdeveloped awareness of their bodies and poor psychosocial adjustment. An improvement in the psychological aspects, especially in self-confidence, together with an increased level of physical fitness made it considerably easier for the children to integrate into their home environment. The combination of many types of activities allows them to choose one that they can join in successfully [2].

Since a great number of programmes include many forms of treatment – drug therapy, breathing exercises, group therapy, residential placement and others – in addition to physical activity, it is difficult to single out just which is the most important. If, however, in the comprehensive care of an asthmatic child, the psychological gains of a training programme bring about an improvement in his life, the use of that programme would certainly seem to be justified.

Compliance of the asthmatic patient with his medical treatment is a recurring problem, but we have found that physical activity programmes can often be responsible for an improvement of the patient's attitude towards correct and adequate medication. Teaching the child about his medication, when and what to take, how to use a peak flow meter and what the results mean, all help him to assess his need for medication.

ALTERNATIVE TO POSTURAL DRAINAGE?

The asthmatic child frequently has an excess of bronchial secretion that may be difficult to mobilise. Physical activity and normal play (when the patient is well medicated, or at least not bronchospastic) is used by some and should be used by more therapists since activity causes bronchodilatation and an increase in ventilation which assist in the removal and expectoration of secretions. Physical activity may be used in conjunction with, or instead of, the more traditional postural drainage in selected patients and is less time-consuming, more natural, and far more fun for both the therapist and the patient.

CONCLUSION

Reflections are unfortunately not always possible to substantiate with hard facts, but certain conclusions may nevertheless be drawn. The emphasis on physical activity as a form of treatment is certainly not a generally accepted approach outside specialised centres. Many hospitals may recognise the value of physical activity, yet few use this knowledge in any practical manner. It appeared that many children with chronic asthma would have benefited considerably from an opportunity to participate in a controlled exercise programme under secure medical guidance. The physiotherapist's role in the treatment of asthma remains conventional in most centres. Physiotherapists could and should be more active in using physical activity in their treatments and physiotherapy schools could and should take more initiative in encouraging this aspect of treatment.

The multidisciplinary approach is essential in the total care of patients with such a complex disease as asthma. But this approach is only possible when members of the hospital team learn to communicate with each other and to accept that different disciplines can complement one another in helping these children to function to the best of their abilities.

References

1   Graff-Lonnevig V, Bevegard S, Erikson BO et al.
     Two years follow-up of asthmatic boys participating in a physical activity pro-
     gramme. Actu Paediatr Scand 1980; 69: 347–352
2   Oseid S, Kendall M, Bjørstad-Larsen K, Selbokk R,
     Physical activity programmes for children with exercise-induced asthma.
     In Eriksson BO, Furberg B, eds.
     Swimming Medicine IV 1978: 42.
     Baltimore: University Park Press

DISCUSSION

REEVES
(Lincoln, UK)

Miss Kendall said that she regarded public swimming pools as unsuitable for some asthmatics. Would she comment further on this as it has certainly not been my experience.

KENDALL

I did say that this would exclude some children from continuing swimming in their home environment. Many people think that chlorine is the cause, but I think that they come into contact with allergens in some swimming pools. We have had many patients who have learned to swim at our Institute and have become keen and good swimmers, but when they have returned home they have been unable to continue because the available pool has proved unsuitable.

EDWARDS
(Loughborough,
UK)

I cannot think of any problem that we have had with public pools either with the children with eczema or with the asthma getting worse when the children get into a different environment. It may be that their premedication needs adjusting, either in dosage or type; but if this is adequate and you ensure that they do actually take the premedication before they enter the pool, there should be no problems.

STRUNK
(Denver, USA)

So that Miss Kendall's comments about swimming pools do not get out of perspective, I would just like to say that swimming is not the best exercise for every asthmatic. We should consider what the child likes to do and can do and what facilities are available. Just because swimming is good for most asthmatics does not mean that it is the only activity a child can do as a continuing exercise or training programme. At the National Jewish Hospital we try to individualise the choice so that the child will do something that he will be able to do, and want to do, for the rest of his life.

ANDERSON (Camperdown, Australia)	You referred to the use of pre-exercise medications which we also practise at the Royal Prince Alfred Hospital. However, do you also use non-pharmacological methods for preventing exercise-induced asthma such as a mask, or pre-exercise sprints or the refractory period?
KENDALL	We use masks only in cold weather and only if the child wants to use them. We would never use them as a substitute for premedication. But all our children at the Institute are severe asthmatics. We do not see the milder ones at all.
BURGE (Birmingham, UK)	A number of the children I see are socially deprived and I think there would be problems integrating them with a group. How often does Miss Lid have problems of this nature and does she have children who fail in the exercise groups?
NYSTAD LID	I do not force any child to take part in an activity. A child may stand on the side-lines and look at the other children for some time. I also take children individually to see what activities they can manage and then I choose an activity especially suited for the child when starting with a group.
GILLAM (Victoria, Australia)	First, I would like to stress what others have said and that is that warm-up is beneficial for all children — I think sometimes we become rather paranoid about trying to get objective results. Secondly, the importance of interval-type activities has been stressed but the demonstrations I have seen were no different from any other physical education class. Do you agree that it is most important to avoid continuous activity in some children?
NYSTAD LID	I agree. But if you look at children playing, they have natural intervals so this does not really create problems. Children play by chosing natural activities with natural intervals.

KENDALL

Interval training has sometimes been misunderstood as implying that the child has to sit down — that he does a spurt of exercise and then has to sit and rest. This is something that we definitely try to avoid. We try to make the intervals a natural occurrence — for example, a ball game is a natural form of interval training. If you sit a patient down in the middle of an activity programme that is supposed to be fun and tell them to watch their breathing or their heart rate, you are continually reminding them that they are asthmatic. You are contradicting the aims of the treatment session.

LINDSAY
(Camperdown, Australia)

As Miss Kendall pointed out, quite frequently some children in a training group are obviously not training. That is a problem with group activities if one of the objectives for individual children is to improve their aerobic capacity. Unless you are careful the lazy child will not increase his heart rate and maintain it at that level sufficiently long to get a training effect. What you get is no training effect in some children and some training effect in others, and whether you like it or not that is what happens in games. Goal keepers and wingers, for instance, can play in a game without any aerobic fitness at all. So how do you ensure that within a group all individuals get a training effect?

KENDALL

I agree entirely. I have asked many children at Voksentoppen if they play football and they say that they do. But when I ask them where they play, it is always in goal — practically every football team in this country must have a goalie who is an asthmatic. In our treatment programmes we never leave the children alone; we always have at least one, and preferably two, people with the group who are aware of which children are inclined to be lazy or lacking in motivation and they try to help them into activities in the nicest possible way.

FINAL COMMENTS

OSEID
(Chairman)

Dr Morisbak's paper was of great importance in showing the role that can be played by professionals. For a long time doctors were the only people to prescribe exercise and they had not the faintest idea about exercise physiology or even what exercise was. Dr Morisbak has suggested how to attract those people who really should be helping us with these programmes.

EDWARDS
(Loughborough,
UK)

Since we started encouraging this type of programme our experience has grown enormously, particularly in the past 12 months, in that there are now more than 50 groups in the United Kingdom and they are led by a wide variety of people. We have encouraged co-operation between different professionals, although we have always insisted that there is a doctor at the centre of the group because he has to assess the children and adjust their treatment. But the real skill lies in encouraging the backward child to come forward. This really depends on the group leader and I think we are learning that it is the trained teacher or physiotherapist who can do that better than any doctor. Each in their own way contributes their own skills but it is their skill in encouraging children, however backward, to participate that makes for eventual success.

FITCH
(Nedlands,
Australia)

Swimming classes for asthmatics have been held in Sydney since about 1965, and in Western Australia since 1974. Each State in Australia now has asthma swimming classes. In Victoria, where they have a Government-provided recreation facility for the asthmatics, they are particularly well organised. I believe these classes should be conducted entirely by the physical education profession. We use these classes to overcome the lack of activity in asthmatics who cannot move around because of exercise-induced asthma or chronic asthma. Having given the child exertional competence in the pool, we then try to get him or her into the normal physical activity. Finally, I should like to say that both the asthmatic child and the non-asthmatic child will improve their biochemical and physical performance if they train to similar levels of frequency and duration. Asthmatics are no different from anybody else provided you can control them.

PIERSON
(Seattle, USA)

We have adopted another approach in our community, not having an institute like the Voksentoppen Institute. With a few allergists who are interested in the problem of exercise-induced asthma, we have approached the physical education teachers and the school nurses and shown them how children with exercise-induced asthma can perform normally in the school setting with adequate premedication. Once they understand the nature of the problem and become motivated to take care of these patients, we have found them to be very helpful.

HAIDER
(Bury, UK)

Our asthmatic children are first assessed in the hospital — clinically and immunologically and their pulmonary function tested. They are then allocated to the community clinics near their homes which are run on an open-door basis. Parents meet together and discuss among themselves as well as with a specially trained health visitor and school nurse. The discussion group is then joined by the paediatrician. More than two years ago we formed an asthma patients (and parents) association. This is a self-help group. They educate themselves with the help of different specialists, such as doctors, physiotherapists, physical instructors, and so on. They also arrange weekly swimming sessions for these children in the local swimming baths.

OSEID

The approaches to what we call exercise vary from training once a week to once a day or even three times a day. I feel this is something that has to be standardised — or at least guidelines on the prescription of exercise for asthmatics must be provided. I know that Professor Alan Morton who is a co-worker with Dr Fitch has given some thought to this and I would ask Dr Fitch to comment.

FITCH   Alan Morton is a professor of physical education, a former national rugby player, and a former asthmatic. His approach to this problem has been published [references 28 and 31 in my paper]. It includes consideration of such aspects as warm-up and cooling-down; duration, frequency and intensity of exercise and until what age (Morton has said throughout life); type of exercise; exercise loading; pre-exercise medication; and medication to reverse exercise-induced asthma.

Warm-up   The point that Dr Lindsay made about warm-up was that it should be scientifically evaluated — though he was not necessarily saying that everybody should have to have a two-degree increase in rectal temperature before he can take part in any physical activity.

Duration   Professor Morton recommended 30–40 minutes per session, but if the asthmatic was very unfit he might need to begin with a 15-minute session. This means 15 minutes of activity and does not include the rests inbetween. The duration of 30–40 minutes can, of course, be considerably lengthened, though this depends on the intensity of the activity — if you are exercising at a high intensity 30–40 minutes can be quite tiring.

Frequency   This should be four to five times a week, with a minimum of three times a week. I say three times a week because I am aware of the impracticality of bringing people to a centre too many times a week.

Intensity   The start should be made at a low level of intensity with a gradual increase; Professor Morton suggested that the exercise should be based on some type of interval work. I think, however, that the word sprinting as used by Dr Phelan's group is a misnomer. An increase of 25–30 per cent above steady-pace rate is not sprinting — for instance, if you run a steady-pace kilometre in five minutes, it would scarcely be regarded as sprinting to run it in four minutes. We have increased our interval work training up to 75 per cent above steady pace and I still would not regard that as sprinting. I believe interval work is definitely superior and, moreover, underlies virtually every ball game. You run around, you get the ball, then you have a rest until the ball comes your way again — unless, of course, you are the goal keeper, when you might not touch the ball at all. It does not matter whether the interval work is in the swimming pool, in the gymnasium or anywhere else.

Type of exercise The games and activities should be of the asthmatic's own choice; they should be pleasurable not something he is made to do. Nevertheless Professor Morton did make the point that perhaps all asthmatics should, at some stage, take part in swimming training as this was a good and useful way to get back to activities if the asthmatic was, for example, sick at any time.

Exercise loading and premedication Professor Morton's views on these aspects agree with what we have been saying throughout this meeting.

OSEID

A most important point brought out by Dr Fitch is that exercising once or twice a week is not sufficient to have a physical effect. I want to stress this because otherwise we will end up by believing that we are doing something good to the children physically when we are doing nothing of the kind. This is not to say that exercising once or twice a week might have psychological and social benefit and be worthwhile on that account, but in physical terms more intense training is required.

INDEX